Medicine, Society, and Faith in the Ancient and Medieval Worlds

Printed in the United States
3417

MEDICINE, SOCIETY, AND FAITH IN THE ANCIENT AND MEDIEVAL WORLDS

DARREL W. AMUNDSEN

The Johns Hopkins University Press
BALTIMORE AND LONDON

To my beloved Jeanne, whom God has given to me to have and to hold, for better for worse, for richer for poorer, in sickness and in health, to love and to cherish, till death us do part.

© 1996 The Johns Hopkins University Press
All rights reserved. Published 1996
Printed in the United States of America on acid-free paper
05 04 03 02 01 00 99 98 97 96   5 4 3 2 1

The Johns Hopkins University Press
2715 North Charles Street
Baltimore, Maryland 21218-4319
The Johns Hopkins Press Ltd., London

ISBN 0-8018-5109-2
ISBN 0-8018-6354-6 pbk
Library of Congress Cataloging-in-Publication Data will be
found at the end of this book.
A catalog record for this book is available from the
British Library.

Contents

Preface

As I look back over the first two and one-half decades of my career, especially that aspect covered by the "publications" and "papers presented" sections of my *curriculum vitae*, I realize how little control I had at any point in charting the course of my scholarship.

As an undergraduate classics major, I was intent on writing my senior seminar paper on the graffiti of Pompeii as a source of social history. The topic of the age of Greek and Roman girls at menarche, which was resolutely imposed upon me by my professor, who promised me publication in a highly reputed journal if I found anything worthy of note, was far removed from anything of even the remotest interest. Little could I have known the effect that this frustrating and (I was convinced) irrelevant assignment would have on the subsequent direction of my scholarship.

When I was a first-year graduate student in a seminar on Isidore of Seville, the surprisingly rewarding research that I had done in the medical and legal texts relevant to female puberty led me on to Isidore's *De medicina* and the legal codes of the Visigoths. The result was a published paper entitled "Visigothic Medical Legislation," which attracted the attention of the organizer of an international symposium on "Society, Medicine, and Law" in Jerusalem. His invitation to participate stimulated me to go back to Roman law in order to understand the Romans' concept of tort as it applied to professional liability. So intrigued was I by the historical relationship of medicine and law that I published several more papers in that area. I had found a niche in which I was eager to stay. Indeed, if I had been left to set my own course, I might well have made it my field of research. But that was not to be.

In the 1960s what was later dubbed the bioethics movement quickly gained national attention. It had been generated and stimulated by a variety of factors. Developments in medical technology had dramatically increased public interest in some aspects of medical ethics. Additional catalysts appeared. Burgeoning demands for consumers' rights, coupled with the civil rights movement, had stimulated a patients' rights movement. Feminism, the "new morality," and the sexual revolution had brought the issue of abortion into public discussion and debate. Liberalized abortion laws had not only increased the intensity of the debate but also raised public awareness of demands for the "right to live," and the "right to die." These issues were made ever more perplexing by increasingly efficient medical technology.

Bioethical issues continued to receive much attention from the media, to provide the basis for litigation and a focus of much political debate, to add vigor to already active tensions between Western monotheisms and secular medicine, to revivify tensions that had been latent for some time, and to create new areas of potential conflict; indeed, to be discussed by nearly everyone from the man in the street to that byproduct of the bioethics movement, the bioethicist.

Late in 1974, because of the work I was doing on medicine and law, I was asked to contribute three articles—histories of medical ethics in the ancient Near East, Greece and Rome, and early Christianity through the Middle Ages—to the *Encyclopedia of Bioethics,* which was then in its formative stages. Before I was invited to write these articles, if anyone had asked me whether I had any interest in medical ethics and its history, I would likely have replied, "Only as they relate to the history of medicolegal issues." Hence it was quite unexpectedly that I found myself addressing a broad range of related issues that I would otherwise never have pursued. Some, however, proved sufficiently interesting to engage me further. For instance, I researched one matter in which my work in the history of medical ethics had stimulated my interest: the ethical standards of physicians during the plague epidemics of the late Middle Ages (see chapter 10, below).

Just as I was finishing this study, Robert Veatch of the Hastings Center invited me to prepare, for their "Death and Dying" research group, a paper in which I was to attempt to answer the question of whether the ostensible duty to strive at all costs to prolong or sustain life had its roots in

"Hippocratic" medicine and, if my conclusion was negative, to seek to locate and explain the origins of this ethical imperative (see chapter 2, below).

The work that I was doing in the history of medical ethics was repeatedly bringing me face to face with puzzling features of the history of the relationship of medicine and Christianity. I had recently sought to clarify the position of the medieval Catholic Church on medical and surgical practice by clerics (see chapter 8), when I was invited to be a visiting scholar at the College of Physicians of Philadelphia. With rich collections of incunabula and early printed editions available there and in Washington, D.C., I was able to explore much more deeply the extensive efforts of late medieval moral theologians to define the ethical and religious duties of physicians (see chapter 9).

An invitation to contribute a paper to an issue of the *Bulletin of the History of Medicine* honoring Owsei Temkin on his eightieth birthday brought to mind an extended conversation I had had with that most gracious and distinguished scholar a few years earlier, when I had given a seminar on medicine and early Christianity at the Johns Hopkins Institute of the History of Medicine. Hence I was confident that an essay on medicine and faith in early Christianity (see chapter 5) would treat a subject in which he was interested (as his recently published and richly perspicacious *Hippocrates in a World of Pagans and Christians* was later to demonstrate).

It was about this time that Lutheran General Hospital of Park Ridge, Illinois, invited me to join the long-term study of religion and medicine that was later to be called Project X: Health/Medicine and the Faith Traditions. During my period of association with Project X, I was commissioned to pursue various aspects of the history of the relationship of medicine and religion. One of these ventures was an effort to weave into a colorful tapestry the many disparate strands of medicine and medieval Catholicism (see chapter 7). While I was working with Project X, H. Tristram Engelhardt, Jr., editor of the series Philosophy and Medicine, with which I had been involved in various scholarly endeavors, invited me to participate in symposia on the ethical questions regarding defective newborns (see chapter 3) and suicide and euthanasia (see chapter 4).

As I glance back over the pages of this preface, I am struck afresh by how fortunate I was in having been forced or invited into scholarly endeavors to which my own designs, interests, and imagination would never have directed me. And when Jacqueline Wehmueller expressed interest, on behalf of the Johns Hopkins University Press, in publishing a selection of some of my previously printed essays, I regarded this as an excellent incentive in mid-career for thinking retrospectively about the direction and scope of my scholarship, and also as an opportunity to provide a more enduring format for some papers that had been originally published for highly specialized audiences.

The process of choosing the essays to be included in this volume took some amusing turns. The final form resulted in a short selection of papers that share some common themes. Chapters 2 and 3 are the only essays that deal with the classical world. Their function is introductory and propaedeutic to the main focus of the volume, which is Christianity and medicine. Chapter 6, on the renegade quasi–father of the church Tatian, is, in a sense, an extended footnote to chapter 5. It was presented at the International Congress on Ancient Medicine in Its Socio-cultural Context held in Leiden and will see almost simultaneously its initial publication in a book derived from that congress and its reprinting in the present volume. Chapter 11, "The Moral Stance of the Earliest Syphilographers, 1495–1505" was written specifically for the present volume, as was chapter 1, "Body, Soul, and Physician," in which I introduce and muse upon the themes that unite the remaining ten chapters.

As the final shape of the volume became clear to the anonymous external reader to whom various batches of vying essays had been sent, I was cautioned that "care must be taken when presenting historical essays which describe issues that are of current concern." I agree wholeheartedly. But several of the essays that appear in this volume were commissioned papers that were written in response to invitations from scholars who were very active in the bioethics movement. They wanted objective appraisals by an historian who they hoped possessed neither a personal agenda nor a desire to read present problems into the past.

Let me conclude by relating some of the principles that have undergirded the essays in this volume. I should first acknowledge that, as I am a philologist with training in history, my concerns, although initially textual, have always become broadly contextual. Further, I have profited from the methodological insights of those historians who appear to be frustrated anthropologists, sociologists, or psychologists.

We who are historians should eschew our propensity to a patronizing presentism by striving to know the culture that we are studying as intimately and deeply as is humanly possible. We should be driven by a passion to grow in our understanding and appreciation of who the objects of our studies were. We ought continually to ensure that as much as possible we leave at the threshold of our historical investigations our subjective baggage of personal biases and prejudices. The closer the issues that we are investigating are to our own hearts, the more cautious we should be lest we be motivated by an agenda to demonstrate something to be true about the past simply because we want it to have been true. And if we ever intentionally or inadvertently, explicitly or implicitly, sit in judgment on, or moralize about, the beliefs and values of the times and places that we are studying, we should do much soul-searching about our motives and be absolutely convinced that we thoroughly and intimately understand even the most subtle nuances of the beliefs and practices of those times and places.

Often, of course, we fall short. It is in the very nature of the historian's craft that we must. We are never free of bias and prejudice. When we research issues dear to our hearts we may have agendas that are effectively hidden even from ourselves. Nor can we ever enter into another ethos so completely that we can claim to know it from the inside, especially if it is temporally distant and culturally distinct from our own. And if we are, in fact, becoming more and more intimately acquainted with the society that we would love to visit with much greater immediacy than the historian's tools provide, then as we grow, we look back occasionally on our own scholarship and see how much we have grown in, say, the last decade or two. If there is nothing in an essay or book we published early in that period that we would not now write differently and with greater understanding, we are less to be admired for our early competence than pitied for our present blind conceit.

Hence in chapter 1 I shall introduce the essays that follow not only by describing the common themes that give cohesion to this volume but also by discussing some of the differences of interpretation that have arisen between my earlier and later essays. If the differences were glaring I should never have consented to their being reprinted. If there were no differences I should regret my lack of growth.

A plethora of themes arise and are given varying degrees of attention in these essays. Two, however, loom much larger than all the others: (1) the disputed boundaries of Christianity and medicine (and the question of the propriety of medicine for Christians); (2) respect for human life, that is, a principle of sanctity of human life (including the duty to treat or to attempt to sustain the life of the ill). Chapter 1 provides a conceptual and historical framework for these themes.

Acknowledgments

The eleven essays in this volume were not a manuscript looking for a publisher. Chapters 2 through 10 had been previously published and would have remained isolated from each other were it not for the initiative of others. So my first acknowledgment of gratitude is to the Johns Hopkins University Press, especially to Jacqueline Wehmueller, who suggested this venture to me. She complements her competence with a graciousness and a patience that are truly supererogatory. I also wish to express my thanks to the anonymous referee who read all the essays that were considered for inclusion in this volume, especially for his or her insightful criticism of the early drafts of chapters 1 and 11.

My boyhood friend Gary B. Ferngren, with whom I would play Roman soldier and Jewish zealot when our peers were cowboys and Indians, is my most honest and perspicacious critic. As colleagues, collaborators, and brothers-in-law, we work together so closely in our scholarship that the end result is little different whether labeled Amundsen; Ferngren; Amundsen and Ferngren; or Ferngren and Amundsen. I am richly blessed having him as my closest friend.

I owe a special debt of gratitude to H. Tristram Englehart, Jr. Behind the scenes on several highly significant occasions, showing a confidence and trust in me far greater than I had earned, he has recommended that I be entrusted with scholarly opportunities that have invariably proven to be richly rewarding.

During my two and one-half decades at Western Washington University, the Bureau for Faculty Research has been very supportive of my scholarly endeavors. Three deans have been especially encouraging and helpful: the late Herbert C. Taylor, Jr., James W. Davis, and Peter J. Elich. To them I extend my appreciation.

Over the years during which the essays contained in this volume were written, several very efficient secretaries have spoiled me with their tireless kindness: Marilyn Lyon, who has throughout been the patient recipient of my nearly indecipherable manuscripts; Valerie Worthen, for a short but significant period; and then Kathie Loftin, during the last three years. To them I extend my sincere thanks as well as to Peggy Reynolds, who became involved at the very end of this project.

To my friend and former student Otto Walfred Mandahl, Jr., I am deeply grateful for his labor of love that has resulted in the thorough indexes for this volume.

As this volume neared production, I was favored with the help of Miriam L. Kleiger as manuscript editor. Her persistent competence and good taste have sheltered the reader from my inadvertent ambiguities, stylistic inconsistencies, and infelicitous expressions. Any that remain should be attributed to my stubbornness rather than to her oversight.

I also wish to acknowledge the help rendered by two former students of mine, Desiree McCollough, who adapted the notes from their original, varied formats, and Shannon Waterman, whose attentive scrutiny of the page proofs revealed several errors that had eluded earlier readers.

Chapters 2 through 10 are reprinted with the kind permission of their publishers. All appear as originally printed (other than a few minor alterations, primarily for consistency of style of both text and citations) except for chapter four, "Suicide and Early Christian Values," which I have abridged for the present volume. They originally appeared as follows:

—Chapter 2: "The Physician's Obligation to Prolong Life: A Medical Duty without Classical Roots," *Hastings Center Report* 8, no. 4 (1978): 23–30.

—Chapter 3: "Medicine and the Birth of Defective Children: Approaches of the Ancient World," in *Euthanasia and the Newborn: Conflicts about Saving Lives*, ed. R. C. McMillan, H. T. Engelhardt, Jr., and S. F. Spicker (Dordrecht: Reidel Publishing Co., 1987), 3–22. © 1987 by D. Reidel Publishing Company.

—Chapter 4: "Suicide and Early Christian Values," in *Suicide and Euthanasia: Historical and Contemporary Themes*, ed. Baruch A. Brody (Dordrecht: Kluwer Academic Publishers, 1989), 77–153. © 1989 Kluwer Academic Publishers.

—Chapter 5: "Medicine and Faith in Early Christianity," *Bulletin of the History of Medicine* 56 (1982): 326–50.

—Chapter 6: "Tatian's 'Rejection' of Medicine in the Second Century," in *Ancient Medicine in Its Socio-Cultural Context,* ed. Ph. J. van der Eijk, H.F.J. Horstmanshoff, and P. H. Schrijvers (Amsterdam and Atlanta: Rodopi, 1995), 2:377–92.

—Chapter 7: "The Medieval Catholic Tradition," in *Caring and Curing: Health and Medicine in the Western Religious Traditions,* ed. Ronald L. Numbers and Darrel W. Amundsen (New York: Macmillan Publishing Co., 1986), 65–107.

—Chapter 8: "Medieval Canon Law on Medical and Surgical Practice by the Clergy," *Bulletin of the History of Medicine* 52 (1978): 22–44.

—Chapter 9: "Casuistry and Professional Obligations: The Regulation of Physicians by the Court of Conscience in the Late Middle Ages," *Transactions and Studies of the College of Physicians of Philadelphia* n.s. 3 (1981): 22–39, 93–112.

—Chapter 10: "Medical Deontology and Pestilential Disease in the Late Middle Ages," *Journal of the History of Medicine and the Allied Sciences* 32 (1977): 403–21.

ONE

Body, Soul, and Physician

Religions have historically provided constructs for understanding the place of humanity within the total structure of reality. That reality has included awesome powers that were superior to man, to whose whim and caprice he thought himself to be vulnerable, and on whose mercy he placed his hopes. This held true for pantheistic animists and polytheists who worshipped a multitude of supernatural beings, for pantheistic monists who worshipped a deified Nature under which was often subsumed a diverse spectrum of spiritual entities, and for monotheists who worshipped a single Deity who, as the Creator, was regarded as transcendent but also immanent in his intimate involvement in his creation. Religions have typically provided not only inclusive constructs of reality but also a modus vivendi: rules that governed man's relationship with the supernatural and the mechanisms whereby he could attempt to win the favor or avert the disfavor of spiritual beings. Hence we can say that a major role of religion has been to provide for man's well-being in the broadest sense.

Medicine typically has had well-being, in the sense of physical (and perhaps mental) health, as its sole telos. By "medicine" we mean (1) the substances, mechanisms, and procedures for restoring and preserving health and physical wellness; and (2) those who employed such substances, mechanisms, and procedures, in at least one of their recognized roles in their society, in order to assist people who availed themselves of their expertise. So medicine's role has been like that of religion but much more limited: to restore to health those who were beset by sickness or hampered by dysfunction or injury; in some instances to succor those whose health medicine could not restore; and to preserve health through prophylaxis or regimen.

Since religion has historically been concerned with well-being in an all-encompassing sense, and medicine has been concerned with well-being in a much more limited sense, it should not be at all surprising that there have always existed both tensions and compatibilities between medicine and religion.

The relationship between medicine and religion may be depicted by the four following configurations:

I. Medicine is subsumed under religion. In a monolithic society, most of whose members adhere to one religion, this model prevails. Religion's all-inclusive concern with humanity's well-being provides the exclusive context for medicine's much more limited concern with the well-being of the body. There are two variations of this model as it applies to a monolithic society:

A. Tensions between medicine and religion are entirely latent, and a compatibility prevails that is possible only when the aims of medicine are entirely subordinated to those of religion, as is the case in a monolithic society in which both the nosological and the therapeutic models are religious or magico-religious (i.e., pre-rational speculative). This construct and model I(B), below, include, as subject to religion, all aspects of what we may call medical ethics, that is, all moral considerations that arise not only in the arena of crisis and care but also in the total biological spectrum from conception to death. Once naturalistic nosological and therapeutic models developed and were popularly accepted, model I(A) could no longer prevail.

B. Ecclesiastical authorities in a religiously monolithic society such as that of medieval Europe attempt to ensure uniformity of belief and practice by striving to subordinate medicine in all its aspects to religion. This is not to suggest that medieval European ecclesiastics wished to impose religious nosological and therapeutic models. Indeed, their understanding of disease was essentially naturalistic, and their therapies were typically naturalistic as well. But their belief in the sovereignty of God as the Final Cause, in his freedom to intervene in natural processes, and in the subtle trickery of evil powers that draw people away from God by healing them directly or luring them to rely on naturalistic models without reference to, or dependence on, him, motivated ecclesiastical authorities throughout the Middle Ages to subordinate medicine to the prevailing Christian construct of reality and to Christian ethics. There is an additional variation of model I:

    C. All aspects of medicine are subordinated to the religious beliefs of certain groups. In a pluralistic society, members of certain religious groups regard a subordination of all aspects of medicine to their religious beliefs as the only acceptable model. Obviously the difference between what they regard as the only acceptable model and the model that prevails in society is productive of much tension.

II. Religion and medicine are partially separated. In this model, medical ethics are still subordinate to religion. The roots of this model go back to the earliest naturalistic explanations of health and disease in classical Greece. Nurtured by the "Enlightenment," it reached full bloom in the mid- to late nineteenth century with the scientific revolutions that established as medicine's foundational sciences anatomy, physiology, biochemistry, pathology, and bacteriology. This resulted in a thorough desacralization of nosological and therapeutic models, which made medicine and its practitioners "objective neutrals" far removed from the realm of religion. In this construct, which has been the dominant model in the West until quite recently, the compartmentalization of the realms of medicine and religion were not complete. Those aspects of medicine that were viewed as outside religion's terrain were regarded as thoroughly compatible with religion owing to the coexistence that mutual irrelevance fosters. But in this model there was still an overlap between religion and medicine because Western society was—although not, strictly speaking, monolithic—nevertheless united by a moral consensus. Hence, while nosological explanations and therapeutic methods were thoroughly desacralized, an essentially religious, Judeo-Christian morality governed the realm of medical ethics. In this model the tensions were almost as minimal as in model I(A).

III. Medicine and religion are completely separate. This has been the dominant model for social policy and law in the West for the last few decades. In a pluralistic society that lacks a moral consensus, many people insist that the domains of medicine and religion must be kept distinct and separate. Medical ethics is defined by the lowest common moral denominator and regulated by econometrics and cost-benefit analysis, or so it seems to religious opponents of this model. Owing to this total compartmentalization of medicine and religion, there are, of course, enormous tensions between those who promote this model and members of religious groups who regard model I(C) or model II as the only acceptable model. We should note in this regard, however, that there are some today, albeit a small minority, who on religious grounds regard model III as the only acceptable model, because (as discussed below) they are convinced that it is totally inappropriate for them to be involved in, or to avail themselves of, any aspect of the realm of medicine (for an example of which, see the second paragraph below). Or, perhaps more likely, they might opt for model I(A), the model in which all disease and dysfunction are explained by a religious nosology and dealt with by employing religious mechanisms.

IV. Religion is subsumed under medicine. In this model, which America is rapidly approaching, the realm of medicine is expanding to include therapy for virtually every perceived personal or social ill, inadequacy, or dysfunction. In this therapeutic society, religion is being redefined and absorbed by medicine. This is the ultimate realization of the World Health Organization's definition of health: "Health is a state of complete physical, mental, and social well-being, not simply the absence of illness and disease."[1] And it is a resacralization of society in the cocoon of a new spirituality, a therapeutic spirituality that, as an inversion of model I(A), is really very similar to it. Such a construct is anathema to those who regard its exact antithesis, model I(C), or, perhaps, model II, as the only acceptable relationship of medicine and religion.

The concerns of those who are, on religious grounds, opposed to model IV, involve the boundaries of medicine and religion, as does the following. Infrequently, yet with regularity, we encounter news reports of parents who refuse to allow medical treatment of their children who will otherwise almost certainly die. Judicial decisions to intervene, or less commonly, not to interfere, always arouse a great deal of interest since— although typically the parents are members of a religious group on the fringes of Christianity—an aspect of the right of self-determination is being tested. Religious groups that range from liberal to conservative are embarrassed by these highly publicized cases because the total denial of secular medicine evinced by such parents is discordant with the historical position of the three Western monotheisms. There is, however, an enduring concern on the part of some monotheists that the "God of the gaps" has been conceptually excluded from much of the arena of health care by naturalistic, one-dimensional explanations of disease and models of healing.

However, there are other categories of tension between medicine and religion today. Such old issues as abortion, and active and passive euthanasia, remain ubiquitous. The ethical conundrums created by spectacular advances in medical technology, such as in vitro fertilization, fetal-tissue research, organ transplants, genetic engineering, and life-support systems, must (in the opinion of many people) be brought back within the purview of religion.

The bioethical issues that involve the relationship of medicine and religion may be subsumed under two rubrics: (1) the boundaries of medicine and religion; and (2) respect for human life (i.e., the principle of the sanctity of human life). It is to some aspects of these two categories as they have arisen in the first fifteen centuries of the history of Christianity that I shall now direct my attention.

The Boundaries of Medicine and Christianity

The influence of classical culture on the theology and practice of early Christianity and the reactions of Christians to classical culture have long been a source of fruitful scholarly discussion. The grist for modern scholars who are concerned with this issue is the patristic literature devoted to asserting the uniqueness of the Christian gospel, on the one hand, and the salubrious points of harmony between Judeo-Christian revelation and the best features of classical culture, on the other. There is considerable diversity within early Christian literature on such matters. Nevertheless, it is reasonable to speak of "the Christian position" when by that we mean, as David Lindberg defines it, "the 'center of gravity' of a distribution of Christian opinion, for great variety existed."[2] This variety is rendered much more controversial when the literature of those groups that were declared heretical by the orthodox community is included and then juxtaposed with the latter's responses. The line between orthodoxy and heresy was often drawn on the basis of the extent to which the theology of any group was perceived as having been derived from pagan constructs that were deemed inherently incompatible with Judeo-Christian revelation.[3]

Specific aspects of classical culture, especially pagan philosophical systems, have been isolated for special scrutiny by those who have sought to understand how early Christians were influenced by, and sometimes reacted against, a predominantly pagan and hostile environment.[4] Sometimes ancient "science," as a subset of philosophy, has been the focus of their attention.[5] Now and then, secular medicine's role in the theology and practice of the early church, of particular Christian sects, and of individual church fathers has evoked specialized studies by a variety of scholars.[6] I suggest that six fundamental principles must be propaedeutic to further discussion of the place of health, sickness, healing, and the art of medicine in early Christianity in general and in the theology of individual church fathers in particular.

First, all church fathers shared the basic presupposition that God's creation was essentially good. One may reasonably assert that any ostensibly Christian writer who classified all created matter as inherently and intrinsically evil was *eo ipso* not Christian. To insist that such radical dualism as that of the Gnostics, the Manichees, and some Docetists belongs within the broad range of early Christian beliefs that in the aggregate can be regarded as normative is to make of early Christianity something so amorphous as to be infinitely malleable.[7]

Second, all church fathers held that although humanity and all of nature are fallen, God has provided for man to sustain himself through the proper use of nature. Within the history of Christianity, there have been dramatic changes in what has been regarded as the proper use of nature for man's benefit. And at all times there has been considerable variation within the broad boundaries of Christianity. Since self-denial, and particularly asceticism, is exceedingly rare today among Christians and within Western society generally, the spiritually motivated desire (expressed in the vast majority of early Christian sources) that Christians should not pamper the body at the expense of the soul or be consumed with the material and temporal to the detriment of the spiritual and eternal may seem severe and is often misunderstood today.[8]

Third, all patristic sources who say anything about medicine share the assumption that the use of physicians and the art of medicine are not *essentially* and *intrinsically* inappropriate for Christians.

Fourth, all church fathers who write on medicine and physicians also place significant limitations on Christians' recourse to them. One must not rely exclusively on them. One must rely on God as the source of the skill of the physician and of the efficacy of the medicine, for God may choose to heal through them, to heal without them, or to withhold healing.

Fifth, the sentiment, commonly held by Christians today, that all healing comes from God, whether directly, through prayer, or through the use of medicine and the skill of physicians, cannot be accurately attributed to any extant source from the patristic period. All the church fathers were unequivocal in their conviction that healing sometimes came from evil sources. Satan and his minions, that is, demons (and early Christians regarded the multitude of pagan deities as demons) were able to heal. No church father dismissed the pagan healing cults as frauds or denied that demons effected cures. Asclepius was a demon to be taken very seriously indeed. Furthermore, the church fathers never denied the efficacy of magic. Granted, they regarded some practitioners of magic as charlatans and tricksters. But they never denied the demonically based power of magic, since they knew that many pagans employed magic efficaciously for a variety of purposes, including the healing of disease.

Sixth, the church fathers were convinced that the art of medicine could be used for egregious and sinful ends.

Thus far I have made some very dogmatic assertions. I have made them unequivocally. Moreover, I have reached a point in my study of medicine in the early church at which I feel confident not only in underscoring their accuracy but in making an additional assertion: no Christian document from the patristic period entirely condemns, *on theological grounds,* the Christian's use of physicians and medicine.[9]

These six basic presuppositions, which I am convinced that all church fathers shared, may be categorized as three positive principles followed by three negative positions. The positive principles are: (1) since the world as God created it is good, matter is not inherently evil; (2) God provided in nature for man's sustenance; and (3) physicians and their art may be used beneficially by Christians. The negative positions, assumptions that qualify these principles, are sometimes implicit but usually glaringly explicit in our sources. (1) There are significant limitations on the occasions and extent to which the Christian should use the services of physicians and medicines. (2) God is by no means the source of all healing, for much healing comes through spiritually pernicious sources such as the demonic healing cults and demonically empowered magic. And (3) the art of medicine can be used for evil purposes.

I am also convinced that the foundational presuppositions regarding the appropriate place of medicine in God's creation that are seen in the patristic sources are without exception found in medieval Catholic sources as well. The same tensions continued, as did the compatibilities. In spite of strongly expressed uneasiness about some aspects of the use of medicine found in primary sources, no Christian document from the Middle Ages entirely condemns, on theological grounds, the Christian's use of physicians and medicine.

Nevertheless, because many scholars approach the texts with the assumption that patristic and medieval Christianity were inherently hostile to, and suspicious of, medicine, they read such presuppositions into their sources or rely on other scholars who do so. I have been guilty of the latter. In chapter 2, "The Physician's Obligation to Prolong Life: A Medical Duty without Classical Roots," which was published in 1978 while I was still relying primarily on secondary literature for my understanding of the place of medicine in early Christianity, I remarked, quite in passing, "Many early Christians and church fathers . . . insisted that God . . . either inflicts or permits disease and the practitioner of the secular healing arts thus works against divine purposes. Wide acceptance by Christians of the medical art as consonant with the sanctified life of faith took centuries."[10] I was in very good company, however, as I shared this undercurrent of misunderstanding that has sometimes seriously, and at other times only slightly, distorted modern scholarly perceptions of the acceptability of secular medicine to the early church.

Many scholars, as early as Adolf Harnack in 1892 and as late as Vivian Nutton in 1985,[11] have viewed early Christianity as a religion of physical healing. In Nutton's words, "From its inception Christianity offered itself as a direct competitor to secular healing."[12] In the paper just cited, Nutton refers to the conclusions that I reached in "Medicine and Faith in Early Christianity" as "far too bland,"[13] and in another essay published the same year, he writes that while I had

strongly argued that, on the whole, Christianity was favorable to medicine, or at any rate, not hostile—a conclusion with which I would agree—yet this argument is rather too bland, and misleading on one important point. As Harnack long ago showed, Christianity is a healing religion *par excellence*. The New Testament emphasizes the power of Christ and his apostles to cure diseases, and this was one of the features that secured for Christianity the primacy among competing religions. Similarly, Ramsay MacMullen[14] has recently pointed to the crucial significance of healing miracles in securing the allegiance of intellectual doubters and of the ordinary people to Christianity. Yet this Christian healing was not that of the doctors. It succeeded where they had failed, often over many years and at great expense; it was accessible to all; it was simple. It was a medicine of prayer and fasting, or of anointing and the laying on of hands. The power to heal was given to Christian elders, and they were to be consulted first in all cases of illnesses.[15]

In a recent paper Gary Ferngren has conclusively demonstrated that early Christianity was not a religion that offered freely to all the healing of physical ills. Although the New Testament emphasizes the miracles of Jesus and, to a lesser extent, those of the apostles as substantiating proofs of the truth of Christianity, the role of healing miracles within the Christian community and as part of the evangelistic enterprise during the second and third centuries was so minor as to be nearly negligible.[16] If early Christianity had been "a direct competitor to secular healing" as a predominantly healing cult, *tension* would be too bland a word to use for the relationship between it and secular medicine: "open hostility and conflict" would have to be used. Furthermore, it is interesting to note that it is not until the fourth century that reports of miraculous healings are frequently encountered. With the rise of the cult of saints and relics in the later part of that century, they become commonplace. If the assumptions of certain scholars are correct, we have the peculiar puzzle that the tensions between Christianity and medicine were diminishing in intensity at the very time during which the frequency of miraculous healings was dramatically increasing, that is, at a time when competitiveness between the two healing alternatives should have been exacerbated.

Further study in which I have engaged since writing "Medicine and Faith in Early Christianity" has intensified my certainty that the conclusions articulated there are correct. One deficiency in my understanding of the issues at that time, however, was corrected when I concentrated a decade later on the question of why Tatian had felt compelled to condemn the field of pharmacology. It was only then that I came face to face with the obvious fact that early Christians did not see God as the source of all healing, believing that evil forces healed as well.

The assumption of Christian hostility to medicine has thoroughly conditioned scholars both to accept the most negative interpretation of texts and to impose some equally negative ones of their own.[17] I shall give two examples from an article by Fridolf Kudlien, an excellent classical scholar who should, however, speak with considerably less certainty about early Christianity. Some patristic sources condemn physicians' performing abortions but none more colorfully and forcefully than Tertullian in chapter 25 of *De anima*. Some scholars use such sentiments as evidence of a Christian denunciation of medicine per se, which, of course, they are not. Tertullian also excoriated physicians who were reputed to have practiced vivisection (ibid., 10), which seems to provide further evidence for his supposed rejection of physicians and their art. Given the vitriol of Tertullian's denunciation both of these procedures and of those who practiced them, it is easy to understand why some scholars have exaggerated his position into a blanket rejection of secular medicine. It is more difficult, however, to excuse the carelessness of Hans Schadewaldt, who attributes to Tertullian the following statement: "Pharmacy in all its forms is due to the same artificial devising. If anyone is healed by matter because he trusts in it, all the more will he be healed if in himself he relies on the power of God. . . . Why do you not resort to the Lord of superior power, but choose rather to heal yourself like a dog with grass, or a deer with a snake, a hog with river crabs, or a lion with monkeys?" Schadewaldt cites page 19 of Harnack's "Medicinisches aus der ältesten Kirchengeschichte," where one finds a footnote that begins with a reference to Tatian, switches to Tertullian, and then, four lines later, returns to Tatian and concludes with a forty-seven-line quotation from Tatian's *Oratio ad Graecos*. Twenty-four lines into this quotation begins the section that Schadewaldt wrongly attributes to Tertullian.[18] Kudlien specifically cites this exact passage in Schadewaldt as his authority for the bold statement that Tertullian "attacks not only Pagan physicians . . . but medicine per se."[19]

After Kudlien adopts Schadewaldt's misattribution of Tatian's words to Tertullian, he includes Tatian among those "whose hostility against physicians and medicine is almost outrageous." He goes on to say that Tatian "argued that one is not allowed to cure diseases since they are sent from God, so that to take medicine would make you an atheist."[20] This is a most interesting jumble of misunderstandings of the attitudes not only of mainstream early Christianity, but even of such a renegade as Tatian, to the nature of disease and healing. Kudlien begins his article by referring to what Ludwig Edelstein has called "the Christian glorification of disease," which seems to have tempered much of what Kudlien writes about Christianity in the article's closing pages. It would be as difficult to locate any early Christian source that simply and unqualifiedly attributes all disease directly to God as it would be to find one that without qualifications attributes all disease to demons. If disease was regarded as caused by demons, to seek healing would have been appropriate if the right means were used. However, if God was credited with being the ultimate cause of disease under the broad rubric of divine sovereignty, it did not follow that to seek healing through appropriate means would be fighting against God's will. Granted, even some of the church fathers who were most liberally disposed to Christians' using medicine (e.g., Basil of Caesarea) held that when a Christian was sick, he should seek to determine why God sent or permitted the affliction before he sought a cure. That is, of course, a long way from maintaining that to attempt to cure diseases is to resist God, who sent or permitted them. Even those exceedingly few extreme ascetics who may legitimately be said to have glorified disease did not encourage such an attitude in others. Some, who refused to seek any kind of healing of their own ills, employed the secular art of medicine to minister to the ills of others.[21]

That the same individual could with equanimity refuse medical care for himself when ill, but administer medicines to the ill as an expression of Christian charity, is one of many examples of the complex and subtle ambiguities that characterized the relationship of medicine and Christianity at least through the end of the Middle Ages.

Without an adequate understanding of these ambiguities, one will almost inevitably reach erroneous conclusions about that relationship. Even the compatibilities will be misunderstood. An example is the misreading of medical-spiritual metaphors, which early and medieval Christian authors were very fond of employing. Thus clerics are described as *medici spirituales* or *medici animarum*. They must be *medici periti*, expert physicians, who can astutely diagnose and treat diseases by applying first the most gentle herbs, then, if necessary, harsher medicines, and finally, as a last resort, painful cautery or surgery. There is practically no end to the rich variety of metaphors of which these authors avail themselves. It is painful to see scholars misreading such passages as applying to the body rather than to the soul, to *medici corporum* rather than to *medici animarum,* and hence as evidence of Christian enthusiasm for secular medicine, whether practiced by secular physicians or by clerics.[22]

By the late Middle Ages the existence of a recognized medical profession whose monopoly was guaranteed by both state and church, whose responsibilities were defined and, as much as possible, enforced by the church, and whose medical theory was not discordant with orthodox theology and whose techniques were not religiously illicit, was useful in providing a traditionally acceptable, nonspiritual source of healing clearly distinct from the sometimes magical alternatives feared by ecclesiastical authorities. Yet this alliance of the church with orthodox medicine as practiced by a recognized and licensed profession still remained uneasy. For the propensity of the sick was to neglect their duty to God, that is, to make use of medicine and not desire the help of God. This is a frequently repeated concern throughout the first fifteen hundred years of Christianity (and well beyond), where the attitude criticized was one of independence, a belief that one was able to maintain or restore one's health without reference to one's Creator. The church could exhort, threaten, and plead against that attitude but could not effectively regulate or control the attitudes of the sick or of physicians toward the medical art, which was itself regarded not only as being a gift of the Creator but also as having a dangerous potential to lure people away from submission to him.

Respect for Human Life, or the Principle of the Sanctity of Human Life

It is revealing to study the iconography of the "death chamber" in Western civilization from the late Middle Ages to the present. Initially, the dominant characters besides the dying person are spiritual beings—angels and demons—who contend for his soul, while the clergy provide solace and administer the sacraments. Present but in the background are physicians, helplessly hovering in the shadows, obligated to be there in spite of their inability to cure. This picture gradually gives way to a scene in which the dominant figures are physicians and nurses. Spiritual forces are gone; so, often, are the clergy, but if they are present they are as inconspicuous as the physicians in the earlier depiction. Finally, a new picture emerges. The clergy are gone; so, for the most part, are the physicians and nurses. In their place are various medical apparatus. The patient is alone.

These scenes of the moment of death illustrate some aspects of the issues that I wish to discuss under the rubric of respect for life. By the late Middle Ages physicians were increasingly expected to be involved with the dying patient. They had not always been. Indeed, in classical antiquity, taking on a case that could not be successfully treated was regarded as the physician's ethical duty by virtually no one. Many would have regarded a physician who took on a hopeless case as acting un-ethically, being propelled by mercenary motives or a desire to experi-ment at the expense of his patients. Likewise, if a patient's condition became hopeless, no one would have regarded the physician as obli-gated to stay with him until the end; if he did stay, many would castigate him for the same reasons. After all, the physician's role was to attempt to cure the ill (or to provide prophylactic advice to the healthy). Most probably would have asked what business he had with the dying.[23]

Such was also the attitude throughout the early Middle Ages. The advent of Christianity created no change in this aspect of medical deon-tology. But Christianity did introduce moral obligations that were quite alien to the Greek and Roman ethos. One of these was an obligation to care—not an obligation to cure, but an obligation to care—a categorical imperative to extend compassion in both word and deed to the poor, the widow, the orphan, and the sick. This was a truly revolutionary change in attitudes toward the sick, and we continue to feel its effects. As Henry Sigerist observed, Christianity introduced

the most revolutionary and decisive change in the attitude of society toward the sick. Christianity came into the world as the religion of healing, as the joyful Gospel of the Redeemer and of Redemption. It addressed itself to the disin-herited, to the sick and the afflicted, and promised them healing, a restoration both spiritual and physical. . . . It became the duty of the Christian to attend to the sick and poor of the community. . . . The social position of the sick man thus became fundamentally different from what it had been before. He assumed a preferential position which has been his ever since.[24]

To Sigerist's generally valid observations three qualifications must be made.

First, Christianity was not predominantly a religion of physical healing.

Second, although Christianity demanded of its adherents a practical charity that, as Sigerist so well expressed it, gave to the sick man "a preferential position which has been his ever since," it did not en-courage the seriously ill to cling desperately to life. To go to extreme lengths to forestall death in cases where little or nothing can be done is clearly denounced in early Christian literature as tantamount to blas-phemy. But the fact that Christians were encouraged to trust in the sovereign will of God and to place their destiny in his hands in such circumstances must not be construed as evidence that they placed a low value on human life and employed suicide or active euthanasia when afflicted with extreme suffering.

Just how incisively some modern scholars have severed themselves from their Judeo-Christian roots became clear to me when I was asked to write a study of suicide (including active euthanasia) and early Christian values (an abridged version of which is printed as chapter 4 of the present volume). I had accepted the invitation convinced that the undertaking would be straightforward and relatively uncomplicated. If I had limited myself to analyzing the primary sources, I would have presented a relatively short and quite uncomplicated study. But, for better or worse, I thought that it would be interesting to see just what conclusions anyone who wished to peruse the recent literature on suicide would derive about early Christian attitudes toward suicide. What I found shocked and amazed me. Misunderstandings of the most basic tenets of Christianity and an ignorance of patristics, not to mention the New Testament, had embued some modern scholars with highly distorted assumptions about early Christian attitudes toward suicide. Their basic presuppositions may be summarized as follows:

1. Early Christianity was a depressing religion whose adherents were so burdened by sin, guilt, and hopelessness that many of them committed suicide in despair; alternatively, it was an ecstatic religion that induced its followers to seek martyrdom or suicide in order to gain heaven.

2. So great was the contempt of early Christians for their sinful flesh that some killed themselves in order to escape it.

3. The lack of evidence that any Christians except Judas killed themselves for the reasons given above presents no problem. Christians who were willing to die for their faith, some eagerly, others even volunteering, had such a low regard for their own lives that suicide would have been natural to them. After all, martyrdom is suicide too, as is any willingness to die for any cause.

4. People thus disposed would not have hesitated to kill themselves to escape from suffering, especially that due to illness, and most especially that due to painful and terminal illness. And they would happily have assisted each other in this endeavor. Unfortunately for these scholars, there is no example of a Christian committing suicide in the face of painful or terminal illness during those centuries.

5. It was Augustine who turned everything on its head by introducing a thoroughly negative perspective on suicide and active euthanasia, a perspective with which Christianity has been grievously saddled until the late twentieth century.

Why should some recent scholars, none of whom is a specialist in New Testament and patristic studies or even in Greco-Roman history, have such significant misunderstandings of the very essence of early Christianity and early Christian history? It is inconceivable that their colleagues in an earlier generation, say forty years ago, would so thoroughly have misconstrued the spirit of early Christianity. Is it because Western society has so consciously cut itself off from its Judeo-Christian roots that many people who are educated in the West now know little more about Judeo-Christian tradition and values than they do, for example, about Buddhism?

We in the humanities can no longer assume an accurate understanding of the most basic aspects of our Western heritage either by our colleagues or by our students. About ten years ago I asked a class of fifty students, evenly divided among freshmen, sophomores, juniors, and seniors, who Abraham was. Only four of fifty had any recollection of having heard of him. The same feeling of disbelief that I experienced then I felt afresh when reading recent assessments of early Christian attitudes toward suicide.

The majority of our students have been cut off from the Judeo-Christian roots of Western civilization. Not merely our students but some of our colleagues as well have little understanding of this tradition. Although they have academic credentials in abundance, they are as uneducated or miseducated in such matters as are the majority of their students. Unfortunately, this does not always prevent them from speaking or writing with confident assertiveness about a subject of which they have a distorted view. Hence much contemporary scholarship is vitiated by merely trendy but wrongheaded misconceptions about the most basic foundations of Judeo-Christian history and thought.

It is not just those who are outside their fields of competence when dealing with Christian history and theology who are saying some truly remarkable things about suicide in early Christianity. Recently some scholars trained in theology and the history of Christianity have forced under the broad semantic umbrella of "voluntary death" early Christians' attitude that "to die is gain," their willingness to die for their faith (a few even actively seeking martyrdom), their contempt for death, their lack of attachment to this life, and their eager anticipation of heaven. Arthur Droge and James Tabor, for example, in *A Noble Death: Suicide and Martyrdom among Christians and Jews in Antiquity,*[25] take this "voluntary death" to be the moral equivalent of suicide and active euthanasia (as well as doctor-assisted suicide). Hence the enthusiastic endorsement on the back of the book's dust jacket by Derek Humphrey, founder of the Hemlock Society: "This book will upset traditional Christian views about the right to choose to die." But although early Christians actively cared for the sick and indeed gave to the sick, in Sigerist's words, a preferential position that has been theirs ever since, *there is no evidence that this preferential position of the sick included an expedited "final exit."*

The third qualification that must be made to Sigerist's statement is that Christianity's imperative of providing charitable care to the destitute does not appear to have initially imposed on physicians any sense of obligation to take on hopeless cases or to stay with those patients whose condition had become hopeless. Granted, the Christian qua physician should be compassionate. But the physician qua physician had no obligation to minister in any way to the dying. This view gradually underwent a significant change during the course of the high and late Middle Ages.

A small number of treatises that deal with medical ethics have survived from the early Middle Ages.[26] They are part of a genre at least as old as the Hippocratic Corpus. Most of the attention in these treatises is directed toward traditional concerns such as the physician's character and basic etiquette. Nevertheless, we see in them a blending of Hippocratic etiquette with Christian morality, particularly charity.

Beginning with the anonymous Salernitan treatise entitled *De adventu medici aegrotum,*[27] the treatises on medical ethics of the late Middle Ages reached their apogee in the writings of such physicians and surgeons as Bernard Gordon, William de Congenis, William de Saliceto, Arnald of Villanova, Jan Yperman, Henri de Mondeville, John Arderne, and Guy de Chauliac.[28] Their ethical observations remain loyal to the traditional concerns of the genre and preserve the early medieval blending of classical medical etiquette with Christian ethics. A new pragmatism, however, is present, a pragmatism born of the realities of medical practice by secular, although Christian, practitioners in a society starkly different from that of the monastic authors of the early medieval medical literature. Although no mention of guilds or universities appears in this literature, its tone and emphasis, when dealing with basic qualifications and responsibilities of physicians, demonstrates that the practice of medicine was considered to be a privilege that not only was restricted to those who met requirements for training and skill but also brought responsibilities to those exercising the role of physician or surgeon. There is no outright statement of the physician's obligation to his immediate community. Yet the obligation to the Christian community at large, an obligation to extend medical charity to the poor and destitute, occurs with emphasis. Although not stated as a specific obligation, treating dangerous and even desperate cases is generally not discouraged as it had traditionally been. While it is occasionally warned against, so infrequent are these warnings in comparison to advice on what to tell the critically ill patient and his relatives or friends, that one must conclude that there was a growing tendency to take on dangerous or even hopeless cases.

This tendency seems to have been the product of two possibly complementary sources. The first is itself the very basis for medical practice in the late Middle Ages. A specific authority (whether royal, ecclesiastical, or municipal) granted to a select few the privilege of practicing. That privilege, although perhaps respected elsewhere by other authorities, was limited to a specified region. The authorities who granted what was essentially a monopoly were also (in theory) responsible for protecting that monopoly. The contents of the documents either requesting or granting the privilege to exercise a monopoly in supplying medical or surgical service within the community demonstrate that responsibilities were clearly recognized as being attached to the privilege of holding a monopoly. While there is a compelling need for a thorough study of medical and surgical guild ethics in the late Middle Ages, and although conditions undoubtedly varied enormously, nevertheless some examples from London in the fourteenth and fifteenth centuries probably are reasonably representative.

In 1369, three surgeons were appointed as master surgeons of the City of London. They swore before the mayor and aldermen

that they would well and faithfully serve the people, in undertaking their cures, would take reasonably from them, etc.,[29] would faithfully follow their calling, and would present to the said mayor and aldermen the defaults of others undertaking cures, so often as should be necessary; and that they would be ready, at all times, when they should be warned, to attend the maimed or wounded, and other persons etc.; and would give truthful information to the officers of the city aforesaid, as to such maimed, wounded, and others, whether they be in peril of death or not, etc. And also, faithfully to do all other things touching their calling.[30]

The stated duties of these master surgeons are to three different groups: (1) their profession; (2) the people; and (3) the state. (1) They are to do all things faithfully that pertain to their calling. (2) They are well and faithfully to serve the people, be available to attend those who need their services, and charge them reasonable fees. (3) In a super-visory capacity, they are to report to the appropriate officials the failings of their fellow surgeons; and in a forensic capacity they are to give truthful information to the officers of the city concerning the maimed, the wounded, and others. This tripartite responsibility is the fundamen-tal principle of medieval craft guild ethics.

Madeleine Pelner Cosman writes that this document "implies, though it does not state, that patients who have desperate wounds or are in danger of death must be shown to the masters. Later documents [1390 and 1424], in fact, state that responsibility precisely."[31] The oath of the master surgeons of 1390 is almost identical to that of 1369, except that the master surgeons swear to be ready "to examine persons hurt or wounded, and others, etc."[32]

In 1423 a petition was addressed by representatives of the physicians and of the surgeons of London to the mayor and aldermen requesting that a joint *collegium*, or guild, of the two crafts be authorized.[33] Medical practice was to be under the aegis of two surveyors of medicine and sur-gical practice under two masters. The two houses were to be united under one rector of medicine. George Unwin, the great historian of English guilds, writing in the early twentieth century, says of the document under consideration that it illustrates "the best spirit of professionalism at this period of London history." He summarizes its contents as follows:

Their rules were meant to ensure that all practitioners in both branches should be duly qualified, if possible, by a University training, and they sought to provide a hall where reading and disputation in Philosophy and medicine could be regularly carried on. No physician was to receive upon himself any cure [i.e., case], "desperate or deadly," without showing it within two or three days to the Rector or one of the Surveyors in order that a professional consultation might be held, and no surgeon was to make any cutting or cauterization which might result in death or maiming without similar notice. Any sick man in need of professional help but too poor to pay for it, might have it by applying to the Rector. In other cases the physician was not to charge excessive fees, but to fix them in accordance with the power of the sick man, and "measurably after the deserving of his labour." A body composed of two physicians, two surgeons, and two apothecaries, was to search all shops for "false or sophisticated medicines," and to pour all quack remedies into the gutter.[34]

Most important for our concerns, physicians taking on "desperate or deadly" cases were required to consult the appropriate authorities within the collegium. Such cases involved not only special considerations but special obligations as well.

In 1493 an agreement was entered into between the Barbers' Company and the Surgeons' Guild. Although the two corporations were not united by this agreement, they were to choose two wardens from among the barber-surgeons and two from the surgeons. These four wardens were to have jurisdiction over all surgical matters in the city and over all surgeons practicing in London, whether of the Barbers' Company or the Surgeons' Guild, or of foreign provenance. They were to be responsible for examining outsiders who wished to practice and bringing to the mayor anyone illegally practicing surgery. The wardens also would be available for the mandatory consultation in cases liable to result in death or maiming. They were not to force any surgeon to leave a case under his care, "but that yche of them be redy to helpe eche other w^t counsell or deed, y^t worship profyte and the honeste of the crafte, and helpyng of the seke be had and done on all sydis."[35]

As with the oath of 1369, discussed above, but with a somewhat different arrangement of emphases, this last sentence, quoted from the agreement of 1493 entered into by the Barbers' Company and the Surgeons' Guild, gives in a nutshell the foundational principles of medieval medico-surgical guild ethics: (1) that each guild member be ready to help the other with counsel or deed; (2) that he have a regard for the profit (i.e., the well-being) and honor of the guild; and (3) that he help the sick "on all sides." It is essential to keep the order of these principles in mind if we are properly to understand the thrust of the guild movement as it affected the development of medical ethics.

The guilds were functional organizations that were inherently selfish and designed to promote and protect the special interests of their members. They were companies of brethren united, more often than not, by a common economic activity, which was viewed as being best served by the subordination of individual to group or corporate interests. The well-being and honor of the craft depended upon the mutual cooperation of its members. If guild members practiced cooperation and were mindful of the honor of the guild, then they could effectively render the services or produce the commodities that were their central economic function. Achieving all three of these, in late medieval urban life, hinged upon the authority of the craftsmen, merchants, professors, physicians, or surgeons to perform their functions unmolested by those who would illicitly meddle in their affairs. Thus an exclusive right to fill a particular role was sought; and in exchange for the privilege of holding a protected vocational status, the guild would guarantee as a sine qua non a level of expertise in the production of its commodity or in the rendering of its service. It also accepted the responsibility to police and to supervise its own members, in respect to both their qualifications (that is, training leading to licensure) and their performance. Regulations governing the minutiae of conduct, both within the guild and in relationships with customers or the community, varied considerably from guild to guild and from city to city. But the obligation to ensure competence and quality seems to have been a constant and essential feature.

In the late Middle Ages, the conviction was very strong that every man must have his *officium* (his office or calling) and that commensurate with his calling there were certain duties and obligations incumbent upon him that were distinctly and ontologically attached to his officium. That one responsibility of physicians and surgeons was to service the sick of the community *indiscriminately* would probably have seemed self-evident.

The second source of the growing tendency to take on dangerous or hopeless cases is the increasing theological emphasis in the late Middle Ages that the physician should do all he could to cure until the end, or nearly the end, and that he had a right to receive his fee under such circumstances. One finds in the casuistic literature the seed of what was later to blossom into a medical duty to prolong life. This is discussed in detail in chapter 9. Late medieval moral theologians strongly articulated the view that the physician is religiously obligated to extend care to a rich miser even if the latter both refuses to pay and resists treatment. Additionally, some moral theologians maintained that even if a patient should refuse to call a confessor the physician must not desert him, since succor must be given to those who are in danger regardless of how stubborn they are. While this is still far from an imperative to prolong life, it is a significant change from what had been traditional medical attitudes and practice.

It appears that by the late Middle Ages the Judeo-Christian principle of the sanctity of life was wedded to the socio-religiously defined expectations attached to those entrusted with the privileged monopoly of medical and surgical practice. In the earliest-published essay reprinted in this volume (chapter 10), I had asserted that in the late Middle Ages the "physician acted totally within the strictures of accepted ethics by refusing to treat a patient for whom the physician had no hope of recovery. The only criticism that contemporaries could make would be that he was in error to regard the condition as untreatable." It should be obvious that I would not now make such a categorical statement. Conditions and consequent expectations were changing. By the late sixteenth century, the simple desertion of incurables by physicians must have become relatively rare. Francis Bacon writes that "in our times, the physicians make a kind of scruple and religion to stay with the patient after he is given up."[36] He levels no criticism against their continued attendance on the terminally ill, but castigates physicians for failing to give more diligence to finding cures for conditions thought incurable.

This very basic change in attitudes toward the responsibility of a physician to his patient is neatly illustrated by contrasting the positions of two popes, one from the late twelfth century and the other from the mid-eighteenth century. Both have to do with the question of a physician's entering holy orders. In the late twelfth century, Pope Clement III responded to a physician who requested admission to holy orders but was troubled that, as a result of his medical practice, he might have unknowingly incurred an irregularity that would, if known, be an obstacle to his admission to orders. Clement replied that he should search his memory to ensure that he had never, even unintentionally, harmed a patient by any treatment that he had administered.[37] When Pope Benedict XIV addressed the same question in the mid-eighteenth century, he stated that physicians who wished to enter orders should first obtain a dispensation *ad cautelam,* that is, as a precaution, since they could never be absolutely certain that they had always employed every means at their disposal for those patients who died under their care.[38] There is a vital change here: while in the twelfth century the concern was with possible harm inflicted on a patient actively, in the eighteenth it was with harm that resulted passively. In the first case, the question was, Did you ever harm patients by the treatment you gave them? In the second, it was, Did you ever harm patients by failing to give them the treatment you should have given? These two documents by themselves prove nothing, but they illustrate a very fundamental change both in physicians' sense of responsibility to their patients and in popular expectations, a change rooted, at least in part, in a redefinition of medical practice from a right to a privilege.

So it is well before the advent of modern medicine that physicians were saddled with the expectation that they must do all that they could to cure a patient and that they not desert the patient *in extremis.* Hence, beginning with the late Middle Ages, they were depicted as lingering in the background in the death chamber, able to do nothing, but still obligated to be there. The major change since then is in the capacity of the medical profession to cure disease and prolong life, and in the often-unrealistic expectations of society that physicians should be able to perform miracles. This has in part resulted from a changed view of nature. Granted, since the time of Hippocrates and Plato dispute has intermittently arisen over the question of whether the physician works with or against nature in the treatment of illness. Francis Bacon's plea that physicians seek to prolong life by finding cures for supposedly incurable conditions has blossomed into an attitude that in such a quest it is "man against nature"—the "conquest" of disease involving the use of human ingenuity to thwart nature's purposes. Nevertheless, the principle of the sanctity of life had long before been allied with the physician's obligation to do all he could for the patient and to stay with him to the end.

A duty to attempt to treat the terminally ill, or at least not to desert them, is rendered significantly more complex in the face of epidemics of virulently contagious diseases. Chapter 10, "Medical Deontology and Pestilential Disease in the Late Middle Ages," seeks to answer the question of whether medieval physicians, beginning with the Black Death of 1348–49, were possessed of an ethical imperative to treat plague victims. When I wrote that essay, the issue was merely an historically interesting academic question. This is no longer the case.

For more than thirty years a *pax antibiotica*—to use John D. Arras' apt expression—has existed, at least in the Western world.[39] Virtually every life-threatening *communicable* disease has been conquered either by immunization or by efficacious treatment. Although the specter of that noncommunicable killer, cancer, looms large in our consciousness, and we impatiently await another medical miracle, we have long been accustomed to enjoy freedom from reasonable fear of deadly communicable diseases. This environment has fostered an absence of such fear not only among the public generally but also among physicians. For the first time in human history, a generation of physicians has arisen who practice their art in an environment that has become, if not entirely risk free, at least free from the risk of contracting life-threatening communicable diseases. In the past decade, however, that cozy security has been devastated by what has become known as HIV infection, and AIDS.

The responses to this new plague have been varied and revealing. Some AIDS activists have become exceedingly demonstrative in demanding what some regard as supererogatory efforts by medical research facilities to find a cure for AIDS and by the government to fund their efforts.[40] Others have moralized AIDS, seeing it as a judgment of God on the homosexual community and, to a lesser extent, on users of intravenous illicit drugs. Indeed, an opinion poll taken by the Los Angeles Times Syndicate in November 1987 suggested that 43 percent of Americans regarded AIDS as God's punishment for moral decline.[41] But even those who moralize AIDS have come to recognize that the spillover of the disease into society at large makes the moral ambiguities of this syndrome great enough to render clearcut pronouncements of divine retribution difficult.

The response of the medical community has been mixed and, in some respects, troubling. Although studies have shown only a minute occupational risk of infection, some physicians have refused to give care to seropositive patients. A relatively prominent surgeon, Dudley Johnson, publicly announced that he would not perform "long operations" on anyone who tested seropositive. Ninety-one percent of the surgeons responding to a poll conducted by *Cardiovascular News* regarding Johnson's announced intention shared his opinion.[42] Physicians refusing to care for AIDS patients became sufficiently vocal and numerous to provoke the American Medical Association to condemn such conduct and Surgeon General C. Everett Koop to denounce them as "a fearful and irrational minority."[43] Early in 1992 a survey (conducted by Charles Lewis of the University of California—Los Angeles) of 202 internists in private practice in Los Angeles County revealed that 48 percent refuse HIV-infected patients.[44] Another survey found that 50 percent of 1,121 American physicians would refuse if given a choice.[45] To complicate matters even further, some physicians have expressed a willingness to treat only seropositive patients who contracted HIV "innocently," that is, other than through homosexual activity or sharing needles in illicit drug use.[46] It is interesting to note that distinct nuances in some recent studies suggest a philosophical tolerance, however limited and highly qualified, of nearly every justification for refusing to treat the seropositive other than a moralizing one.[47]

We have, then, at least four negative reactions to AIDS patients by some members of the medical community: (1) a flat refusal to treat any under any circumstances; (2) a refusal to engage in any long or complex procedures; (3) a refusal to treat if the physician is able to avoid treating; and (4) a refusal to treat those whose mode of contracting AIDS the physician regards as morally opprobrious. Even if only a relatively small minority of physicians have taken any of these positions, it is obvious that there is at present a crisis of medical ethics precipitated by the AIDS epidemic, and that this crisis is likely to increase in seriousness as the number of AIDS patients increases and until a cure for AIDS is developed. Should AIDS suddenly disappear, the ramifications of the negative positions taken by what could be a sizable minority of physicians may be enormous. One positive effect of AIDS, however, is that it has stimulated ongoing analyses of some crucial and foundational aspects of medical ethics by representatives of various disciplines.[48]

One of these disciplines is history. Seldom do scholars explore the question of whether physicians are ethically obligated to treat patients who are HIV positive without attempting first to derive some understanding of the issues from history, usually from the intersecting of the history of medical ethics with that of epidemiology. It is, of course, unlikely that history can provide anything that could be reasonably claimed as a binding precedent. It should, however, be able to furnish more than interesting, but in the final analysis irrelevant, anecdotes. Is there an ethico-historical antecedent of AIDS? Surely none that is exact. Plague is much more dissimilar than similar to it. Syphilis is a more likely candidate. There are some suggestive parallels. But the congruities should not be pushed too far.

It was indeed the AIDS "epidemic" that stimulated me to study the writings of the earliest syphilographers in an effort to determine (1) their moral response both to the disease and to those suffering from it, especially as its venereal mode of transmission became patent; and (2) whether they felt a duty to treat those whose actions had brought the disease upon themselves. The final conclusions to that study, which is only now being put into form for publication as chapter 11 of this volume, were written with a view to answering those questions and with no eye on possible parallels with AIDS. A short and very superficial version of chapter 11, which ostensibly was to cover the first thirty-five years of the syphilis "epidemic," had the ambitious and, I can say in retrospect, presumptuous title, "AIDS, Ethics, and Moral Judgments: The Historical Antecedent of the Syphilis 'Epidemic' of the Renaissance." Fortunately, I was disabused of such lofty interpretive pretensions. If there are any parallels, it is for others to draw them.

NOTES

1. Preamble to the "Constitution of the World Health Organization," in *The First Ten Years of the World Health Organization* (Geneva: WHO, 1958).

2. David Lindberg, "Science and the Early Church," *Isis* 74 (1983): 529.

3. There is an enormous and still-growing volume of scholarly literature that addresses both the conceptual framework and the broad range of issues that arise in any effort to understand the relationship of early Christianity and classical culture. As a starting point, one should peruse the voluminous writings of Adolf Harnack and Jean Daniélou, whose presuppositions, and hence conclusions, generally conflict, at least on the major issues. Reference should also be made to Charles N. Cochrane, *Christianity and Classical Culture: A Study of Thought and Action from Augustus to Augustine* (Oxford: Oxford University Press, 1940); M.L.W. Laistner, *Christianity and Pagan Culture in the Later Roman Empire* (Ithaca, N.Y.: Cornell University Press, 1951); and the various essays edited by Arnaldo Momigliano in *The Conflict between Paganism and Christianity in the Fourth Century* (Oxford: Oxford University Press, 1963).

4. On the impact of pagan philosophy (which constitutes a considerable portion of classical culture) on Christianity, there is also an extensive literature. The works of Werner Jaeger, *Early Christianity and Greek Paideia* (Cambridge: Harvard University Press, 1961); A. H. Armstrong and R. A. Markus, *Christian Faith and Greek Philosophy* (London: Darton, Longman, and Todd, 1960); Henry Chadwick, *Early Christian Thought and the Classical Tradition: Studies in Justin, Clement, and Origen* (Oxford: Oxford University Press, 1966); and H. B. Timothy, *The Early Greek Apologists and Greek Philosophy, Exemplified by Irenaeus, Tertullian, and Clement of Alexandria* (Assen, Holland: Van Gorcum, 1973) constitute a good starting point.

5. John W. Draper, *The History of the Conflict between Religion and Science*, 8th ed. (New York: D. Appleton, 1876); and Andrew D. White, *A History of the Warfare of Science with Theology in Christendom* (New York: D. Appleton, 1896), which are essentially anti-Christian—especially anti-Catholic—polemics, are both still in print in several languages and continue to play a significant role in shaping both popular and scholarly misunderstandings of Christianity's historical relationship with science. Lindberg, "Science and the Early Church" (n. 2), presents both a balanced corrective to Draper and White and a reliable assessment of the current *status quaestionis*. See also Richard A. Norris, *God and World in Early Christian Theology: A Study in Justin Martyr, Irenaeus, Tertullian, and Origen* (London: Black, 1966); and especially D. S. Wallace-Hadrill, *The Greek Patristic View of Nature* (New York: Barnes and Noble, 1968).

6. In addition to chaps. 5 and 6 below, see the literature cited in chap. 5, nn. 1 and 21, to which should be added Owsei Temkin, *Hippocrates in a World of Pagans and Christians* (Baltimore: Johns Hopkins University Press, 1991); Paul Diepgen, *Die Theologie und der ärztliche Stand* (Berlin-Granewald: Dr. Walther Rothschild, 1922); Darrel W. Amundsen and Gary B. Ferngren, "Medicine and Religion: Early Christianity through the Middle Ages," in *Health/Medicine and the Faith Traditions: An Inquiry into Religion and Medicine*, ed. M. Marty and K. Vaux

(Philadelphia: Fortress, 1982), 93–131; idem, "The Early Christian Tradition," in *Caring and Curing: Health and Medicine in the Western Religious Traditions,* ed. Ronald L. Numbers and Darrel W. Amundsen (New York: Macmillan, 1986), 40–64; Gerhard Müller, "Arzt, Kranker und Krankheit bei Ambrosius von Mailand (334–97)," *Sudhoffs Archiv* 51 (1967): 193–216; K. Schweiger, "Medizinisches im Werk des Kirchenvaters Origenes" (Med. diss., Düsseldorf, 1983); and Karl-Heinz Leven, *Medizinische bei Eusebios von Kaisareia,* Düsseldorfer Arbeiten zur Geschichte der Medizin 62 (Düsseldorf, 1987).

7. The categorizing of some individuals and groups, e.g., Marcion and the Marcionites, evokes considerable scholarly disagreement. Marcion is regularly credited with a blanket rejection of physicians and the art of medicine on the basis of his radical dualism and such flimsy evidence as his expunging from Col. 4:14 the designation of Luke as ὁ ἰατρὸς ὁ ἀγαπητός. I have, in fact, taken this position (see chap. 5, below), as have, for example, Harnack, Frings, Schadewaldt (all cited in chap. 5, n. 1); and Fridolf Kudlien, "Cynicism and Medicine," *Bull. Hist. Med.* 48 (1974): 305–19.

8. Although Peter Brown, *The Body and Society: Men, Women, and Sexual Renunciation in Early Christianity* (New York: Columbia University Press, 1988), is concerned primarily with the subject described in the book's subtitle, it offers some interesting observations on the motivations for ascetics' discipline of their bodies. It was not a hatred of the body, but rather a love of the body, because it was to be resurrected, that stimulated measures that seem to us rather harsh. See especially 222–26 and 235–39.

9. Some church fathers (e.g., Origen and pseudo-Macarius) taught that the most spiritually mature Christians should rely entirely on God for the healing of their physical ills but held that medicine and physicians were gifts of God for the succor of the rest of humanity, which indeed included the vast majority of Christians. A very different case is that of Arnobius, who hurled vitriolic barbs against physicians and seems to be typical of a type encountered in most, perhaps all, societies—that is, those whose distrust of physicians knows no bounds. Arnobius' hatred of physicians need be no more an integral part of his Christianity than were the misiatric sentiments of, say, the Spartan king Pausanius (as recorded by Plutarch, *Moralia* 231A) a salient feature of the latter's religious beliefs.

10. See chap. 2, text at n. 55.

11. A. Harnack, "Medicinisches aus der ältesten Kirchengeschichte," *Texte Untersuchungen zur Geschichte der altchristlichen Literatur* 8, no. 4 (1892): 37–152; nearly passim; and Vivian Nutton, "Murders and Miracles: Lay Attitudes to Medicine in Classical Antiquity," in *Patients and Practitioners: Lay Perceptions of Medicine in Pre-Industrial Society,* ed. Roy Porter (Cambridge: Cambridge University Press, 1985), 48–49.

12. Nutton, "Murders and Miracles," 48.

13. Ibid., n. 83.

14. Nutton refers to Ramsay MacMullen, *Paganism in the Roman Empire* (New Haven: Yale University Press, 1982), 95–96, 135.

15. Vivian Nutton, "From Galen to Alexander, Aspects of Medicine and Medi-

cal Practice in Late Antiquity," in *Symposium on Byzantine Medicine,* ed. John Scarborough, Dumbarton Oaks Papers no. 38 (Washington, D.C.: Dumbarton Oaks, 1985), 5.

16. Gary B. Ferngren, "Early Christianity as a Religion of Healing," *Bull. Hist. Med.* 66 (1992): 1–15.

17. It is precisely this false assumption that helped numerous scholars read into the texts of medieval canon law a blanket condemnation of the practice of medicine and surgery by clerics. See chap. 8, below, which was written specifically to correct such misreadings of the legal texts.

18. Hans Schadewaldt, "Die Apologie der Heilkunst bei den Kirchenvatern," *Veröffentlichungen der Internationalen Gesellschaft für Geschichte der Pharmazie* 26 (1965): 126–27.

19. Kudlien, "Cynicism" (n. 7), 317.

20. Ibid., 317–18. It should be noted, however, that this article contains an excellent discussion of Cynicism and medicine. It is only when comparisons with Christianity are made that serious misunderstandings are evident.

21. See, e.g., Susan Ashbrook Harvey, "Physicians and Asceticism in John of Ephesus," in Scarborough, *Symposium* (n. 15), 87–93.

22. As an example of one effort to correct such misinterpretations of an early medieval theologian's writings, see Frederick Paxton, "Curing Bodies—Curing Souls: Hrabanus Maurus, Medical Education, and the Clergy in Ninth-Century Francia," *J. Hist. Med. Allied Sci.* 50 (1995): 230–52.

23. See chap. 2. My opinions expressed there have not changed. My understanding of the issues, particularly as they arise in the Hippocratic Corpus, however, has been significantly enriched by a study that makes some of my remarks appear retrospectively to be a bit facile: Heinrich von Staden, "Incurability and Hopelessness: the Hippocratic Corpus," in *La maladie et les maladies dans la collection Hippocratique: Actes du VIe colloque international Hippocratique,* ed. Paul Potter, Gilles Maloney, and Jacques Desautels (Paris: Editions du Sphinx, 1990), 75–112.

24. Henry Sigerist, *Civilization and Disease* (Chicago: University of Chicago Press, 1943), 69–70. It should be noted that Sigerist, himself an avowed Marxist, did not carry a banner for Christianity, as is graphically illustrated by a passage in his diaries, entered in London on June 8, 1935: "I firmly believe in the fundamental goodness and honesty of man. Give him social security, a chance to work and his share in the goods of life and he has no reason to be wicked. Christianity came into the world as the religion of love, and failed. It was adopted because man was afraid of life. If you are not afraid of this life you need not wait for a hypothetical hereafter. Christianity failed to create satisfactory economic conditions. It did not prevent man from exploiting his fellow-men and therefore sowed hatred instead of love." *Henry E. Sigerist: Autobiographical Writings,* selected and translated by Nora Sigerist Beeson (Montreal: McGill University Press, 1966), 110.

25. Arthur Droge and James Tabor, *A Noble Death: Suicide and Martyrdom among Christians and Jews in Antiquity* (San Francisco: Harper, 1992).

26. They are discussed, with lengthy quotations, by Ernst Hirschfeld, "Deontologische Texte des frühen Mittelalters," *Archiv für Geschichte der Medizin und der*

Naturwissenschaften 20 (1928): 353–71; and Loren C. MacKinney, "Medical Ethics and Etiquette in the Early Middle Ages: The Persistence of Hippocratic Ideals," *Bull. Hist. Med.* 26 (1952): 1–31.

27. See Henry E. Sigerist, "Bedside Manners in the Middle Ages," *Quart. Bull. Northwestern Univ. Med. School* 20 (1946): 136–43.

28. See Mary Catherine Welborn, "The Long Tradition: A Study in Four-teenth-Century Medical Deontology," in *Medieval and Historiographical Essays in Honor of James Westfall Thompson,* ed. James Lea Cate and Eugene N. Anderson (Chicago: University of Chicago Press, 1938), 344–57; E. A. Hammond, "In-comes of Medieval English Doctors," *J. Hist. Med. Allied Sci.* 15 (1960): 154–69; and Luis García-Ballester, "Medical Ethics in Transition in the Latin Medicine of the Thirteenth and Fourteenth Centuries: New Prospects on the Physician-Patient Relationship and the Doctor's Fee," in *Doctors and Ethics: The Earlier Histo-rical Setting of Professional Ethics,* ed. Andrew Wear, Johanna Geyer-Kordesch, and Roger French (Amsterdam: Rodopi, 1993), 38–71.

29. So abbreviated here and elsewhere in the original. Madeleine Pelner Cosman, "Medieval Medical Malpractice: The Dicta and the Dockets," *Bull. New York Acad. Med.* 49 (1973): 26, says that this indicates "that the procedures of investiture and components of commitment were written down incompletely because they were familiar and formulaic."

30. Henry Thomas Riley, ed., *Memorials of London and London Life in the XIIIth, XIVth, and XVth Centuries* (London: Longmans, Green, 1869), 337.

31. Cosman, "Malpractice" (n. 29), 26.

32. The oath of 1390 is in Riley, *Memorials of London* (n. 30), 519–20.

33. The text of the petition is printed in John Flint South, *Memorials of the Craft of Surgery,* ed. D'Arcy Power (London: Cassell, 1886), 299–301.

34. George Unwin, *The Gilds and Companies of London* (London: Frank Cass, 1963), 173.

35. Sidney Young, *The Annals of the Barber-Surgeons of London* (London: Blades, East, and Blades, 1890), 66–69.

36. *The Philosophical Works of Francis Bacon,* trans. R. L. Ellis and J. Spedding, ed. J. M. Robertson (1905; reprint, Freeport, N.Y.: Books for Libraries, 1970), 487.

37. Gregory IX, *Decretales* 1.14.7.

38. Pope Benedict XIV, *De synodo diocesana libri tredecim* 1.13.10.

39. This expression was, to the best of my knowledge, coined by John D. Ar-ras, "The Fragile Web of Responsibility: AIDS and the Duty to Treat," *Hastings Center Rep.* 18, special suppl. (1988): 10.

40. E.g., Charles Krauthammer, "AIDS: Getting More Than Its Share," *Time,* June 25, 1990, 80. See the reaction by Timothy F. Murphy, "No Time for an AIDS Backlash," *Hastings Center Rep.* 21, no. 2 (1991): 7–11.

41. Arras, "Fragile Web" (n. 39), 18.

42. Ibid., 14, 17.

43. "Doctors Who Shun AIDS Patients Are Assaulted by Surgeon General," *New York Times,* September 10, 1987, as cited by Arras, "Fragile Web" (n. 39), 20 n. 34.

44. "Doctors Shun Those with HIV," *USA Today*, February 2, 1992.

45. Ibid.

46. See the discussion by Arras, "Fragile Web" (n. 39), 17.

47. Norman Daniels, "Duty to Treat or Right to Refuse?" *Hastings Center Rep.* 21, no. 2 (1991): 36–46.

48. E.g., in addition to the material cited above, Walter J. Friedlander, "On the Obligation of Physicians to Treat AIDS: Is There a Historical Basis?" *Rev. Infect. Dis.* 12 (1990): 191–203; Daniel M. Fox, "The Politics of Physicians' Responsibility in Epidemics: A Note on History," *Hastings Center Rep.* 18, special suppl. (1988): 5–10; Benjamin Freedman, "Health Professions, Codes, and the Right to Refuse to Treat HIV-Infectious Patients," ibid., 18, special suppl. (1988): 20–25; George J. Annas, "Legal Risks and Responsibilities of Physicians in the AIDS Epidemic," ibid., 18, special suppl. (1988): 26–32; Richard M. Ratzan and Henry Schneiderman, "AIDS, Autopsies, and Abandonment," *JAMA* 260 (1988): 3466–69; Elizabeth Fee and Daniel M. Fox, eds., *AIDS: The Burdens of History* (Berkeley: University of California Press, 1988); Abigail Zuger and Steven H. Miles, "Physicians, AIDS, and Occupational Risk: Historic Traditions and Ethical Obligations," *JAMA* 258 (1987): 1924–28; Edmund D. Pellegrino, "Altruism, Self-Interest, and Medical Ethics," ibid., 258 (1987): 1939–40; and Erich H. Loewy, "Duties, Fears, and Physicians," *Soc. Sci. Med.* 22 (1986): 1363–66. This list could easily be quintupled and it still would provide only a sampling of the extensive and ongoing discussion.

TWO

The Physician's Obligation to Prolong Life: A Medical Duty without Classical Roots

Is the physician's duty to prolong life a modern phenomenon, or does it have its roots in Hippocratic or other strains of classical medicine? First we must ask, what is meant by the phrase "the physician's duty to prolong life"? If this question were put to a physician in classical antiquity, he might reasonably ask whether, by prolonging life, we mean increasing longevity generally; preserving health by prophylaxis; combating curable diseases and injuries; temporarily prolonging the unhealthy life of a terminally ill patient; or refusing to assist in terminating the life of any man with or without his consent, whether healthy or ill, and if ill, whether with a painful but curable or an incurable ailment.

He might also ask what we mean by life. Would we limit the term to useful, productive, happy, and healthy life; to that of the citizen, the foreigner, the freeman, the slave? And of the word *duty* he might quite rightly ask: "Duty to whom? to the patient, even against the patient's wishes? to the medical art or profession? to public opinion, to the state, to religion? to his own conscience, simply as a man, or as a physician?"

This list of hypothetical questions is by no means exhaustive, and of course most of them are still being asked. But there are a few that may seem slightly alien to modern considerations. We should first, at least indirectly, address our attention to these questions, for they will provide us with a heightened awareness of some important differences between the ethos of the classical world and that of modern Western cultures.

The practice of medicine was a right, not a privilege, in classical antiquity. It remained so in the Western world until some geographically limited licensure requirements were instituted beginning in the twelfth century. There was no system of medical licensure, and anyone who wished to could set himself up as practitioner of the healing arts. Therefore, one can speak of a "medical profession" in classical Greece and Rome only in the sense that the phrase designates the aggregate of those who called themselves physicians. This designation does not exclude those medical practitioners or schools of medical theory and practice that seem to us, and may have seemed to some contemporary practitioners, to typify charlatanism rather than medical professionalism. Given this qualification, it should come as no surprise that the phrase "ethics of the profession" can be very misleading. There were no professional standards that were enforceable by law or by inclusive medical organizations. Although certain exclusive medical societies set standards of conduct for their members, at no time was the swearing of any oath or the acceptance of any informal or formal code of ethics required of anyone calling himself a physician and undertaking to treat patients.

This is not to say there were no ethical standards; diverse examples are evident in both medical and lay classical literature. But those that seem consonant with modern medical ethics or appear as "timeless ideals" of medicine may have been held by only an unrepresentative minority of medical practitioners at any given time during the classical period.

What was the physician, the ἰατρός of the Greek, the *medicus* of the Roman? By the most basic definition, he was one who practiced the art of preserving or restoring health. If the primary function of the classical physician was preserving or restoring health, ideally he should be a compassionate man. When I say "ideally," I am thinking in terms of the "ideal" physician as he appears, at least in simile and metaphor, especially in philosophical or political literature. When thus used, the word *physician* was not a neutral term, but denoted a "compassionate, objective, unselfish man, dedicated to his responsibilities." In this manner the good ruler, legislator, or statesman was sometimes called the physician of the state; essentially, the statesman should be to the state what the physician is to his patient.[1]

Although some of the medical literature deals with etiquette, little is said about the "ideal" physician or the moral basis for medical practice. In the Hippocratic Corpus appears the statement "Where there is love of man, there is also love of the art,"[2] which is often cited as if ancient medical ethics were founded upon this lofty principle. Yet it rests in the context of a discussion about fees that is introduced by the admonition "I urge you not to be too unkind." Attempts to find any assertions in the Hippocratic Corpus that would set up philanthropy as an indispensable motivation for practicing medicine are fruitless.[3] Occasional medical sources strongly emphasize that the physician should be moved by love of humanity.[4] But as Galen laments, philanthropy is the inspiration of only a minority of physicians; the majority pursue money, honor, or glory. Proficiency in the art, not one's motivation for practicing, determines whether or not one is a physician.[5] "The motive . . . is a matter of personal choice," as Ludwig Edelstein summarizes Galen's opinion; "it has no intrinsic connection with the pursuit of medicine."[6]

Regardless of the motivation behind engaging in medical practice, an apparently constant ideal was that the physician was "to help, or at least to do no harm," a familiar aphorism found in the Hippocratic Corpus.[7] This famous adage appears in a variety of forms in other classical medical literature and seems to be axiomatic.[8] Although the literature of many cultures, not excluding those of Greece and Rome, is rife with accusations that physicians were using their art to evil ends, it is reasonable to assume that the physicians thus accused were viewed as having acted in violation of an inherent principle undergirding their calling. Thus rhetoricians, when giving examples of contradictions or opposites, were wont to cite the adulterous philosopher, the temple-robbing priest, and the murderous physician.[9] When a physician used the opportunities provided by his relationship with a patient to kill him for political, financial, or other selfish or malicious reasons, not only would he as a physician have been viewed as having acting evilly, but he as a legal persona would have been culpable as an agent of homicide.[10]

Aside from such obvious examples of using the art of medicine to cause harm, were there other activities that would commonly have been so classified? Here we come to the crux of the problem of understanding the ancient physician's conception of his duty to his patients and to the art of medicine. Let us exclude from our discussion the small number of physicians who might have admitted to disagreeing with the proposition that as physicians they should render help, or at least not cause harm. How then would the ancient physician have defined or delimited the terms *helping* and *harming*? Would he have thought it helping or harming (1) to refuse to treat a terminally ill patient if medical intervention would temporarily prolong the patient's life; or (2) to agree to assist a man who for any reason wished to end his life? Now it can be objected that such questions are meaningless. They can only be addressed if fleshed out by specific sets of circumstances of definite cases, real or hypothetical. But if forced to put these two types of action under the rubric of helping or harming, a probably strong, if not overwhelming, majority of ancient physicians would have classified them as "helping, or at least not harming."

Plutarch preserves a favorite saying of Pausanias, king of Sparta from 408 to 394 B.C., to the effect that the best physician was the man who did not cause his patients to linger on, but buried them quickly.[11] Although Pausanias was well known as an excoriator of physicians, his remark represents a quite commonly held attitude. The medical art's two functions were preserving and restoring health, not prolonging life per se.

Plato is perhaps better known than any other classical source for ardently opposing any effort on the part of physicians to prolong the lives of patients who has no chance of regaining their health.[12] Plato, at least within the context of the *Republic,* may be an extreme case, for there his concern was much more with eugenics than with the personal worth of the individual. But aside from utopian literature, there is abundant evidence that, at least among the Greeks of the fifth century B.C. and later, health was considered both a virtue and an indicator of virtue.[13] Health was an ideal, indeed the highest good, set above beauty, wealth, and inner nobility. Health was a goal in itself, for without health all else was without value. The statement in the Hippocratic Corpus that without health nothing avails, neither money nor any other thing,[14] expresses a strong popular, philosophical, and medical view.

Refusing to Treat the Terminally Ill

Let us now directly address the first ethical question posed: Would ancient physicians have thought it helping or harming to refuse to treat a terminally ill patient if medical intervention would temporarily prolong the patient's life? The treatise entitled *The Art* in the Hippocratic Corpus defines medicine as having three roles: doing away with the sufferings of the sick, lessening the violence of their diseases, and refusing to treat those who are overmastered by their diseases, realizing that in such cases medicine is powerless.[15]

Again I emphasize that in classical Greece and Rome there was no system of medical licensure. Bound by no duty to a licensing authority or professional organization, the physician exercised his art at his own pleasure. He sold his services at his own discretion to those who asked and paid for treatment. Lucian emphasizes that the physician should be completely free to treat or to refuse to treat. In one of his treatises he has a physician state that "in the case of the medical profession, the more distinguished it is and the more serviceable to the world, the more unrestricted it should be for those who practice it. It is only just . . . that no compulsion and no commands should be put upon a holy calling, taught by the gods and exercised by men of learning; moreover, it should not be subject to enslavement by the law. . . . The physician ought to be persuaded, not ordered; he ought to be willing, not fearful; he ought not to be hailed to the bedside, but to take pleasure in coming of his own accord."[16] To such a physician, any whim or reason not to treat a particular patient would be a justification not to give treatment. It could be merely a matter of personal sentiment. If, however, the physician were basing his decision whether or not to undertake a case only on the consideration that the treatment he gave would simply prolong the life of a patient for whom there was no hope of recovery, he of course would still be completely free to refuse. No legal or, even in the broadest sense of the word, ethical pressures could compel him to undertake treatment. It was entirely his decision, and regardless of what he decided, he would receive approbation from some medical or lay persons and condemnation from others.

I have already mentioned that in a treatise in the Hippocratic Corpus one role of medicine was to refuse to treat those who are overmastered by their diseases, realizing that in such cases medicine is powerless. This represents a very strong and, in my opinion, prevailing sentiment among ancient physicians. It is one for which precedent could easily have been found in Egyptian and Assyro-Babylonian medicine.[17] And it was a medical sentiment that remained strong throughout most, if not all, of the Middle Ages.[18]

In Greco-Roman medicine, the decision to refuse to treat such a patient was motivated by a variety of factors. If treatment would simply prolong life, the patient's interests would not have been served. Indeed, the physician would have been considered by many physicians and lay persons as having harmed rather than helped the patient. While the patient's interests may have been a partial motivation behind the decision not to treat, the most frequently articulated concern in the medical sources was the possible damage that such a case might cause to a physician's reputation. Many, if not most, of the ethical principles expressed in the medical literature were motivated by the physician's concern for his reputation. Although from a modern vantage point this seems reprehensible, we must remember that the physician's reputation was his only credential.[19] Earning and preserving a good reputation was a precarious enterprise. Charlatans were criticized for avoiding dangerous cases and exaggerating the severity of ailments that yielded easily to treatment.[20] Thus the conscientious physician, although he might shy away from hopeless cases, was urged in the medical literature not to refuse dangerous or uncertain ones.[21] But the decision whether to take on a dangerous case was entirely the individual physician's. Some cases in the therapeutic treatises in the Hippocratic Corpus are introduced with the advice that certain procedures should be allowed *if the physician chooses to attempt treatment.*[22] Indeed, it appears that physicians might have based their decisions on whether they were liable to earn less reprobation from refusing to treat than from agreeing to treat such cases.

If the physician did elect to take on a dangerous case, the importance of the art of prognosis or forecasting became evident. The physician who declared before beginning treatment that the prospects of a cure were only slight thereby avoided responsibility for an unfavorable outcome.[23] The medical literature is divided on the question of whether a physician should withdraw from a case once it became clear that he would be of no meaningful help. Some urged that the physician ought not to withdraw, even if by so doing he might avoid blame.[24] Others felt that he should withdraw if he had a respectable excuse, particularly if continuing treatment might hasten the patient's death.[25]

There is no denying, however, that physicians did sometimes attend cases considered incurable. In the Hippocratic Corpus many diseases that ended in death are described, with no mention of prognosis and with no recommendation to the physician that such cases be undertaken or rejected. In most of these, the medications to be employed are named. It was recognized that it was necessary to deal with incurable complaints in order to learn how to prevent curable states from advancing to incurability, particularly in the case of wounds. Even a cursory look at the *Epidemics* in the Hippocratic Corpus should convince the reader that the author's intention was not to show how to cure. Nearly 60 percent of the cases end in death, and treatment is very seldom mentioned. Such a physician's medical attendance was perhaps designed less for the individual patient's good than for the advancement of medical knowledge.

Opinions certainly varied on the physician's responsibility to undertake treatment of hopeless or dangerous cases. But the following quotation from Celsus represents what appears to have been the mainstream of medical thought: "For it is the part of a prudent man first not to touch a case he cannot save, and not to risk the appearance of having killed one whose lot is but to die; next when there is grave fear without, however, absolute despair, to point out to the patient's relatives that hope is surrounded by difficulty, for then if the art is overcome by the malady, he may not seem to have been ignorant or mistaken."[26] Taking on a hopeless or, under some circumstances, an extremely dangerous case is perhaps the closest issue in ancient medicine to the modern question of employing "extraordinary measures."

Danielle Gourevitch writes of the Greco-Roman physician, "Far from feeling any liability for abandoning his patient, he would feel guilty if he undertook a cure he could not successfully carry out."[27] This is perhaps somewhat overstated. It is true that if the physician were motivated by greed to continue inefficacious treatment, he would be viewed as acting reprehensibly; nevertheless, if he were attempting a novel treatment in an effort to effect a cure, the ethical implications would not be as clearcut.[28] Markwart Michler views the "Hippocratic" admonition to refuse to treat patients overwhelmed by their diseases ("an inhuman attitude") as a taboo finally broken by the authors of the treatises *On Fractures* and *On Joints* in the Hippocratic Corpus. In these works the authors are said to be motivated by a desire to advance knowledge so as to be able ultimately to render more effective treatment to the suffering.[29] The objective even here was not an ethically based imperative to prolong the life of the incurable patient, but rather a very pragmatic desire to increase the boundaries of the art.

Laín Entralgo bases much of his understanding of Greek medical ethics on the idea that the Greek physician's sense of responsibility both to his art and to his patient rested on his *physiophilia*, that is, love of nature. Since, in Laín Entralgo's view φύσις (nature) "was 'divinity' to the Hippocratic doctor, he was deeply and spontaneously conscious of the religious and ethical imperative to respect the limits of his art. . . . The frequency and sternness with which [the] injunction to abstain from therapy is formulated in the *Corpus Hippocraticum* . . . clearly shows that it was not a mere piece of technical advice, but a religious and ethical injunction. Under the influence of his belief about nature, man and his own art, the Greek physician understood that it was his duty to abstain from treating the incurably and mortally ill."[30]

The diverse opinions of many more scholars could be quoted, but to little profit. The issues were usually not wrestled with in the primary sources that have survived, and modern appraisals of ancient attitudes often are not tempered by the consideration that divergent opinions existed side by side in antiquity and that society was not static. There are significant differences between, for example, fifth-century B.C. Athens, third-century B.C. Rome, and the Roman Empire of the first century A.D. The attitudes toward old age and death held by the Athenian gentleman of the fifth-century B.C. were, in certain respects, significantly different from those of a Roman aristocrat of a later period. "Generally speaking, the Greeks judged old age unfavorably. The Romans, however, cherished and respected it."[31]

It is noteworthy that an increased interest in the investigation of chronic diseases and the development of geriatric medicine were probably due in great part to the influence of Roman ideals. I cannot here deal adequately with the sundry issues that impinge upon the ancient physician's willingness to take on dangerous or hopeless cases. I am, however, confident that, although attitudes varied, generally a physician who prolonged, or attempted to prolong, the life of a man who could not ultimately recover his health was viewed as acting unethically.

Assisting in Suicide

We turn now to the second ethical question: would the ancient physician have thought it helping or harming to agree to assist a man who, for any reason, wished to end his life? To this question *probably* a majority of ancient physicians would have given the reply "Helping, or at least not harming." It is absolutely essential that we consider the ancient physician as a functioning member of a highly complex and diverse society whose moral responses arose from ethical foundations sometimes strikingly different from what may seem typical of the Western world today. Except among some groups on the periphery of classical thought, the "sanctity of human life" was an idea partially obfuscated by, or at least subservient to, the belief in the inherent right of the free man to dispose of his life as he saw fit, if not always in its living, at least in its termination.

In neither Greek nor Roman law was suicide a concern of the state, except the suicide of a slave or of a soldier. Indeed, even murder, at least in Greek law, was not a crime against the state (a public offense); it was considered solely a matter between the victim (and his family) and the killer. Although murder was classified as a public offense in Roman law, it did not follow that suicide was viewed as self-murder; instead, it was outside the purview and interest of law. Should a person who wished to commit suicide enlist the aid of a second party, the latter, in rendering such assistance, was not culpable. Turning to extralegal sources, we find few objections in classical literature to suicide in general, fewer still to the suicide of the hopelessly ill.[32] Granted, a few cults or philosophical schools condemned all suicide, regardless of the circumstances. But these were both comparatively small in number and quite insignificant in long-range influence. Christianity is of course an exception, but the rise of its influence corresponds roughly with the decline of classical culture.

Platonists, Cynics, and Stoics considered suicide an honorable alternative to hopeless illness;[33] some philosophers regarded it as the greatest triumph of man over fate.[34] The Epicurean school did not censure suicide, but condoned it under many circumstances.[35] Porphyry wrote a treatise entitled "On Sensible Removal," and some authors went so far as to compose lists of conditions justifying suicide.[36] Pliny, for example, considered pain due to bladder stones, stomach disorders, and headache valid reasons for suicide.[37] Whether or not to commit suicide was completely up to the individual; whether or not to assist in the act was up to the physician, if asked. The literature contains references to physicians cutting the veins of patients, both ill and well, who asked for such a procedure.[38] Poison was even more common than sustained phlebotomy, and various poisons were developed by physicians, who were praised for employing their toxicological knowledge in the production of drugs for inducing a pleasant and painless death.[39] Assisting in suicide was a relatively common practice for Greco-Roman physicians; the very infrequent criticism of such physicians was made *primarily* by sources that would have to be considered atypical of classical thought. The so-called Hippocratic Oath must be placed into such a category.

The Hippocratic Oath: An Esoteric Document

Although scholarly opinion varies considerably as to how many (if any) of the treatises in the Hippocratic Corpus were written by Hippocrates,[40] few (if any) scholars today hold that the Oath that bears his name was written by the historically elusive "father of medicine."[41] Even the date of the composition of the Oath is unknown; some scholars place it as early as the sixth century B.C. and others as late as the first century A.D.[42] It apparently did not excite a great deal of attention on the part of physicians or others earlier than the beginning of the Christian era; the first known reference to it was made by Scribonius Largus in the first century A.D.[43]

Some of the stipulations in the Oath are not consonant either with ethical precepts prevalent elsewhere in the Hippocratic Corpus and in other classical literature or with the realities of medical practice as revealed in the sources. This has inspired a number of attempts either to explain away those inconsistencies or to attribute the Oath to an author or school whose views were, in other respects as well, discordant with those characteristic of classical society.[44] Most significant is Edelstein's theory that the Oath was a product of the Pythagorean school. Edelstein's thesis is tempting and, in my opinion, the most convincing so far advanced.[45] The Pythagorean origin of the Oath, however, should not be considered proved. It is reasonable to say with absolute certainty that the Oath, taken as a whole, is an esoteric document that is often inconsonant with the larger picture of Greco-Roman medical ethics.

Among the stipulations in the so-called Hippocratic Oath are prohibitions of the performance of abortions and the practice of surgery, both of which were common practices of Greco-Roman physicians. Immediately before these two injunctions is the famous passage that reads, "I will neither give a deadly drug to anybody, not even if asked for it, nor will I make a suggestion to this effect."[46] These three prohibitions have at least this much in common: they are inconsistent with values expressed by the majority of sources and atypical of the realities of ancient medical practice.

I do not want to debate the various possible origins of an oath that must be considered esoteric in many of its essentials. But it is known that, while these three prohibitions remained atypical of medical ethics for the entirety of the classical period, during the first and second centuries A.D. a greater sensitivity to two of them began to be evidenced. During the early Christian era some pagan physicians, influenced by the Oath, refused to perform abortions under any circumstances; others would perform them only to preserve the health of the mother, and others would perform them on request for any reason.[47] Some physicians began emphasizing philanthropy as their essential motive and extended philanthropy to include what we may generally term "respect for life."[48] Stressing, on the basis of the Oath, that medicine is the science of healing, not of harming, Scribonius Largus credits "Hippocrates," in condemning abortion, with going "a long way toward preparing the mind of the learners for the love of humanity. For he who considers it a crime to injure future life still in doubt, how much more criminal must he judge it to hurt a full grown human being."[49] He then asserts that unless medicine "strives fully in each of its parts to help those in need, it is not better than promising sympathy to men." Later he writes that the medical art should never be injurious to anyone. But Scribonius' insistence that the physician not harm or be injurious to anyone is just as neutral in respect to the issue of active or passive euthanasia as the Hippocratic aphorism "to help, or at least to do no harm."

Some physicians may have preferred not to assist in suicide, for it could prove to be a messy business, at least from a legal point of view. Physicians were frequently charged with, or at least suspected of, poisoning their patients. Other physicians, however, who may have refused to aid a person in committing suicide, perhaps condemned suicide under all circumstances for philosophical or religious reasons, but such physicians seem to have left few records of their sentiments, much less professional justification.

Aretaeus, who lived in either the first or the second century A.D., can *perhaps* be placed in this last category of physicians. He writes that some patients suffering from a particularly painful disease still shrink from death, while others beg for it. In these cases, he writes, it still is not proper for the responsible physician[50] to cause the patients' death, but it is proper to drug such patients to relieve their anguish.[51] On the basis of the paucity of such statements as Aretaeus' and the plethora of evidence of opposite sentiments, it is safe to conclude that the author of the Oath and perhaps Aretaeus represented a minority opinion on the question of active euthanasia.[52]

Prolonging Life: A Search for the Origins

Does the modern physician's duty to prolong life have its roots in Hippocratic or other strains of classical medicine? The answer to this question must be a qualified "no." The only duty common to probably all Greco-Roman physicians was "to help, or at least to do no harm." Taking on a hopeless case was entirely the prerogative of the individual physician, and few voices would have condemned a refusal, particularly if such a decision were based on the conviction that the patient's unhealthy life would only be temporarily extended. Prolonging the life of a patient who did not want to live would probably have been considered harming the patient and therefore would have been seen as unethical by all, or nearly all, classical physicians, even by those constituting that minority who would not assist actively in terminating a patient's life.

While the physician's duty to prolong life does not have its roots in any strains of classical medicine, the idea of "respect for life" is quite a different matter. Owsei Temkin writes, concerning the so-called Hippocratic Oath and sources expressing compatible attitudes, that "sufficient material has now been gathered to prove the existence of a tradition which, in its uncompromising form, did not sanction any limit to the respect for life, not even therapeutic abortion."[53] This tradition that would sanction no limit to the respect for life appears, in its emphasis, to have been entirely negative: the physician would not actively terminate life by abortion or euthanasia. But it laid no stress, apparently, on the positive correlate that would require the physician actively to prolong life. This negative tradition did indeed become stronger with the rise of Christianity: abortion, suicide, and euthanasia became sins. As Temkin says, "God has given life, and man must not interfere with His purposes."[54] Many early Christians and church fathers, however, insisted that God also either inflicts or permits disease, and that the practitioner of the secular healing arts thus works against divine purposes.[55] Wide acceptance by Christians of the medical art as consonant with the sanctified life of faith took centuries. While abortion, suicide, and euthanasia became sins, the prolonging of life did not become either a virtue or a duty.

If the duty to prolong life is not found in classical medicine, where might we begin to look for it? Francis Bacon (late sixteenth, early seventeenth centuries), in his *De augmentis scientiarum*, divides medicine into three offices: the preservation of health, the cure of diseases, and the prolongation of life. He then writes that "the third part of medicine which I have set down is that which relates to the prolongation of life, which is new, and deficient; and the most noble of all."[56] He protests that physicians have not recognized the significance of the "new" branch of medicine but have confused it with the other two. He urges physicians to investigate means of developing a regimen designed to contribute to longevity.

Coming closer to our subject, in the same work Bacon writes that physicians "in their inquiry concerning diseases . . . find many which they pronounce incurable, some at their commencement, and others after a certain period."[57] At first sight he may seem to be castigating physicians for refusing to treat patients with incurable diseases. But this is not his concern here. Rather, his criticism is directed against the lack of concern with finding cures for conditions regarded as incurable. He exhorts "some physicians of eminence and magnanimity" to produce "a work on the cure of diseases which are held incurable . . . since the pronouncing of these diseases incurable gives a legal sanction as it were to neglect and inattention, and exempts ignorance from discredit."[58]

Expanding his discussion of the deficiencies of the medical art and profession of his day, Bacon writes that he considers it "to be clearly the office of a physician, not only to restore health, but also to mitigate the pains and torments of diseases; and not only when such mitigation of pain, as of a dangerous symptom, helps and conduces to recovery; but also when, all hope of recovery being gone, it serves only to make a fair and easy passage from life. For it is no small felicity which Augustus Caesar was wont so earnestly to pray for, that same *Euthanasia* [Bacon's emphasis]; which likewise was observed in the death of Antoninus Pius, which was not so much like death as like falling into a deep and pleasant sleep."[59]

Bacon then levels another criticism against the profession: "But in our times, the physicians make a kind of scruple and religion to stay with the patient after he is given up, whereas in my judgment if they would not be wanting to their office, and indeed to humanity, they ought both to acquire the skill and to bestow the attention whereby the dying may pass more easily and quietly out of life. This part I call the inquiry concerning *outward Euthanasia* [Bacon's emphasis], or the easy dying of the body (to distinguish it from that Euthanasia which regards the preparation of the soul); and set it down among the desiderata."[60] So, at least in the estimation of Bacon, the medical profession of his day was deficient owing, among other things, to its lack of concern with finding cures for supposedly incurable conditions and with finding and applying means for making death less unpleasant. He uses the term *euthanasia* in its etymological meaning, that is, an easy death, probably devoid of any implication of expediting death.

Most germane is Bacon's assertion that, in his time, "the physicians make a kind of scruple and religion to stay with the patient after he is given up." What is Bacon saying? What, if his statement is taken at face value, are these physicians, who feel obliged to stay with their patients after they are given up, doing? It is difficult to say how fair and objective Bacon is being here. He might very likely be saying that, on the one hand, physicians declare patients terminally ill who are suffering from diseases that the medical art has declared incurable without giving adequate attention to attempting to find a cure. But, on the other hand, physicians feel obligated to continue treating such patients for whom medical science holds out no hope, although they do not feel any compulsion to provide the means of an easy and felicitous death.

Now the statement that "the physicians make a kind of scruple and religion to stay with the patient after he is given up" can be taken to imply a sense of duty on the part of physicians to make an attempt, however inept or futile, to prolong the lives of terminally ill patients or simply not to desert them. Even if it means only the latter (and I do not so limit it), it is still a significant step toward the former. Bacon claims no recent origin for this scruple. But such a statement as his would most certainly not have been made, at least not commonly, in classical antiquity or during the greater part of the Middle Ages. It is my opinion that there were significant changes in the ethical bases for medical practice during the late Middle Ages, roughly from the twelfth through the fifteenth centuries. Many converging factors played roles in the formation of medical professionalism in a relatively "modern" sense of the word: the development of guilds, which, in exchange for the right to hold a monopoly in providing a service or commodity, were bound to adopt and enforce ethical codes; the creation of universities (which were themselves guilds); the institution of medical licensure requirements in some areas; and very importantly, the increasing importance of the Catholic Church as a factor in moral and ethical definition. Canon lawyers and moral theologians, including casuists and authors of *summae confessorum* and confessional manuals, directed considerable attention to defining and classifying the sins, both of omission and commission, as well as the moral obligations of various professions. Needless to say, the medical profession excited a great deal of their interest.

I have only begun to scratch the surface of the vast quantity of relevant primary sources, but I have found some tantalizing hints in certain authors. For example, the fifteenth-century moral theologian and casuist

Saint Antoninus of Florence, in his *Summa theologica,* devotes a lengthy section to the medical profession. In it are such statements as these: "Even if the sick man forbids any medicines to be given to him, a physician called by him or by his relatives, can treat the patient against the patient's will, just as a man ought to be dragged against his will from a house that is about to collapse,"[61] and "Succor must be given, following the rule of charity, to those who are in danger, however stubborn they may be."[62]

I must stress that these two quotations by themselves prove nothing but are merely a sliver from a vast beam of primary evidence begging to be investigated by the historian of medical ethics. For it is there that I am reasonably certain that solutions can be found for, or at least significant light shed upon, many problems in the development of medical ethics. One of these problems is of course the question of the origin of the physician's duty to prolong life, a duty that does not, except in its negative side, have direct roots in classical medicine, but was, in my opinion, probably well established by the seventeenth century.

NOTES

1. See, e.g., Thucydides, *The Peloponnesian War* 6.14; Euripides, *The Phoenician Women* 893; Plato, *The Statesman* 293A–C; idem, *Laws* 862B, 720D–E (cf. *Gorgias* 464B); idem, *Republic* 342D; Aristotle, *Nicomachean Ethics* 1180b; idem, *Politics* 1287a; pseudo-Demosthenes, *Against Aristogeiton* 2.26; Aeschines, *Against Ctesiphon* 225 f. Compare Cicero, *Republic* 1.62, 5.5; idem, *De oratore* 2.186; idem *Disputationes* 3.82. Even epigraphy yields an example: *Supplementum epigraphicum Graecum* 10.98.14.

2. *Precepts* 6.

3. P. Laín Entralgo, *Doctor and Patient,* trans. F. Partridge (New York: McGraw-Hill, 1969), argues that the Greek physician's relationship with his patients was based on a combination of *philantropia* and *philotechnia* (17 ff.). Later he maintains that "a careful study of the Hippocratic writings leads to the conclusion that Hippocrates and his direct and indirect followers were 'philanthropists' *avant la lettre*" (245 n. 1). His thesis, unfortunately, rests upon his belief that "there is an 'instinct to help' at work in human nature, moving a man to succour the sick" (45).

4. E.g., Scribonius Largus (in Karl Deichgräber, *Professio medici: Zum Vorwort des Scribonius Largus,* Abhandlungen der Akademie der Wissenschaften und der Literatur, no. 9 [Mainz, 1950]); and James H. Oliver and Paul Lazarus Maas, "An Ancient Poem on the Duties of a Physician," *Bull. Hist. Med.* 7 (1939): 315–23. For a discussion of the changing attitudes in classical antiquity toward philanthropy as the basis for medical practice, see Fridolf Kudlien, "Medical Ethics and Popular Ethics in Greece and Rome," *Clio Medica* 5 (1970): 91–121, especially 91–97.

5. Galen, *De placitis* 9.5.

6. Ludwig Edelstein, "The Professional Ethics of the Greek Physician," in *Ancient Medicine: Selected Papers of Ludwig Edelstein,* ed. Owsei Temkin and C. Lilian Temkin (Baltimore: Johns Hopkins Press, 1967), 336.

7. *Epidemics* 1.11.

8. See the discussion by C. Sandulescu, "*Primum non nocere:* Philological Commentaries on a Medical Aphorism," *Acta Antiqua Hungarica* 13 (1965): 359–68.

9. For the motif of the physician as a poisoner, see Quintilian, *Institutio oratoria* 7.2.17 f., 2.16.5; Calpurnius Flaccus, *Declamationes* 13; pseudo-Quintilian, *Declamationes minores* 321; Libanius, *Progymnasmata* 7.3.

10. See Darrel W. Amundsen, "The Liability of the Physician in Classical Greek Legal Theory and Practice," *J. Hist. Med. Allied Sci.* 32 (1977): 172–203; and idem, "The Liability of the Physician in Roman Law," in *International Symposium on Society, Medicine, and Law,* ed. H. Karplus (Amsterdam: Elsevier, 1973), 17–31.

11. Plutarch, *Moralia* 231A.

12. Plato, *Republic* 406C, 407D, 408B; cf. Euripides, *The Suppliant Women* 1109 ff. (quoted by Plutarch in his "Consolation to Apollonius," *Moralia* 110C); Aristotle, *Rhetoric* 1361b; Demosthenes, *Third Olynthiac* 33.

13. See, e.g., Ludwig Edelstein, "The Distinctive Hellenism of Greek Medicine," in *Ancient Medicine* (n. 6), 386 f.; Werner Jaeger, *Paideia: The Ideals of Greek Culture,* trans. G. Highet (New York: Oxford University Press, 1944), 3:44 f. For a discussion of health as the greatest good by a late classical source, see Sextus Empiricus, *Against the Ethicists* 48 ff.

14. *Regimen* 3.69; cf. Herophilus in Sextus Empiricus, *Adversus mathematicos* 11.50.

15. *The Art* 3; cf. *Diseases* 2.48.

16. Lucian, *Disowned* 23, in vol. 5 of Lucian's works, trans. A. M. Harmon, K. Kilburn, and M. D. Macleod (Cambridge: Harvard University Press, 1913–67).

17. See Darrel W. Amundsen, "History of Medical Ethics: Ancient Near East," in *The Encyclopedia of Bioethics* (New York: Free Press, 1978).

18. See Darrel W. Amundsen, "History of Medical Ethics: Medieval Europe," in *Encyclopedia of Bioethics;* and idem, "Medical Deontology and Pestilential Disease in the Late Middle Ages," *J. Hist. Med. Allied Sci.* 32 (1977): 403–21, especially 414 ff.

19. See Ludwig Edelstein, "Hippocratic Prognosis," in *Ancient Medicine* (n. 6), 76 f.; and idem, "The Hippocratic Physician," in ibid., 88 ff.; Henry E. Sigerist, *A History of Medicine,* vol. 2 (New York: Oxford University Press, 1961), 305.

20. E.g., in the Hippocratic Corpus, *Precepts* 7; Celsus, *De medicina* 5.26.1C (quoted below); Menander, *Phanium* 497K. See also Babrius, *Fables* 75, and Ausonius, *Epigrams* 4, for the motif of the deserted patient who recovers and encounters his physician. There is a slightly variant rendition attributed to Aesop: see *Fables of Aesop,* trans. S. A. Handford (Baltimore: Penguin, 1954), no. 189.

21. E.g., in the Hippocratic Corpus, *Precepts* 7; *Ancient Medicine* 9; *On Joints* 69; cf. *The Art* 8; Paulus Aegineta 6.88; Ctesias in Oribasius, *Collectionum medicarum reliquiae* 8.8.

22. E.g., *Diseases* 3.7; *Internal Affections* 12.

23. What responsibility a physician may have felt is open to discussion. There are many passages in the Hippocratic Corpus where the concern with incurring blame is expressed. (See, e.g., *On Joints* 67; *Decorum* 14; *Ancient Medicine* 9.) Gert Preiser, "Uber die Sorgfaltspflicht der Ärzte von Kos," *Mededizin-Historische Journal* 5 (1970): 1–9, maintains that there seems to have been no liability for the physician in Greek law. Thus, although the concern with the use of prognosis as a means to protect the physician from accusations suggests legal liability, Preiser holds that this concern was motivated by a professional responsibility based upon the "Hippocratic physician's" broad conception of his duty to his *techne*. I have attempted elsewhere to demonstrate that Greek, or at least Attic, law allowed for the prosecution of the dolose, incompetent, or negligent physician, as did Roman law. See note 10, above, both articles cited.

24. See Edelstein, "Professional Ethics of the Greek Physician" (n. 6), 323; and idem, "Hippocratic Physician" (n. 19), 90 ff.

25. E.g., in the Hippocratic Corpus, *On Fractures* 36; cf. *Aphorisms* 6.38; *Prorrhetic* 2.9.

26. Celsus, *De medicina* 5.26.1.C, trans. W. G. Spencer (Cambridge: Harvard University Press, 1935–38).

27. Danielle Gourevitch, "Suicide among the Sick in Classical Antiquity," *Bull. Hist. Med.* 43 (1969): 503.

28. See pseudo-Quintilian, *Declamationes maiores* 8, where both sides of the question are argued.

29. Markwart Michler, "Medical Ethics in Hippocratic Bone Surgery," *Bull. Hist. Med.* 42 (1968): 297–311.

30. Laín Entralgo, *Doctor and Patient* (n. 3), 48.

31. Edelstein, "Distinctive Hellenism of Greek Medicine" (n. 13), 381. Edelstein's statement is generally true; but it would be an easy task to cull from Greek literature sentiments of reverence for old age and from Roman sources statements of the opposite opinion.

32. There is an extensive literature on the history of suicide. A classic study is Rudolf Hirzel's "Der Selbstmord," *Archiv für Religionswissenschaft* 11 (1908): 75–104, 243–84, 417–76. David Daube's "The Linguistics of Suicide," *Philos. Public Affairs* 1 (1972): 387–437, is well worth consulting for its historical perspective. Gourevitch's article "Suicide" (n. 27), is of the most immediate relevance for the subject under discussion.

33. See especially Hirzel, "Der Selbstmord" (n. 32), 279 ff. A very cogent expression of the Stoic attitude toward suicide is Seneca's *Letters to Lucilius* 77. See also Diogenes Laertius, *Lives of the Eminent Philosophers* 4.3, 6.18, where criticism is directed against those who would cling to life when suffering from disability or extreme pain.

34. Hirzel, "Der Selbstmord" (n. 32), 279 n. 1. It should be noted that Plato, for example, condemned suicide as opprobrious if one is "not compelled to it by the occurrence of some intolerable and inevitable misfortune" (*Laws* 873C). On the origin of the famous prohibition in the *Phaedo*, see J.C.C. Strachan, "Who Did Forbid Suicide at *Phaedo* 62 B?" *Classical Quart.* 20 (1970): 216–20.

35. See Ludwig Edelstein, "The Hippocratic Oath," in *Ancient Medicine* (n. 6),

17. Aristotle argues in *Nicomachean Ethics* (1138a) that since the law does not expressly permit suicide, it forbids the act. Aristotle is concerned here with a citizen acting unjustly toward the state by thus depriving his city of a useful citizen. Elsewhere he unequivocally condemns the cowardice of one who kills himself simply to escape from poverty or love or pain (*Nicomachean Ethics* 1116a). It is very doubtful, in my opinion, that Aristotle would extend this castigation to the terminally ill suicide.

36. For some examples, see Gourevitch, "Suicide" (n. 27), 509 ff.

37. Pliny the Elder, *Historia naturalis* 25.7.23.

38. See, for example, Tacitus, *Annals* 15.69. Cf. Suetonius, *Life of Lucan.*

39. See Gourevitch, "Suicide" (n. 27), 508.

40. For a discussion of the problem, see Ludwig Edelstein, "The Genuine Works of Hippocrates," in *Ancient Medicine* (n. 6), 133–44; and G.E.R. Lloyd, "The Hippocratic Question," *Classical Quart.* 25 (1975): 171–92.

41. Savas Nittis' thesis that Hippocrates himself composed the Oath in Athens between March and October of 421 B.C. is unconvincing; see Savas Nittis, "The Authorship and Probable Date of the Hippocratic Oath," *Bull. Hist. Med.* 8 (1940): 1012–21.

42. Ludwig Edelstein dates the composition of the Oath to the middle to late fourth century B.C.. Edelstein, "Hippocratic Oath" (n. 35), 55 ff.

43. Scribonius Largus, *Professio medici*, p. 24 in the edition cited in n. 4.

44. Edelstein's discussion of the Oath (originally published in 1943) includes a summary of previous scholarly treatment.

45. Much has been written on the Oath since Edelstein's monograph, and several leading scholars have questioned the validity of his central thesis of the Pythagorean origin of the Oath. See, for example, Kudlien, "Medical Ethics" (n. 4); and Karl Deichgräber, *Der Hippokratische Eid* (Stuttgart: Hippokrates-Verlag, 1955), especially 40.

46. I have followed Fridolf Kudlein's translation. Kudlien, "Medical Ethics" (n. 4), 118 n. 47.

47. So writes Soranus, *Gynaecia* 1.60.

48. For a discussion, see Owsei Temkin, "The Idea of Respect for Life in the History of Medicine," in *Respect for Life in Medicine, Philosophy, and the Law,* by Owsei Temkin, William K. Frankena, and Sanford H. Kaddish (Baltimore: Johns Hopkins University Press, 1977), 1–23.

49. Scribonius Largus, *Professio medici*, p. 24 in the edition cited in n. 4.

50. The subject under discussion here is intestinal obstruction. This phrase (τῷ ἀρχιητρῷ δὲ οὐ θέμις πρήσσειν) is significant for two reasons.

—The expression οὐ θέμις is roughly equivalent to the Latin *ne fas*, meaning "morally wrong," "contrary to divine law," "in violation of what is customarily accepted," or simply "not proper." How strongly Aretaeus is here using the word, and what moral overtones are implied, are open to interpretation. θέμις without the negative is used in the next clause where he says that it "is proper" to drug the patient. In another instance he writes that the physician "is not able to make the ill [sc., those suffering from atrabiliousness] entirely well. For then the physician would be mightier than God. But it is proper [θέμις] for the physician to bring about the absence of pain and both regressions and latencies of diseases" (Corpus Medicorum Graecorum 2.158, lines 6 ff.). Elsewhere he writes that "it is not proper [οὐδὲ ... θέμις] to drink from a pool or from a river by mouth" (ibid., 86, line 29, where the subject is elephantiasis). Thus we should hesitate to interpret Aretaeus' statement quoted in the text as an extremely strong moral injunction.

— This is the only instance where Aretaeus uses the term ἀρχιητρός (Ionic for ἀρχιατρός), a word that usually means an official physician (either a court physician or a community physician). It also appears to have been used generally to mean a "responsible practitioner," and indeed, in Liddell and Scott's *Greek-English Lexicon*, this passage of Aretaeus is the only example cited to illustrate this meaning. In roughly the score of instances where he employs a word for "physician," Aretaeus uses ἰητρός (Ionic for ἰατρός). Indeed he uses ἰητρός in this same passage when stating what procedures the physician ought to follow when dealing with patients suffering from intestinal obstruction. Thus the clause may be translated, "It is *not proper* for a *responsible* physician to do this," and would then not be nearly as condemnatory as might appear at first sight. Indeed he probably is merely saying that a responsible physician should not perform euthanasia, at least when dealing with the ailment under consideration, while the less responsible and average physician might very well do so.

51. Corpus Medicorum Graecorum 2.133, lines 10 ff. In another passage Aretaeus, when discussing the treatment of inflammation of the lungs, writes that "if you give a drug to a patient at the height of choking and at the point of death, you would be responsible for his death in the opinion of the common people" (ibid., 120 lines 8 f.). Aretaeus' concern here seems to be less with the ethical issue than with reputation and possible legal implications.

52. There are three other sources sometimes cited as evidence for opposition to active euthanasia in classical antiquity.

— A passage in the Oxyrhynchus Papyri (no. 437, third century A.D.) where the Oath is quoted as the basis for the rejection of giving poison.
— A problematic passage in a metrical oath of unknown date: οὔτε τις ἂν δώροις με παραιβασίην ἀλεγεινὴν ἐκτελέειν πείσειε καὶ ἀνέρι φάρμακα δοῦναι λυγρά. A possible translation is "nor would anyone bribe me to alleviate a painful condition by giving baneful drugs (i.e. poison) to a man [sc., a patient]" (Corpus Medicorum Graecorum 1.1, pp. 5 f., lines 15 ff.). Owing to some ambiguity in the Greek, the exact relationship between τις and ἀνέρι is uncertain. If τις refers to a third party, then the swearer of this oath is refusing to give poison to a patient when asked by someone other than the patient. If ἀνέρι has a pronominal force, to which τις is antecedent, then he is refusing to give poison to the person requesting it for himself. It is ambiguous and may well have been intended to be ambig-

uous. (I wish to thank Ronald Kotrc of the College of Physicians of Philadelphia for discussing this passage with me.)

— A statement made by a physician in *The Golden Ass,* a novel written by Apuleius in the second century A.D. The statement can be interpreted as a condemnation of medical assistance in effecting euthanasia or as simply an assertion that the medical art should not supply the means for murder. On this passage see Temkin, "Respect for Life" (n. 48), 4; Darrel W. Amundsen, "Romanticizing the Ancient Medical Profession: The Characterization of the Physician in the Graeco-Roman Novel," *Bull. Hist. Med.* 48 (1974): 325; Gourevitch, "Suicide" (n. 27), 506 f.; and Edelstein, "Hippocratic Oath" (n. 35), 13 f. and nn. 23 and 24.

53. Temkin, "Respect for Life" (n. 48), 5.

54. Ibid., 16.

55. E.g., Arnobius, *Adversus gentes* 1.48; and Tatian, *Oration to the Greeks* 18. See Victor C. Dawe, "The Attitude of the Ancient Church toward Sickness and Healing" (Th.D. diss., Boston University School of Theology, 1955), especially 153 ff.

56. Francis Bacon, *De augmentis scientiarum,* in *The Philosophical Works of Francis Bacon,* trans. R. L. Ellis and J. Spedding, ed. J. M. Robertson (1905; reprint, Freeport, N.Y.: Books for Libraries, 1970), 485, 489.

57. Ibid., 487.

58. Ibid.

59. Ibid.

60. Ibid.

61. Antoninus of Florence, *Summa theologica* 3.7.2.3, my translation. The context is a discussion of the physician's obligation to treat the miser who, because of the expense, refuses to allow himself to be treated.

62. Ibid., 3.7.2.4, my translation. Some interpreters of canon law had rigidly maintained that a physician sins mortally who treats a patient who has not first confessed. Antoninus here maintains that such an opinion is too harsh, and justifies his position by the statement quoted in the text.

THREE

Medicine and the Birth of Defective Children: Approaches of the Ancient World

So diverse are the varied strands of ancient Greek and Roman cultures that it is dangerous—indeed, probably irresponsible—to speak of any universal ancient attitudes and practices, unless significant qualifications are placed upon any assertions other than the most specific and limited. In attempting accurately to describe—or, more correctly, to reconstruct—the response of people in antiquity to the defective newborn, it is necessary first to provide the broader context of values that informed, or actually formed, that response. And that broader context of values involves such issues as human worth, human dignity, the value of life, and human rights, inalienable and otherwise.

In the introduction to his very perspicacious monograph *Human Value: A Study in Ancient Philosophical Ethics*, John M. Rist maintains that the view that such rights as "the right to life, to have enough to eat, to live without fear of torture or degrading punishments, the right to work or to withold one's labour," or any other rights, "are the universal property of men as such was virtually unknown in classical antiquity." He further asserts that classical antiquity had no theory "that all men are endowed at birth (or before) with a certain value . . . though some of its philosophers took certain steps toward such a theory."[1]

It is especially in the literature of political philosophy that theories of human value are developed. The most famous representative of this genre is Plato's *Republic*, which must be supplemented by the *Statesman* and the *Laws* to provide a thorough picture of Plato's conception of human value within the ideal state. Does the ideal state exist for its inhabitants, or do the latter exist for the sake of the state? It seems as though both are true in Plato's view. Private worth, which is possession of the virtues, will inevitably lead to the seeking of the public good. While personal worth or value is always manifest in one's social utility, and is thus contributory to the common good, Plato seems to hold that personal worth is the *telos* of the ideal state (as the best environment for growth in personal virtue), rather than that the state is the telos of personal value. But the relationship is transparently circular, cause and effect, means and end being inextricably interwoven.

Within Plato's ideal state, failure to contribute renders one worthless. And there are levels of worth; some people are superior to others. The Guardian class, of course, has an intrinsic value that exceeds that of slaves, whose only value is in their material contributions to the state. But slaves aside, even among the Guardian class there are grades of worth. Although Plato views men and women of the Guardian class as fully equal, the qualities of this class are starkly masculine, suggesting that the most virtuous (i.e., valuable) women are those who are most like men in their developed character. The children of superior adults clearly possess a potential worth that increases as they come closer to maturity. However, children's worth is not intrinsic but only potential, and children are valued in proportion to their approximation to the ideal adult. They must be malleable, disposed to virtue, and physically fit.

Plato's concern for healthy children is clearly seen in his marriage regulations. The maximum number of superior adults should couple with others of equal worth. The number of inferior types coupling with others of similar value should be kept at a minimum. Since adults who are too young or too old produce less vigorous children than do those who are of ideal age for procreation, people should be prevented from having children except during their ideal years for producing robust offspring.[2] Indeed, the purpose of marriage is first to produce children to ensure the continuity of the state, and second to improve human stock.[3]

In a society in which absolute value is always seen through the grid of social value, those who are physically defective, or at least those who are chronically ill, should not be kept alive by diet, drugs, and regimen, since such people will likely reproduce similarly wretched offspring and be of use neither to themselves nor to society.[4] Indeed, the only legitimate claim to medical care is the continued social usefulness of the one desiring care.

Aristotle's view of human value is expressed in a variety of his works, ranging from the biological to the political and ethical. He clearly postulates a hierarchy of worth within the species. Men with fully developed virtue(s) are most fully human, and thus of the greatest value both to themselves and to society. There are, of course, gradations within this group. All other humans are, by comparison, defective by nature or in their present state. Those who are defective by nature include especially those whom Aristotle calls "natural slaves," that is, individuals who have a capacity to acknowledge reason but not to conceptualize or to engage in rational activity. They are somewhat like domesticated animals: defective by nature. Also defective by nature, but having considerably greater range of capacity for virtue than natural slaves, are those women who themselves are not natural slaves. They are naturally defective by virtue of being women but yet, in unnatural or unusual circumstances, may demonstrate a kind of female excellence. But at the best they are defective males.

Quite distinct from natural slaves and women are children. Children may be natural slaves—a condition not immediately discernible—or female, and thus limited in potential. But all male children, except for those who prove to be natural slaves, are potentially virtuous men, therefore potentially fully human. Children, however, resemble natural slaves and animals more than they do virtuous men, because they lack the developed capacity for rational thought and behavior.

For both Plato and Aristotle, then, human value is primarily social value and is determined by potentiality.[5]

Do the positions taken by Plato and Aristotle reflect the values of classical society? The answer to that question must be a highly qualified, yet hearty, affirmative; qualified, because there was a tremendous diversity of values in classical antiquity; a hearty affirmative for two reasons: (1) No pagan, whether philosopher or jurist, appears to have asked whether human beings have inherent value, or possess intrinsic rights, ontologically, irrespective of social value, legal status, age, sex, and so forth. (2) Connected with the first reason is a fundamental, though primitive and residual, principle that, as Thrasymachus expresses it, "justice is the will of the stronger." Rights are recognized only by their enforceability. It was against the idea that might makes right that various philosophers, including Plato and Aristotle, reacted. Power must be checked by justice, justice being essentially the definition and enforcement of rights. Rist observes that, "instead of starting with a consideration of human rights, or of basic rights, [the ancients] start with theories of power and of how power shall be tempered by justice. As their thought proceeds, they come to recognize that certain types of people, for various reasons, are in fact possessed of rights. . . . The moral problem is not viewed in terms of enlarging or protecting the rights of the weak, but of controlling and rationalizing the power of the strong."[6]

Rist's comments certainly appear valid when one considers the various legal systems of classical antiquity. Among the Greeks the exclusivistic atmosphere of the polis fostered a definition of rights focusing on citizens—more on males, who possessed the franchise, than on females, who did not. The rights of adult male citizens' dependents (wives, to a certain degree, and children) and human possessions (slaves) were essentially developed with a view to protecting the rights of the adult males on whom those persons depended or to whom they belonged. This prevailed even in the highly developed law of the Roman Empire, though its more cosmopolitan character is reflected in its extension of various, if limited, rights to a broader spectrum of society than had typically been the center of Greek attention. Yet the emphasis remains on the rights of the adult male citizen primarily, with a variety of rights defined for women (these rights essentially comprising limitations of their fathers' or husbands' power and authority), and even for slaves (slight limitations being placed on the absolute power of owners).

Human Value and Newborns

In part, some of the changes that we see during the early centuries of the empire were the result of what some have hailed as a growing humanitarianism, a by-product of a sentiment not of egalitarianism, but at least of the brotherhood of man, proclaimed especially by the Stoicism of this period. This found its way into the medical ethics of probably a minority of physicians in an ethic of respect for life that condemned both abortion and active (although not passive) euthanasia, and a broader sentiment of generosity and altruism, a philanthropy predicated upon the unexpressed and ill-defined feeling that somehow people have a value to which our compassion is owed.

Even this pagan humanitarianism, however, was not grounded on a principle of inherent value of life. A stand against abortion and active euthanasia by the probably Pythagorean author of the so-called Hippocratic Oath, and by such physicians as Scribonius Largus and Soranus, both of whom lived in the early empire, was based less upon an idea of inherent value or sanctity of life than on an abhorrence of a physician's using his art in actively terminating life (fetal or otherwise); and especially in the case of abortion, an enduring, if not always articulated principle that value is more potential than ontological.

The strongly held idea that human value is acquired rather than inherent was nearly pervasive in classical antiquity, even among those pagans who condemned abortion. It was so central to ancient conceptions of value that a fully developed principle of sanctity of human life was never achieved in pagan society. This is particularly easily demonstrated by considering the status of newborns and their treatment. Once more I quote John Rist:

> It was almost universally held in antiquity that a child has no intrinsic right to life in virtue of being born. What mattered was being adopted into a family or some other institution of society. Both Plato and Aristotle, as well as the Stoics, Epicurus, and presumably Plotinus, accept the morality of the exposure of infants . . . on eugenic or sometimes on purely economic grounds. . . . We see here further clear evidence of the ancient view that somehow value is acquired, either by the development of intelligence or by the acceptance into society. There is no reason to think that the philosophers made substantial advances on the assumptions of the general public in this regard.[7]

Rist is absolutely correct in this assertion. Some clarification, however, is necessary. Is it misleading to say that in antiquity the attitude that "a child has no intrinsic right to life in virtue of being born" was "almost universal?" There were indeed some pagans who did condemn exposure[8] of healthy children for any reason: is Rist referring to these by his qualifying "almost"? That would imply that such individuals condemned exposure of healthy infants on the grounds that there is an "intrinsic right to life in virtue of being born." Or is Rist suggesting that there were some—that few permitted by his "almost"—who unequivocally condemned all infanticide, including exposure of healthy infants and the disposal of the defective? If there actually were any pagans in the second of these categories, they most certainly had not formulated an ethic of intrinsic human value, any more than had those who were in the first category. His "almost" cannot include any—even the most humanitarian—pagans, not even those who were adamant in condemning abortion.

Although Rist's first qualifier, the adverb *almost* can be misleading, his second qualifying phrase is more helpful, namely, that various philosophers accepted the morality of exposure of infants "on eugenic or sometimes on purely economic grounds." If we take the term *eugenic* in a broad sense, we can apply it to the disposal of defective infants, as distinct from the exposure of healthy infants for economic (or other non-eugenic) reasons. These two categories must be kept distinct if we are to understand the response of pagans in classical antiquity to defective infants.

First of all, it can be categorically asserted that there were no laws in classical antiquity, Greek or Roman, that prohibited the killing, by exposure or otherwise, of the defective newborn. Further, it is unlikely that there actually were any laws that classified exposure (as distinct from other forms of killing) of the healthy newborn as parricide or homicide, or prohibited the practice on other grounds, except, perhaps, in some limited regions or under unusual circumstances before the Christianization of the Roman Empire. If any such law or laws existed, there appears to have been little or no effort to enforce them.[9]

As already mentioned, there were some pagans who opposed the exposure of healthy infants. Aristotle implies in the *Politics* that there was in Greece some sentiment against exposure of healthy infants or traditions hostile to the practice, when he recommends that, if there are already too many children, abortion—before sensation (πρὶν αἴθησιν)[10]—be practiced in those regions where "the regular customs hinder any of those born being exposed" (ἐὰν ἡ τάξις τῶν ἐθῶν κωλύῃ μηδὲν ἀποτίθεσθαι τῶν γιγνομένων).[11] The second-century B.C. historian Polybius criticizes the practice of child exposure, which he saw as one of the causes of the serious depopulation of Greece that occurred in the second century B.C., attributing the act to people's "pretentious extravagance, avarice and sloth."[12] The Stoic philosopher Epictetus, who lived in the late first and early second centuries A.D., criticizes Epicurus for approving the exposure of children, saying that even a sheep or a wolf does not abandon its own offspring. His argument is that we ought not to be more foolish than sheep or more fierce than wolves, but rather should yield to our natural impulse to love our own offspring.[13] It is significant that he uses στέργειν here, the obvious word for having "natural affection," as distinct from other Greek words that are translated by the English word *love*.

Many of the examples of condemnation of child exposure found in classical authors are in descriptions of the practices of other cultures. The novelist Heliodorus (third century A.D.), in *An Ethiopian Romance*, has an Ethiopian gymnosophist say that he found and reared an exposed girl "because for me it is not permissible to disregard an imperiled soul once it has taken on human form. This is a precept of our gymnosophists."[14] These attitudes were divergent enough from typical classical values that some authors were sufficiently intrigued to tickle their readers by relating such strange customs of exotic peoples. Others who decried various practices of their own societies describe the contrasting purity of other cultures. Tacitus, a contemporary of Epictetus, does both. He finds it remarkable that among the Germans it was regarded as shameful to kill any "late-born" child, that is, an unwanted child.[15] He uses nearly an identical sentence when he attributes the same peculiarity to the Jews, a people whose customs he usually finds strange and obnoxious.[16]

That Jews of Tacitus' time regarded the killing of infants as a reprehensible act, violating sacred law, is evident from the writings of Philo Judaeus[17] and Josephus.[18] Relying on the writings of Hecataeus of Abdera (sixth/fifth centuries B.C.), Diodorus Siculus remarks that Moses required the Jews "to rear their children" (τεκνοτρόφειν),[19] and says virtually the same thing about the Egyptians, that is, that they are required "to raise all their children" (τὰ γεννώμενα πάντα τρέφουσιν).[20] Oribasius (personal physician to Julian "the Apostate") maintains that Aristotle also attributed this same practice to the Egyptians (τὸ τρέφειν πάντα τὰ γινόμενα).[21] And the geographer Strabo (first centuries B.C./A.D.) asserts that the Egyptians most zealously observe the custom of raising every child who is born (τὸ πάντα τρέφειν τὰ γεννώμενα παιδία).[22]

The expressed or implied motivations behind these condemnations of exposure differ. Epictetus obviously regards exposure as a violation of natural law. Polybius regards those who engaged in it as selfish and immoral. Tacitus says that the Germans held this practice (as well as any limitation of the number of their children) as *flagitium* (a disgraceful or shameful deed) and says of the Jews that they saw it as *nefas* (contrary to divine law, impious), a word much more charged with moral principle than that descriptive of German sentiment. Josephus maintains that it was forbidden by the Law, and Philo condemns it as murder, a perversion of natural law. Diodorus Siculus implies that the Jews were motivated to condemn the practice by a desire to increase their population, the motive specified by the same author for the Egyptians' forbidding the act. And Heliodorus' imaginary Ethiopian gymnosophist regarded it as morally wrong, at least for his exclusive group of gymnosophists.

The Killing of Defective Newborns

These instances of condemnation of child exposure, or of infanticide in the broader sense of the word, whether by some few Greeks or Romans or by exotic peoples, both Jews and pagans, can be taken to include the condemnation of the killing of the defective newborn, and not only the exposure of healthy infants. There is no qualifying phrase introduced by "except." The statements are generally quite specific and seem to imply that all that are born are raised, the word translated "raised" meaning "nourished," and the word translated "born" either the word commonly used for giving birth, or else the word for becoming or coming into existence. These phrases certainly would, on the surface, seem all-inclusive. Aristotle, you recall, recommends early abortion as a means of population control in the event that "regular customs hinder any of those born being exposed."[23] Such a statement seems inclusive, even in the English translation. But it most certainly is not, for it follows directly on this: "As to exposing or rearing the children born, let there be a law that no deformed child shall be reared" (περὶ δὲ ἀποθέσεως καὶ τροφῆς τῶν γιγνομένων ἔστω νόμος μηδὲν πεπηρωμένον τρέφειν).

Aristotle, in writing the *Politics,* is describing "the best state." As we have just seen, in such a state he thinks there should be a law that no deformed child should be reared. While the practice of exposing or killing deformed infants was, as we shall see, common enough in classical antiquity, suggesting a law that would make it mandatory was not by any means typical. Quintus Curtius, writing in the first century A.D., thought it was worthy of note to inform his readers that at the time of Alexander the Great it was supposedly the custom in part of India not to permit parents to determine whether their children should be reared; the decision was in the hands of "those to whom the charge of the physical examination of children had been committed. If these have noted any who are conspicuous for defects or are crippled in some part of their limbs, they give orders to put them to death."[24] This sounds very similar to the well-known custom ascribed to the Spartans in Plutarch's *Life of Lycurgus:* "Offspring was not reared at the will of the father, but was taken and carried by him to a place . . . where the elders . . . officially examined the infant, and if it was well-built and sturdy, they ordered the father to rear it . . . but if it was ill-born and deformed, they sent it to . . . a chasm-like place at the foot of Mount Taÿgetus, in the conviction that the life of that which nature had not well-equipped at the very beginning for health and strength, was of no advantage, either to itself or to the state."[25]

The explanation given for this practice is a concern for eugenics. We can assume the same in the case of Aristotle's ideal state and the supposed custom in India. Another feature that they have in common is that the parents have no say in the matter. Both of these aspects are present in a passage from Plato's *Republic:* "The offspring of the inferior, and any of those of the other sort who are born defective, they will properly dispose of in secret, so that no one will know what has become of them."[26] This passage has been the focus of much controversy, with some scholars maintaining that it has nothing to do with exposure.[27] Irrespective of that debate, we need to step back for a moment and look at the vocabulary in these four passages used to describe the infants in question.

The child is described as ἀνάπηρον (maimed, crippled) by Plato. Aristotle uses a related word, πεπηρωμένον, meaning essentially the same thing. The text of Quintus Curtius is somewhat corrupt, but the basic meaning is "defective" or "crippled." Plutarch uses two terms, the first of which, ἀγεννές, is quite unusual, having the meaning "unborn" or "uncreated," *perhaps* "grossly deformed"; the second, ἄμορφον, means "misshapen" or "disfigured." Aside from the fact that the vocabulary is frustratingly imprecise, we should note that there appears to be nothing superstitious in the procedures or decision making described. The conditions are assumed to be natural defects, of no numinous or ominous character. The situation changes when we look at the Roman scene.

The first-century B.C. historian Dionysius of Halicarnassus attributes to Romulus, the legendary founder of Rome, the following law. Explaining how Romulus had made the city large and populous, Dionysius maintains that "he obliged the inhabitants to bring up all their male children and the first born of the females, and forbade them to destroy any children under three years of age unless they were maimed or monstrous from their very birth. These he did not forbid their parents to expose, provided they first showed them to their five nearest neighbors and these also approved."[28] Irrespective of the very questionable historicity of this "law," an important element is introduced. There are two different categories of defective infants here: ἀνάπηρον, the same word that Plato used, translated as "maimed," and τέρας, a noun denoting a sign or wonder, a marvel, a portent, or anything that serves as an omen, as, for instance, here a strange creature or monster. What is probably meant is a grossly deformed infant, perhaps the type implied by Plutarch's word ἀγεννές. The significant difference is that Plutarch's adjective is devoid of superstitious meaning, while the word τέρας is supernatural to the core. While the infant in Plutarch's account is probably no more or less grotesque than that in Dionysius', the response that each elicits is different, the response at least of the two authors as revealed in their choice of vocabulary.

Much more common in Roman than in Greek society was the occurrence of *prodigia* (in Greek, τέρατα, plural of τέρας), unnatural and inexplicable events, such as the birth of a lamb with five legs, a human hermaphrodite, and the like. While some prodigia on record are so bizarre that their historicity must be discounted, many, perhaps most, are well within the realm of possibility, especially after exaggeration is subtracted from the account. A prodigium had enormous significance; it was itself a message from the supernatural powers, more often than not a warning, eliciting a communal fear and guilt in Roman society, particularly during the Republican period. The message had to be discerned by *haruspices* (soothsayers), the unnatural thing destroyed, and a *piaculum*, that is, an expiatory rite, performed. Consider the following event, which occurred in 207 B.C., as recorded by the first-century B.C. historian Livy:

Relieved of their religious scruples, men were troubled again by the report that at Frusino there had been born a child as large as a four-year-old, and not so much a wonder for size as because . . . it was uncertain whether male or female. In fact the soothsayers summoned from Etruria said it was a terrible and loathsome portent; it must be removed from Roman territory, far from contact with earth, and drowned in the sea. They put it alive into a chest, carried it out to sea and threw it overboard. The pontiffs likewise decreed that thrice nine maidens should sing a hymm as they marched through the city.[29]

Such events abound in the extant literature.[30] The motivations for the killing of such newborns are different from the primarily eugenic concerns of the other authors whom we have considered thus far. The response to prodigia is rooted in some very deep-seated fear, guilt, and shame that are only slightly evident in the response to the birth of sickly, maimed, or moderately deformed infants. The maimed, the deformed, and the monstrous constitute a continuum that can accommodate both superstitious and eugenic concerns. A law requiring the killing of deformed infants would include so-called monstrous births as well, motivated perhaps by both eugenic and superstitious responses. Such seem to underlie a law in the ancient Twelve Tables, a code thought to have been compiled in Rome in the fifth century B.C., to which Cicero alludes. This law required that a *puer ad deformitatem* be killed quickly.[31] While modern translators render this as "terribly deformed," that seems stronger than the Latin, which appears to accommodate the entire continuum described above.

The continuum broadens when we consider a passage in a treatise written by the first-century A.D. Stoic philosopher Seneca: "Mad dogs we knock on the head; the fierce and savage ox we slay; sickly sheep we put to the knife to keep them from infecting the flock; unnatural progeny we destroy; we drown even children who at birth are weakly and abnormal. Yet it is not anger, but reason that separates the harmful from the sound."[32] Here we see *portentosi*, that is, unnatural or monstrous births; *debiles*, that is, sickly or weak infants; and *monstrosi*, that is, deformed or abnormal newborns. We should note that Seneca is neither recommending nor condemning this practice. He simply gives it as an example, along with several others, of violence or ostensibly destructive activity, in which his society engaged as a matter of course, that did not involve anger or hatred but was motivated by a concern for individual or social good. The two sentences immediately preceding the section quoted say, "Does a man hate the members of his own body when he uses a knife upon them? There is no anger there, but the pitying desire to heal."

It should be clear that in Roman culture the killing of defective newborns was common, and was even apparently required in the case of those infants so grossly deformed or unusual as to appear to be *portentosi* or monstrous births. For Greece, however, we have seen only the anomalous conditions in Sparta and the "ideal" practices suggested by Aristotle and Plato. These really tell us little about conditions in Greek society during the classical period. There is, however, a passage in Plato's *Theaetetus* that is very revealing. The man whose name supplies the title for this dialogue has suggested that knowledge is nothing more than perception. Socrates wishes to subject this "brain-child" to examination to see whether it is worth rearing. Socrates had earlier warned him that that was precisely what he was going to do once Theaetetus gives birth to his idea:

I suspect that you, as you yourself believe, are in pain because you are pregnant with something within you. Apply, then, to me, remembering that I am the son of a midwife and have myself a midwife's gifts, and do your best to answer the questions I ask as I ask them. And if, when I have examined any of the things you say, it should prove that I think it is a mere image and not real, and therefore quietly take it from you and throw it away, do not be angry as women are when they are deprived of their first offspring. For many, my dear friend, before this have got into such a state of mind towards me that they are actually ready to bite me, if I take some foolish notion away from them, and they do not believe that I do this in kindness.[33]

After Theaetetus elaborates his theory, Socrates says, "Shall we say that this is, so to speak, your newborn child and the result of midwifery? Or what shall we say?" Theaetetus replies, "We must say that, Socrates." Socrates then continues: "Well, we have at least managed to bring this forth, whatever it turns out to be; and now that it is born, we must in very truth perform the rite of running around with it in a circle—the circle of our argument—and see whether it may not turn out to be after all not worth rearing, but only a wind-egg, an imposture. But, perhaps, you think that any offspring of yours ought to be cared for and not put away; or will you bear to see it examined and not get angry if it is taken away from you, though it is your first-born?"[34] First of all, it is self-evident that the whole comparison would be sheer nonsense unless a custom prevailed of disposing of defective newborns, even defective first-borns, at least at Athens at that time. Second, we may note that mothers typically were angry when their first-born was taken from them. Apparently they were better able to cope with losing a defective infant if they already had at least one healthy child. Third, it is evident that the examination of a newborn infant was part of a midwife's responsibilities. There is relatively little attention given in ancient medical literature to the duties of midwives. However, Soranus, a physician who lived in Rome in the first and second centuries A.D., wrote a gynecological treatise—the best that has survived from antiquity—that was designed for midwives. A passage in this treatise is entitled "How to Recognize the Newborn That Is Worth Rearing." It reads:

Now the midwife, having received the newborn, should first put it upon the earth, having examined beforehand whether the infant is male or female, and should make an announcement by signs as is the custom of women. She should also consider whether it is worth rearing or not. And the infant which is suited by nature for rearing will be distinguished by the fact that its mother has spent the period of pregnancy in good health, for conditions which require medical care, especially those of the body, also harm the fetus and enfeeble the foundations of its life. Second, by the fact that it has been born at the due time, best at the end of nine months, and if it so happens, later; but also after only seven months. Furthermore by the fact that when a woman puts it on the earth it immediately cries with proper vigor; for one that lives for some length of time without crying, or cries but weakly, is suspected of behaving so on account of some unfavorable condition. Also by the fact that it is perfect in all its parts, members and senses; that its ducts, namely of the ears, nose, pharynx, urethra, anus are free from obstruction; that the natural functions of every [member] are neither sluggish nor weak; that the joints bend and stretch; that it has due size and shape and is properly sensitive in every respect. This we may recognize from pressing the fingers against the surface of the body, for it is natural to suffer pain from everything that pricks or squeezes. And by conditions contrary to those mentioned, the infant not worth rearing is recognized.[35]

While this passage from Soranus gives concrete evidence for what was undoubtedly a common practice both in Greek and Roman cultures, it is not, strictly speaking, a medical pronouncement upon the decision-making processes involving the care of the defective newborn. It is written on the assumption that a defective infant is *eo ipso* not worth rearing. The question is simply how to determine most easily and efficiently which infants are worth rearing. Even this was a question seldom addressed by ancient medical authors. It was a midwife's concern—which is why we encounter this guidance in a gynecological treatise written for midwives. Not that medical authors, as well as natural philosophers, were uninterested in why some infants were born defective, and how to try to prevent this. Various intriguing suggestions were advanced and theories developed that are not germane to this study.

Two conclusions can now be drawn. One is that the *care* of defective newborns simply was not a medical concern in classical antiquity.[36] The second is that the morality of the killing of sickly or deformed newborns appears not to have been questioned, at least not in extant sources, either by nonmedical or by medical authors. Interestingly enough, Soranus, who was atypical of the ancient medical authors in condemning abortion, not only raises no objection to the rejecting of defective newborns but also, as we have seen, quite dispassionately provides the criteria to be used by midwives in determining which newborns are worth rearing.

The Christian Principle of the Sanctity of Life

I have earlier asserted that the idea that human value is acquired rather than inherent was so central to ancient conceptions of value that a fully developed principle of the sanctity of human life, one that includes even the defective newborn, was never achieved in pagan antiquity. For apparently no pagan raised the question of whether human beings have inherent value, or possess intrinsic rights, ontologically, irrespective of social value, legal status, age, sex, and so forth. The first espousal of an idea of inherent human value in Western civilization depended on a belief that every human being was formed in the image of God. We shall return shortly to this principle of *imago Dei* as a basis for inherent human value.

It is unlikely, however, that the earliest Christians formulated a concise definition of human value based upon the concept of imago Dei. The condemnation of acts that would later be viewed as violations of the rights that accrue to a person as one formed in God's image were, in the earliest Christian literature, part of a broad moral indignation against those aspects of Greco-Roman culture which stand in the starkest contrast to the most basic principles of the gospel of love, mercy, compassion, and salvation from sin to holiness and purity. All aspects of pagan brutality and immorality were condemned; they seemed to early Christian apologists to be common and related features of a society that was viewed as corrupted to its very core by the disease of sin. Apologists condemned in the same breath gladiatorial shows, grossly cruel executions conducted as spectator sports, abortion, infanticide, and a broad and imaginative variety of sexual deviations. Some apologists saw abortion as a sexual crime, in that it was done to destroy the results of a sexual act that was lust when engaged in for a purpose other than procreation. Infanticide had the same motive as did exposure, except that the latter created a potential for another sexual sin, incest, since exposed children often ended up in brothels.[37]

So common, indeed universal, among Christians in the early centuries of Christianity was the condemnation of abortion and infanticide, including exposure,[38] that I shall only mention a few features. Some apologists point out that the practice of infanticide among the pagans is not surprising, in light of a tradition of the sacrifice of infants in various cults—a practice in which some cults still engaged, although it was strictly forbidden by law; and a practice, incidentally, of which early Christians were themselves slanderously accused. Further, these apologists claim, the pagan myths are full of tales of infanticide, which set a precedent of approbation. Further, some early church fathers contrast active infanticide with exposure, asserting that exposing a baby to cold, hunger, and carnivorous animals is more cruel than simply strangling it. But, they tell us, many pagans, thinking that it is impious to kill the infant with one's own hands, kill it by the less messy means of a slow death out of their sight.

None of the early Christian condemnations of infanticide make any reference to the condition of the baby, whether it is healthy or defective, or consider a possible eugenic motivation for the active or passive killing of a newborn. But while I asserted that the relatively rare instances of pagan condemnations of exposure would not have included the killing of the defective, I shall maintain even more categorically that early Christian condemnation of exposure and other forms of infanticide would have included any and every form of infanticide, active or passive, of newborns, whether they be healthy, sickly, or deformed.

There are three reasons that immediately come to mind for this attitude. The first, which I shall mention only in passing, is the significantly different attitude of Christianity to children generally. In classical society, even in its more humanitarian movements, children were essentially viewed as potential adults, their value residing in what they would become. We moderns, in a child-oriented society, generally do not appreciate just how revolutionary was Jesus' teaching that unless you become as little children you cannot enter the kingdom of God. Second, the social thrust of early Christianity was demonstrably and spectacularly oriented to helping the helpless, caring for the destitute, and succoring the deprived.

The third reason requires a little more space than the first two. I made reference earlier to the concept of people being created in God's image as ultimately providing the basis for a Christian theology of human value. I shall leave aside such questions as the relationship of image and likeness of God and the extent to which these concepts are entangled by patristic authors with the Platonic conception that likeness to God is the telos of human endeavor. The earliest Christian apologist who seems to imply the concept of imago Dei as a basis for the condemnation of abortion and infanticide is Clement of Alexandria (second century).[39] Even if the imago Dei may be defaced by human will, obstinacy, and sin, such could not be the case with the fetus and the newborn infant. Such an assertion obviously would include the sickly and deformed newborn. But what of the extreme end of the continuum of which I spoke earlier, the monstrous or grossly deformed?

Augustine, in the *City of God*,[40] comments on the tremendous diversity among people, enormous racial differences, and whole tribes of people who seem to us to be monstrous. He then says,

If whole peoples have been monsters, we must explain the phenomenon as we explain the individual monsters who are born among us. God is the Creator of all; He knows best where and when and what is, or was, best for Him to create, since He deliberately fashioned the beauty of the whole out of both the similarity and dissimilarity of its parts. . . . I know men who were born with more than five fingers or toes, which is one of the slightest variations from the normal, but it would be a shame for anyone to be so silly as to suppose that, because he did not know why God did this, the Creator could make a mistake in regard to the number of fingers on a man's hand. Even in cases of greater variations, God knows what He is doing, and no one may rightly blame His work. . . . It would be impossible to list all the human offspring who have been very different from the parents from whom they were certainly born. Still, all these monsters undeniably owe their origin to Adam.[41]

Later in the same work, Augustine says that pagans mock the idea of the resurrection of the dead, referring to various physical defects as well as "all the human monstrosities that are born" and then asking, "What kind of resurrection will there be in cases like these?"[42] Augustine, in his *Enchiridion,* specifically addresses the question of the resurrection of the grossly deformed, or human "monstrosities":

Concerning monsters which are born and live, however quickly they die, neither is resurrection to be denied them, nor is it to be believed that they will rise again as they are, but rather with an amended and perfected body. God forbid that the double-membered man recently born in the East—about whom most trustworthy brethen, who saw him, have reported, and Jerome the priest, of holy memory, left written mention—God forbid, I say, that we should think that at the resurrection there will be one such double man, and not rather two men, as would have been the case had twins been born. And so all other births which, as having some excess or some defect or because of some conspicuous deformity, are called monsters, will be brought again at the resurrection to the true form of human nature, so that one soul will have one body, and no bodies will cohere together, even those that were born in this condition, but each, apart, for himself, will have as his own those members whose sum makes the complete human body.[43]

The imago Dei, with its attendant value, rights, and responsibilities, attached in early Christian thought to the newborn, whether healthy or sickly, maimed, deformed, or monstrous, indeed to that whole continuum of the defective, in vivid contrast to the attitudes and practices of pagan antiquity. The Christian concept of imago Dei provided both the basis and the structure for the idea of inalienable rights and of intrinsic human value that has prevailed in Western society nearly until the present.

NOTES

1. John M. Rist, *Human Value: A Study in Ancient Philosophical Ethics* (Leiden: E. J. Brill, 1982), 9.

2. Plato, in the *Republic,* recommends that women not bear children before age twenty (460E), but in *Laws* he sets the age at sixteen (785B). Aristotle recommends eighteen as the minimum age (*Politics* 1335a). Their concern is with eugenics.

3. Plato, *Laws* 773D, 783D–E.

4. Plato, *Republic* 407D–E, 410A.

5. For a discussion of Plato's and Aristotle's views on human value, see M. P. Golding and N. H. Golding, "Population Policy in Plato and Aristotle: Some Value Issues," *Arethusa* 8 (1968): 345–58; and Rist, *Human Value* (n. 1).

6. Rist, *Human Value* (n. 1), 131.

7. Ibid., 141–42.

8. The prevalence of exposure in classical antiquity has been debated by modern scholars. For some specialized studies see H. Bennet, "The Exposure of Infants in Ancient Rome," *Classical J.* 18 (1923): 341–51; H. Bolkestein, "The Exposure of Children at Athens and the ἐγχυτρίστριαι," *Classical Philol.* 17 (1922): 222–39; A. Cameron, "The Exposure of Children and Greek Ethics," *Classical Rev.* 46 (1932): 105–14; D. Engels, "The Problem of Female Infanticide in the Greco-Roman World," *Classical Philol.* 75 (1980): 112–20; R. H. Feen, "Abortion and Exposure in Ancient Greece: Assessing the Status of the Fetus and 'Newborn' from Classical Sources," in *Abortion and the Status of the Fetus,* ed. W. B. Bondeson and H. T. Engelhardt, Jr. (Dordrecht: D. Reidel, 1983), 283–99; M. Radin, "Exposure of Infants in Roman Law and Practice," *Classical J.* 20 (1925): 337–42; and L. Van Hook, "The Exposure of Infants at Athens," *Trans. Amer. Philol. Soc.* 51 (1920): 134–45. Engels' assessment appears correct: "After careful analysis of the literacy evidence, earlier studies concerning the exposure of children (and any resultant infanticide) have established that the practice was of negligible importance in Greek and Roman society" (Engels, "Female Infanticide" [n. 8], 112). It has been popularly assumed that the exposure of female newborns was extremely common. Engels convincingly argues that the high level of female infanticide assumed for classical antiquity by some scholars would have produced demographic consequences of a catastrophic nature. It is, of course, important to bear in mind that exposure is an ambiguous word, and that very likely exposure, unless excessive, may well have affected the population relatively little since probably the majority of exposed infants were reared. Sometimes exposure is infanticide; sometimes it is simply abandonment.

9. J. W. Jones writes of ancient Greece generally that "neither Greek public opinion nor Greek law frowned on the practice [of exposure], if the exposure was not delayed beyond a few days after birth" (*The Law and Legal Theory of the Greeks* [Oxford: Clarendon, 1956], 288). Thebes, during the early centuries of the Christian era, may possibly be an exception, if Aelian (*Varia historia* 2.7) can be trusted (for which see Feen, "Abortion and Exposure" [n. 8], 289). Speaking only of Athens, A.R.W. Harrison says that while "there seems general agreement that there was probably no explicit enactment conferring the right to expose," nevertheless there is "no reason to doubt that the father had this absolute discretion and that the right of exposure was more than a purely formal one"

(*The Law of Athens: The Family and Property* [Oxford: Clarendon, 1968], 71, and n. 1). Putting this in other terms, he says that an Athenian father's right to expose his child is "perhaps better expressed as the absence of a duty to introduce it into the family" (73), or "the right to expose should perhaps be thought of as the absence of a duty to rear" (74, and n. 2). The assertion made by the late-second-century or early-third-century A.D. physician-philosopher Sextus Empiricus, in his *Outlines of Pyrrhonism* 3.211, that "Solon gave the Athenians the law . . . by which he allowed each man to slay his own child" can be confidently rejected (Harrison, *The Law of Athens* [n. 9], 71, and n. 2). It can be categorically asserted that the Athenian father never "enjoyed a power remotely resembling the Roman father's *ius vitae ac necis*" (74), that is, "power of life and death" over his children. That power is, of course, the well-known Roman father's *patria potestas*. The question of the legality of exposure in Roman law is entangled in the complexity of the changing patria potestas during the imperial period as well as the development of laws governing the parental reclaiming of exposed children reared by others, either as free children or as slaves, and the sale of free newborns as slaves. The Roman father's authority to put his children to death appears not to have been rescinded until the reign of the first Christian emperor, Constantine, who in 318 promulgated a law concerning parricide, that is, the killing of parents and children (*Codex Justinianus* 9.17.1). In 374, Valentinian enacted a statute concerning homicide which made the killing of an infant a capital offense (*Codex Justinianus* 9.16.7). In the same year he issued another statute that seems unambiguously to forbid exposure of infants. It begins, "Unusquisque subolem suam nutriat. Quod si exponendam putaverit, animadversioni quae constituta est subiacebit" (Everyone should support his own offspring, and anyone who thinks that he can expose his child shall be subject to the penalty prescribed by law [*Codex Justinianus* 8.51.2]). While this seems clear enough, is the penalty referred to here that of Constantine's law of 318 concerning parricide, or is there an even earlier law to which this legislation of 374 has reference? This question is raised in great part by a statement made by the great Roman jurist Paul in his *Sententiae* (third century): "Necare videtur non tantum is qui partum praefocat, sed et is qui abicit et qui alimonia denegat et is qui publicis locis misericordiae causa exponit, quam ipse non habet" (Not only he who strangles a child is held to kill it, but also he who abandons it, or denies it food, as well as he who exposes it in a public place for the purpose of arousing the pity which he himself does not feel. [The better manuscripts read *praefocat* = strangle; some read *perfocat* = smother. *Digest* 25.3.4]). Paul is here obviously defining *necare*. The exact significance of the passage for the right of the Roman father to kill his children—or to expose them—cannot be dogmatically asserted. For a discussion, see Radin, "Exposure of Infants" (n. 8). On *patria potestas*, see W. W. Buckland, *A Text-Book of Roman Law from Augustus to Justinian*, 2d ed. (Cambridge: Cambridge University Press, 1952), sec. 38.

    10. On which see J. M. Oppenheimer, "When Sense and Life Begin: Background for a Remark in Aristotle's *Politics* (1335b24)," *Arethusa* 8 (1975): 331–43.

11. Aristotle, *Politics* 1335b, trans. H. Rackham (Cambridge: Harvard University Press, 1932).

12. Polybius, *The Histories* 36.17, trans. W. Paton (Cambridge: Harvard University Press, 1922–27).

13. Epictetus, *Discourses* 1.23.

14. Heliodorus, *An Ethiopian Romance,* trans. H. Thackeray (Ann Arbor: University of Michigan Press, 1957), 61.

15. Tacitus, *Germania* 19.

16. Tacitus, *The Histories* 5.5.

17. E. R. Goodenough, *The Jurisprudence of the Jewish Courts in Egypt: Legal Administration by the Jews under the Early Roman Empire as Described by Philo Judaeus* (Amsterdam: Philo, 1968), 115–16.

18. Josephus, *Against Apion* 2.24.

19. Diodorus Siculus, *Library of History* 40.3, trans. C. H. Oldfather (Cambridge: Harvard University Press, 1933–57).

20. Ibid., 1.80.

21. Oribasius, *Collectiones medicae,* ed. I. Reader (Amsterdam: Hakkert, 1928–33), 4:99–100.

22. Strabo, *Geography,* 172.5.

23. Aristotle, *Politics* (n. 11), 1335b.

24. Quintus Curtius, *History of Alexander* 9.1.25.

25. Plutarch, *The Parallel Lives: Life of Lycurgus* 16, trans. B. Perrin (Cambridge: Harvard University Press, 1914–26).

26. Plato, *Republic* 460C, trans. P. Shorey (Cambridge: Harvard University Press, 1930–35).

27. See, for example, J. J. Mulhern, "Population and Plato's *Republic,*" *Arethusa* 8 (1975): 265–81.

28. Dionysius of Halicarnassus, *Roman Antiquities* 2.15, trans. E. Cary (Cambridge: Harvard University Press, 1937–50).

29. Livy, *Histories* 37.27, trans. B. O. Foster, E. T. Sage, A. C. Schlesinger, and R. M. Geer (Cambridge: Harvard University Press, 1919–59).

30. For an interesting discussion, see W. den Boer, "Prodigium and Morality," in his *Private Morality in Greece and Rome: Some Historical Aspects* (Leiden: E. J. Brill, 1979), 93 ff.

31. Cicero, *Laws* 3.8.

32. Seneca, *On Anger* 1.15, in *Moral Essays,* trans. J. W. Basore (Cambridge: Harvard University Press, 1928–35).

33. Plato, *Theaetetus* 151B–C, trans. H. N. Fowler (Cambridge: Harvard University Press, 1921).

34. Ibid., 160E–161A.

35. Soranus, *Gynecology,* trans. Owsei Temkin (Baltimore: Johns Hopkins Press, 1956), 79–80.

36. For an interesting discussion of the minor role of pediatrics in ancient medicine, see R. Etienne, "Ancient Medical Conscience and the Life of Children," *J. Psychohist.* 4 (1976–77): 127–61.

37. See, e.g., Justin Martyr, *The First Apology* 27; Tertullian, *Apology* 9; Clement of Alexandria, *Christ the Educator* 21; and Lactantius, *The Divine Institutes* 6.20.

38. See, e.g., Minucius Felix, *Octavius* 30; Justin Martyr, *The First Apology* 27; Lactantius *The Divine Institutes* 5.9; Tertullian, *Ad nationes* 1.15; idem, *Apology* 9; idem, *The Didache* 2; *The Epistle of Barnabas* 19.5; and *The Epistle to Diognetus* 5.6. For a discussion, see I. Giordani, *The Social Message of the Early Fathers,* trans. A. Zizzamia (Boston: St. Paul Editions, 1977), 243–52.

39. Rist, *Human Value* (n. 1), 162–63.

40. Augustine, *City of God* 16.8.

41. Augustine, *City of God,* in *Writings of Saint Augustine,* various translators (Washington, D.C.: Catholic University of America Press, various dates), 7:502–3.

42. Augustine, *City of God* 22.12, vol. 8, p. 459, in the edition cited in n. 41.

43. Augustine, *Enchiridion* 87, in *Writings of Saint Augustine* (n. 41), 4:442–43.

FOUR

Suicide and Early Christian Values

The development of an early Christian position on suicide presents some interesting problems for the historian. In two respects it resembles the ethics of abortion: First, Scripture is silent about both.[1] Second, arguments against the moral permissibility of either, formulated inferentially from Scripture by the church fathers, are easily rejected as being heuristic. Suicide, however, differs from abortion in that while even the earliest non-canonical Christian literature denounces abortion in unequivocal terms, condemnations of suicide by the early church fathers are relatively rare and hardly unequivocal.

There are at least three reasons for the comparative rarity and the equivocal nature of these condemnations. First, such condemnations of suicide by the church fathers as are extant were not part of the broad moral condemnation leveled by early Christian authors against what they regarded as the depravity of pagan society. The moral indignation of the early Christian community, particularly as it was directed against abortion and infanticide, received much of its vigor from the perceived helplessness of the victim, whether a fetus or an infant. Even the occasional condemnation of contraception was motivated in part by concern for the victim (in this case, potential life). So also with gladiatorial combat and extremely cruel executions, in which the pagans needed victims to satisfy their lust for blood. Even acts of sexual immorality were often seen as involving victims, for the greatest indignation of Christian authors was reserved for the forced prostitution of both female and male slaves, helpless victims of pagan depravity; and even outside the brothel, sexual immorality generally involved more than one individual in the act, making it possible that some would be unwilling victims of others' depravity. It is especially the helplessness of the victims of others' sins that increased the extent of moral indignation to the level so frequently encountered in Christian literature. Suicide did not arouse the same kinds of passionate denunciation, for the act was seen not as one in which an innocent party was victimized by another but rather as an act in which one harms only oneself.

Second, the ethics of suicide in early Christianity is more ambiguous than various other ethical issues such as infanticide or abortion. Condemnations of infanticide and abortion by early Christians were unequivocal: no exceptions were even discussed. Furthermore, there was no ambiguity regarding what constituted infanticide or what constituted abortion.[2] But as already mentioned, condemnations of suicide were comparatively rare and were hardly unequivocal. One kind of suicide was approved, at least by some sources: virgins (and even married women) facing sexual assault were lauded by some church fathers for taking their own lives to avoid defilement. Such acts can only be regarded as suicide unless seen through the much later grid of double effect. But some other conditions are exceedingly ambiguous. Is severe asceticism that incidentally but not intentionally results in death suicide? And what of martyrdom? Discussions of what constitutes suicide flourish today. Such discussions often show a lack of precision in defining the English word *suicide* and in delineating the concept usually conveyed by that word. The situation in the ancient world permitted even more confusion, since neither Greek nor Latin had a specific word for suicide.[3]

The third reason for the comparative rarity of condemnations of suicide by the early church fathers is that suicide simply was not a problem for the early Christian community. There is absolutely no evidence in the corpus of Christian literature for the first 250 years of the Christian era that any Christian under any circumstances committed suicide for any reason, unless one should argue that Judas is the one exception. In the absence of even a shred of evidence of suicide by Christians occurring during this period, it is reasonable to assume that suicide did not present itself as a moral problem simply because it was so inherently contrary to Christian values and priorities as not to be considered a viable option for Christians.

Nevertheless, because of the definitional and conceptual ambiguities that have helped to foster the current debate on suicide and that have perhaps been rendered even more muddled by it, one may anachronistically read into ancient sources ambiguities quite alien to the latter's concerns. If one regards as suicide any failure to exploit every conceivable expedient to preserve one's life, one subsumes an exceedingly broad range of motivations, priorities, ideals, decisions, and actions under a rubric that then becomes nearly meaningless. One obscures the past rather than clarifies it when, with one broad and undiscriminating stroke, one labels as suicides *all* who are typically called martyrs. A recent study displays a lack of historical discrimination by grouping into one category Donatist Circumcellions of the fourth and fifth centuries, who persistently attempted to provoke Catholic authorities to put them to death; Christians who, before the legalization of Christianity, refused to blaspheme Christ in order to escape execution; and "the martyrs who *permitted* themselves to be devoured by starving beasts in Nero's arena" (my emphasis).[4] The latter, who were scapegoats put to death after the great fire that destroyed much of Rome in A.D. 64, neither provoked the authorities to execute them nor were allowed the opportunity to recant. Much greater circumspection than this must be used in any serious historical study. Furthermore, one manifests intellectual arrogance of the worst kind when one analyzes a broad range of martyrs and, employing the ephemeral jargon of current psychological models, assures his readers that these martyrs were motivated by self-punitive, aggressive, erotic, masochistic, narcissistic, and exhibitionistic drives.[5] Such mysteries I shall not seek to penetrate.

The various ambiguities mentioned above, combined with some serious misunderstandings of basic tenets of Christianity and an ignorance of patristics, not to mention the New Testament, have led some modern scholars to highly distorted conclusions about early Christian attitudes toward suicide. The following are typical:

There is no condemnation of suicide in the New Testament, and little to be found among the early Christians, who were, indeed, morbidly obsessed with death. . . . The Christian belief was that life on earth was important only as a preparation for the hereafter; the supreme duty was to avoid sin, which would result in perpetual punishment. Since all natural desires tended toward sin, the risk of failure was great. Many Christians, therefore, committed suicide for fear of falling before temptation. It was especially good if the believer could commit suicide by provoking infidels to martyr him, or by austerities so severe that they undermined the constitution, but in the last resort he might do away with himself directly.[6]

Even the most stoical Romans committed suicide only as a last resort; they at least waited until their lives had become intolerable. But in the primitive Church, life was intolerable whatever its conditions. Why, then, live unredeemed when heavenly bliss is only a knife stroke away? Christian teaching was at first a powerful incitement to suicide.[7]

Christianity *invites* suicide in a way in which other major religions do not. . . . The lure exerted by the promise of reunion with the deceased, release of the soul, the rewards of martyrdom, and the attainment of the highest spiritual states, including union with God, all occur in Christianity. . . . Thus the question of the permissibility of suicide arises, though often only inchoately, for any sincere believer in a religious tradition of this sort, whether that individual's present life is a happy one or filled with suffering. Religious suicide is not always a matter of despair; it is often a matter of zeal. The general problem presented by the promise of a better afterlife may be strongest in Christianity, since the afterlife of spiritual bliss depicted by Christianity is a particularly powerful attraction.[8]

Augustine is usually credited with being the architect of the Christian condemnation of suicide. For example: "The early Christian community appeared to be on the verge of complete self-decimation in voluntary martyrdom and suicide until Augustine took a firm position against such practices."[9] "Although there is little reason to think that Augustine's position is authentically Christian . . . it nevertheless rapidly took hold and within an extremely short time had become universally accepted as fundamental Christian law."[10] "St. Augustine was the first to denounce suicide as a crime and thus shaped the later attitude of the Church regarding its sinfulness."[11]

My purpose here is to argue that it is incorrect to suggest that Augustine formulated what then became the "Christian position" on suicide. Rather, by removing certain ambiguities, he clarified and provided a theologically cogent explanation of and justification for the position typically held by earlier and contemporary Christian sources.

The Yale historian George P. Fisher, in the second decade of this century, noted that for the Stoics, who justified suicide under many circumstances, "Life and Death are among the *adiaphora*—things indifferent, which may be chosen or rejected according to circumstances." He then remarked,

How contrary is all this to the Christian feeling! The Christian believes in a Providence which makes all things work together for his good, and believes that there are no circumstances in which he is authorized to lay violent hands upon himself. There is no situation in which he cannot live with honor, and with advantage to himself as long as God chooses to continue him in being.[12]

Fisher perspicaciously grasped the most essential values of early Christianity and as a consequence concluded, "Hence, in the Scriptures there is no express prohibition of suicide, and no need of one."[13]

Fisher's assessment is also valid for the patristic ethos, with one modification: toward the end of the patristic era some sources did approve of one form of suicide, that is, suicide by women to preserve their chastity. Were it not for the fact that patristic literature does in fact include prohibitions of suicide, his conclusion would be equally accurate for post–New Testament Christianity because the most basic Christian values expressed in the New Testament are the same values undergirding and elaborated in patristic literature.

Life and Death in Patristic Thought

To the church fathers, spiritual life was of infinitely greater value than physical life, and spiritual death was much more to be feared than physical death. Indeed, they felt that the Christian should not fear physical death at all, for it would simply be the means whereby he would be brought to those ineffable delights that heaven had in store for him. Numerous examples could be given from patristic sources, but typical is a treatise written by Ambrose (ca. 339–97) entitled *Death as a Good*. Ambrose begins by asserting, "Should death do injury to the soul, it can be considered an evil, but should it do the soul no harm, it cannot."[14] Only Christians have the correct perspective on life and death, and they have always "lamented the longevity of this pilgrimage, since they consider it more glorious 'to depart and to be with Christ.'"[15] After an extensive discussion of a wide variety of related issues, he says, "To the just, death is a harbor of rest; to the guilty, it is reckoned a shipwreck."[16] Then, after quoting Colossians 3:3–4, he begins his concluding paragraph with the exclamation, "Let us therefore hasten to life."[17]

Sentiments identical to those which Ambrose expressed can be found in virtually all the church fathers. Their attitude toward death is nicely described by Peter Brown when he observes that "the early church tended to leapfrog the grave. The long process of mourning and the slow adjustment to the great sadness of mortality tended to be repressed by a heady belief in the afterlife."[18] Hence with great frequency we encounter statements such as the following: "We should rejoice in the death of the righteous" (by Chrysostom [349–407]);[19] and "He who had gone ahead is not to be mourned, though certainly he will be missed" (by Tertullian [ca. 160–

ca. 220]). One's longing for the deceased was to be not a desire for the departed to be here but rather a desire to go and be with them. A few sentences later, Tertullian asserts that "if we bear it with impatience and grief that others have attained their goal, we ourselves do not want to attain our goal."[20] This was frequently given as the mark of the truly committed and serious follower of Christ: a desire to die and be with Christ, demonstrated by a genuine envy for those who have gone "home" already.

The same literature that consistently expressed a yearning for death also consistently expressed a respect for life. The *Shepherd of Hermas,* an anonymous work composed in stages between A.D. 90 and 150, asserts that one who is harassed by distress *(incommoda)* should be assisted, for "many bring death on themselves by reason of such calamities when they cannot bear them. Whoever therefore knows the distress of such a man, and does not rescue him, incurs great sin and becomes guilty of his blood."[21] This passage suggests that the author regarded the suicide of one who resorted to suicide owing to distress as so serious that anyone who could have helped him but failed to do so not only had committed a serious sin but was also guilty of his blood. Early Christians regarded physical life as a gift of God that was so precious that they viewed the care of the sick as a categorical imperative. The gospel as proclaimed in the early centuries of Christianity did not limit itself to the salvation of souls for eternity, but was also directed to salvation within the world. The care of the destitute generally, and particularly of the sick, became a duty incumbent on all believers. Adolf Harnack writes regarding the obligation to visit and care for the sick that "to quote passages would be superfluous, for the duty is repeatedly inculcated."[22] Early Christian literature is indeed rife with such admonitions.[23]

In spite of the sometimes extreme ascetic tendencies of the early church, a central tenet of Christian orthodoxy consistently confirms the inherent worth of life and the moral neutrality of the body. Clement of Alexandria (ca. 155–ca. 220), for example, maintains that those who "vilify the body are wrong. . . . The soul of man is confessedly the better part of man, and the body the inferior. But neither is the soul good by nature, nor, on the other hand, is the body bad by nature."[24] He regarded health as a gift and insisted that the body, as the temple of the Holy Spirit, deserved reasonable care. Clement approvingly quotes Plato's injunction that care must be taken of the body.[25] Tertullian, who can hardly be regarded as effete, says, "I do bathe at the hour I should, one which is conducive to health and which protects both my temperature and my life's blood."[26] The church fathers saw health as a potential good or evil depending on the Christian's use of it. They also saw sickness as a potential good.

Although they thought it proper to desire and to seek the restoration of health when ill, the church fathers regarded excessive concern for the body and a desperate clinging to life as a sad contradiction of Christian values. Cyprian (ca. 200/210–258), writing in Carthage to his fellow Christians while the city was being besieged by plague, was disturbed both by their fear of death and by their efforts to preserve their lives:

What madness it is to love the afflictions, and punishments, and tears of the world and not rather to hurry to the joy which can never be taken from us. . . . How absurd it is and how perverse that, while we ask that the will of God be done, when God calls us and summons us from this world, we do not at once obey the command of His will. We struggle in opposition and resist, and in the manner of obstinate slaves we are brought with sadness and grief to the sight of God, departing from there under the bond of necessity, not in obedience to our will. . . . Why, then, do we pray and entreat that the kingdom of heaven may come, if earthly captivity delights us? . . . Let us be ready for every manifestation of God's will; freed from the terror of death, let us think of the immortality which follows.[27]

Basil of Caesarea (ca. 329–79), instructing his monks about the proper use of the medical art, was governed by principles similar to those that motivated Cyprian. Basil writes, "Whatever requires an undue amount of thought or trouble or involves a large expenditure of effort and causes our whole life to revolve, as it were, around solicitude for the flesh must be avoided by Christians."[28]

In a sermon, John Chrysostom describes a woman who was urged by her Christian friends to employ supposedly efficacious but magical means for the cure of her critically ill child. Chrysostom praises her refusal to resort to such illicit means even though she thought they would restore her child to health. He then laments to his audience the low level of spiritual life and the skewed priorities of so many professing Christians who are little concerned with heaven, although they are willing to undergo anything for the sake of this life. He urges his audience to be ready for death and asks them why they cling to the present life.[29] Similarly, Augustine (354–430) preached that just as the martyrs, even though they loved life, did not cling to it but willingly gave it up when God chose to remove them,[30] so also should those afflicted with seemingly hopeless illness. He points to the irony that so many, when faced with troubles, cry out, "'O God, send me death; hasten my days.' And when sickness comes they hasten to the physician, promising him money and rewards."[31] Augustine was grieved at

what things men do that they may live a few days. . . . If, on account of bodily disease, they should come into the hands of the physician and their health should be despaired of by all who examine them; if some physician capable of curing them should free them from this desperate state, how much do they promise? How much is given for an altogether uncertain result? To live a little while now, they will give up the sustenance of life.[32]

Physical life was worth little to many early Christians. But it was also of inestimable value. The Christian was frequently urged to give his life willingly as a martyr if the only alternative was denying Christ; when sick, although he should seek healing, whether miraculous or medical or both, he should not cling to life but should regard his sickness as potentially the God-given vehicle for his "homegoing." And, under all circumstances, the care of the soul was to take precedence over the care of the body.

Persecution and Martyrdom

The subject of martyrdom in the early church is complex.[33] I cannot deal with the question of why Christians were persecuted but must simply consider reactions to persecution by those who were persecuted or in danger of death. Reactions to persecution took one of four forms: (1) denying Christ (apostatizing); (2) fleeing possible martyrdom; (3) accepting martyrdom when the only escape was denying Christ (i.e., apostatizing); and (4) seeking, provoking, or volunteering for martyrdom.

The third of these was always approved and the first was always condemned by those sources that represent orthodoxy during the patristic era. The major problem posed by apostasy in the face of persecution was whether the Christian community should receive apostates back into fellowship. That controversy, however, lies outside the purview of the present study. When I say that apostasy was consistently condemned by the orthodox community, I am excluding certain heretical groups that were ostensibly Christian. A good example are the Gnostics.

The Gnostic teacher Basilides of Alexandria (early second century) maintained that apostasy—even a light-hearted denial of Christ—was permissible if it would save one's life. A later Gnostic, Heracleon (late second century), taught that what one confessed with one's tongue before men was irrelevant to the condition of one's heart, which only God knows. The reaction of the Christian community to this position was strongly negative. Clement of Alexandria, for example, was totally unambiguous in his denunciation of the Gnostic position: "Now some of the heretics who have misunderstood the Lord, have at once an impious and cowardly love of life; saying that the true martyrdom is the knowledge of the only true God (which we also admit), and that the man is a self-murderer and a suicide who makes confession by death; and adding other similar sophisms of cowardice."[34]

Marshaling other examples would be superfluous: the orthodox community's condemnation of apostasy to escape persecution was unequivocal. Much more troublesome to the early Christian community were the second and fourth responses to persecution: physical flight to avoid death; and seeking, provoking, or volunteering for martyrdom. Of course, these responses are closely related, since it can be and has been argued that refusing the former is tantamount to doing the latter.

Immediately after his condemnation of the Gnostics' glib attitude toward apostasy, Clement writes:

Now we, too, say that those who have rushed on death (for there are some, not belonging to us, but sharing the name merely, who are in haste to give themselves up, the poor wretches dying through hatred to the Creator)—these, we say, banish themselves without being martyrs, even though they are punished publicly. For they do not preserve the characteristic mark of believing martyrdom, inasmuch as they have not known the only true God but give themselves up to a vain death, as the Gymnosophists of the Indians to useless fire.[35]

A few chapters later, he picks up this subject again:

When, again, He [sc. Christ] says, "When they persecute you in this city, flee ye to the other," He does not advise flight, as if persecution were an evil thing; nor does He enjoin them by flight to avoid death, as if in dread of it, but wishes us neither to be the authors nor abettors of any evil to any one, either to ourselves or the persecutor and murderer. For He, in a way, bids us take care of ourselves. But he who disobeys is rash and foolhardy. If he who kills a man of God sins against God, he also who presents himself before the judgment-seat becomes guilty of his death. And such is also the case with him who does not avoid persecution, but out of daring presents himself for capture. Such a one, as far as in him lies, becomes an accomplice in the crime of the persecutor. And if he also uses provocation, he is wholly guilty, challenging the wild beast. And similarly, if he afford any cause for conflict or punishment, or retribution or enmity, he gives occasion for persecution.[36]

We must not suppose that Clement did not hold martyrdom in high esteem and regard it as an obligation if the alternative was apostasy. He writes that the true Christian "when called, obeys easily, and gives up his body to him who asks. . . . In love to the Lord he will most gladly depart from this life."[37] But we do see him adamantly opposed to seeking martyrdom. He demonstrated this attitude in practice by fleeing from Alexandria when persecution struck there.

But not all Christians shared his views. Indeed, Clement's disciple and successor, Origin (ca. 185–ca. 254), as a youth whose father was about to be martyred, wished to present himself to the magistrates for martyrdom. His plans were thwarted by his Christian mother, who hid his clothes to keep him home until the crisis passed. Tertullian, Clement's contemporary, in his *Scorpiace,* written while he was still a Catholic, speaks of the faithful being hunted down like rabbits.[38] The imagery implies that he regarded flight as legitimate. In his treatise *Patience,* written about the same time, he specifies that patience is tested by torture, martyrdom, and the inconveniences of flight.[39] But in his *Ad uxorem,* also written during the same period, he asserts that although flight is permitted as preferable to apostasy, it is not good.[40] This is the first hint of a peculiarity in Tertullian's thought at a time when he was drawing nearer to leaving the Catholic fold for Montanism. After his change of allegiance to this rigorist sect, he wrote his *Flight in Time of Persecution,* in which he denounced, in no uncertain terms, flight from persecution as a denial of Christ and a sign of cowardice. He explains Jesus' command to his disciples to flee when persecuted as applying only to that time and place, "for, if they had been killed right at the beginning, the diffusion of the Gospel, too, would have been prevented."[41]

We must not conclude from this that Tertullian's final, negative position on the question of fleeing from persecution represents simply an extreme position peculiar to Montanism. Others within Catholicism regarded flight from persecution as tantamount to apostasy, or to bribery (to which a fair number had recourse, hence avoiding martyrdom without having to deny Christ by word or by performing pagan rituals). Tertullian, especially as a Montanist, represents a rigorist, Clement a moderate, position on the question. The debate continued well beyond their time, as is well illustrated by the case of Peter, bishop of Alexandria, in the early fourth century. During the Great Persecution (303–12), Peter fled from Alexandria to avoid martyrdom. After the persecution subsided, he returned and composed what may originally have been merely a paschal letter, which was later incorporated into the canon law of the Greek Orthodox Church. In this letter he disparaged those who had volunteered for martyrdom and approved those who had saved their lives by bribery or by flight.[42] Peter's position certainly is not rigorist and is somewhat more liberal than even that of Clement, with whom he shares the opinion that the Christian who does not attempt to escape martyrdom shares moral culpability with the persecutors.

Numerous examples of the contrast between the rigorist and moderate positions could be introduced here. But the contrast between the martyrdoms of Ignatius (in 98 or 117) and Polycarp (between 155 and 160) should be sufficient. In the letters that he wrote while awaiting execution, Ignatius displayed, as W.H.C. Frend says, "a state of exaltation bordering on mania."[43] In his letter *To the Romans,* Ignatius wrote:

I am writing to all the Churches, and I give injunctions to all men, that I am dying willingly for God's sake, if you do not hinder it. I beseech you, be not "an unseasonable kindness" to me. Suffer me to be eaten by the beasts, through whom I can attain to God. I am God's wheat, and I am ground by the teeth of wild beasts that I may be found pure bread of Christ. Rather entice the wild beasts that they may become my tomb, and leave no trace of my body, that when I fall asleep I be not burdensome to any. Then shall I be truly a disciple of Jesus Christ, when the world shall not even see my body. Beseech Christ on my behalf, that I may be found a sacrifice through these instruments. I do not order you as did Peter and Paul; they were Apostles, I am a convict; they were free, I am even until now a slave. But if I suffer I shall be Jesus Christ's freedman, and in him I shall rise free. Now I am learning in my bonds to give up all desires.[44]

His was a case of voluntary martyrdom. Polycarp presents quite a different picture. Yielding to the entreaties of his friends, he withdrew from his city to avoid arrest. Ultimately he was apprehended and, when suffering martyrdom, evinced a moving serenity in the face of death that is quite in contrast with Ignatius' passionate desire for martyrdom.[45]

Both Eusebius and the anonymous, but contemporary, author of the *Martyrdom of Polycarp* record the example of a certain Phrygian named Quintus "who had forced himself and some others to come forward of their own accord. Him the Pro-Consul persuaded with many entreaties to take the oath and offer sacrifice. For this reason, therefore, brethren, we do not commend those who give themselves up, since the Gospel does not give this teaching."[46]

Clement and Peter of Alexandria would agree with this last sentence. Tertullian would not. In his last extant work, addressed to a Roman official named Scapula, Tertullian writes, concerning persecution and martyrdom, that Christians (in this case, Montanists) do not fear these things, but willingly call them down upon ourselves. When Arrius Antoninus [governor of the province of Asia, ca. 184–85] was carrying out a vehement persecution in Asia, all the Christians of the city appeared in a body before his tribunal. After ordering a few to be led away to execution, he said to the rest, "Wretched men, if you wish to die, you have precipices and ropes to hang yourselves." If it should come into our mind to do the same thing here, also, what will you do with so many thousands of human beings . . . giving themselves up to you?[47]

It may very well be that Arrius Antoninus missed the point that this group of Christians was trying to make. Christians were frequently frustrated with the government's inconsistencies in its treatment of them. Only spasmodically were Christians persecuted at the initiative of the government (as distinct from mob action and private accusations). Hence their frustration: "Either clarify your policy and apply it consistently or allow us to live in peace."[48] Aside from the incident described by Tertullian in his letter to Scapula, there is little evidence of groups of Christians presenting themselves en masse before officials.[49] But when it did happen (which was apparently extremely rare) or when individuals or groups volunteered for martyrdom, it undoubtedly smacked of theatrics.

In his invective sketch of Peregrinus, the profligate-turned-Christian-turned-Cynic, Lucian, a second-century Greek satirist, says about Christians, "The poor devils have convinced themselves they're all going to be immortal and live forever, which makes most of them take death lightly and voluntarily give themselves up to it."[50] Although one needs to take satirists with a grain of salt, Lucian's assessment is probably not a significant exaggeration of the sentiments of many pagans who may have regarded Christians as suicidal for their willingness to be martyred. But such pagans, including Lucian and the emperor Marcus Aurelius, who regarded Christians as morbid exhibitionists,[51] would probably have been unaware of how many Christians did in fact unobtrusively flee from persecution to avoid martyrdom. Very likely the majority of Christians who were martyred accepted death "voluntarily" when the only alternative was apostasy. Dying "voluntarily" does not necessarily mean seeking martyrdom. We have already seen that Clement condemns unequivocally those who voluntarily give themselves up to the officials. But he is perfectly consistent when he says that the true Christian "will not forsake his creed through fear of death. . . . in love to the Lord he will most gladly depart from this life. . . . With good courage, then, he goes to the Lord, his friend, for whom he voluntarily gives his body."[52]

Boniface Ramsey asserts that, in patristic thought, "Since martyrdom was a charism, a grace, it could not be demanded as a right; it was a free gift of God."[53] Clement writes that true Christians are "distinguished from others that are called martyrs, inasmuch as some furnish occasions for themselves, and rush into the heart of dangers." By contrast, true Christians, "in accordance with right reason, protect themselves" but, with "God really calling them, promptly surrender themselves, and confirm the call, from being conscious of no precipitancy."[54] Hence, one can be certain that God is calling one to martyrdom only if one has done nothing to precipitate it. During an outbreak of plague in Carthage many Christians were distressed because if they died of the pestilence they would be deprived of the possibility of martyrdom. Cyprian, in addressing their concern, maintained that "martyrdom is not in your power but in the giving of God, and you cannot say that you have lost what you do not know whether you deserved to receive."[55]

The significance of martyrdom varied according to one's soteriology. To some, martyrdom was the only sure means of salvation. Tertullian, in his later years, is representative of this position. To others, martyrdom was one of several means of sanctification leading to salvation. We see this idea heartily emphasized by Clement. Those who held the former position would probably crave martyrdom more than the latter, even though their desire for martyrdom would not necessarily cause them actively to seek it. But even for Clement, martyrdom was the most perfect display of love and was to be desired above any other form of death. Other forms of death could never offer the spiritual glory that martyrdom provided. Hence, for those who ardently wished to depart from this life, any form of death, including suicide, would be an obstacle to that one cherished form of death, martyrdom. Accordingly, those who most wished to die would seek martyrdom if their theology permitted it. Likely the majority of those who wished to quit life held the position most commonly encountered in the literature, namely that seeking martyrdom was wrong. *The very basis for a condemnation of actively seeking that one laudable form of death would* eo ipso *preclude intentionally ending one's own life through some lesser means.*

It is likely that the vast majority of Christians before the legalization of Christianity in 313 not only did not seek martyrdom but held that Christ's admonition to flee when persecuted had an abiding validity. *Those who believed that one should seek by flight to avoid the most glorious and spiritually fulfilling form of death would be very hard pressed to formulate a theological justification for actively seeking to end their lives by their own hand.* Hence, it is not surprising that in the literature extant from the period before the legalization of Christianity, there is absolutely no mention of any Christian, who unsuccessfully sought to provoke pagans to put him to death, resorting to suicide.

Suffering, Sanctification, and the Sovereignty of God

How did the church fathers feel that Christians should regard forms of suffering other than persecution? Were they to inflict suffering upon themselves in pursuit of sanctification? And what of those afflictions that beset humanity generally? Is God sovereign, and if so, how should Christians' appreciation of God's sovereignty affect their understanding of sanctification and, consequently, their response to tribulation? We shall begin by considering self-inflicted suffering.

Asceticism, which is the practice of strict self-denial as a spiritual discipline, was a marked feature of early Christianity beginning in the late second or early third century. Clement of Alexandria was the first Christian author to emphasize asceticism as an ideal on the same level as martyrdom. Later, when Christianity became a licit religion and Christians ceased to be martyred for their faith, the ascetic replaced the martyr in the minds of many Christians as the new spiritual hero. The ascetic way of life in its more extreme forms involved a vilification and abuse of the body by those who had withdrawn from society to engage in a determined effort to subdue indwelling sin. Their self-discipline was regarded as a "daily martyrdom."

Mortification of the flesh (i.e., the carnal mind) and denial of self are stressed in the New Testament. But the asceticism that developed in the late second and early third centuries and gained considerable momentum in the fourth went beyond a simple application of New Testament principles. The climate in which Christian asceticism arose was one in which various classical schools of philosophy extolled simplicity and frugality and in which some pagans yielded to the impulse to experience the "flight of the alone to the alone" and withdrew from society. A few of these became severe ascetics who sought suffering for expiatory, propitiatory, or purificatory ends by abusing their bodies as the prisons of their souls.[56] They were similar in some of their excesses to members of certain heretical groups, such as the Gnostics, Manicheans, and Marcionites (dualists who conceived of matter, including the body, as inherently evil). While the New Testament, particularly Paul, does speak of a dichotomy between flesh and spirit, some Christian ascetics strained the bounds of orthodoxy when they exaggerated this dichotomy by abusing the body for the good of the soul. During these centuries there was only a very fine line between a still orthodox but extreme mortification of the flesh and a dualistic, heretical denunciation of the flesh as inherently evil. Although many church fathers did vilify the body, for the most part their appraisal of the body's worth was tempered by their conviction that it was morally neutral, potentially either a temple or a tomb, and must be subservient to the soul in the latter's campaign against evil.[57] Augustine, who is typically regarded as exemplifying the orthodox spirit in this as in most matters, held that the body is but the slave of the soul. Hence abusing the body accomplishes nothing:

Now it may be asserted that the flesh is the cause of every kind of moral failing, on the ground that the bad behavior of the soul is due to the influence of the flesh. [But] those who imagine that all the ills of the soul derive from the body are mistaken. [For it is] not by the possession of flesh, which the Devil does not possess, that man has become like the Devil: it is by living by the rule of self, that is by the rule of man.[58]

Much that the church fathers say about the body strikes our analgesic ethos as severe. Much of it also appears to contradict their stress on the value of life and on health as a good. For the modern audience this is one of the most enigmatic features of Christianity during the third, fourth, and fifth centuries. All the church fathers whom we have considered thus far regarded most things and most conditions as potentially good or as potentially evil, depending on the Christian's use of, or response to, them. Health could be a good thing, or it could be a bad thing. Likewise with sickness or with any other form or source of suffering. Jerome (ca. 345–ca. 419), for example, writes to a remarkably healthy centenarian that the health of the righteous is God's gift in which they should rejoice, but the health of the unrighteous is Satan's gift to lead them to sin.[59] Hence Jerome tells another correspondent to rejoice not only in health but also in sickness, saying, "Am I in good health? I thank my Creator. Am I sick? In this case also I praise God's will. For 'When I am weak, then am I strong,' and the strength of the spirit is made perfect in the weakness of the flesh."[60] This is a subject to which Jerome's heart warms: sickness can cause people to adjust their priorities. He describes a young lady who was taught by a burning fever, with which she had suffered for nearly thirty days, to direct her attention to more serious pursuits than the pampering of her person, to which, apparently, she had been giving more time than Jerome thought appropriate.[61] Ambrose likewise suggests to a correspondent who had been sick that God had sent the sickness to him for the sake of his spiritual health.[62] And in his treatise *Concerning Repentance* he writes that while sickness restrains one from sin, luxury is a catalyst to sins of the flesh.[63]

How was the Christian to respond when ill? We have already seen that he was encouraged to seek healing but admonished not to cling desperately to life. But was he to aggravate the condition, thereby increasing his suffering and thus supposedly deriving some spiritual benefit? All the church fathers insisted on a practical self-denial and a subduing of the flesh. The extremes of asceticism of which they approved varied. Clement was very mild in that regard compared to Jerome, who, with a hearty fortitude that well matched his often caustic personality, bordered on the severe in the self-denial that he both practiced and preached. In one letter Jerome writes that when one's limbs are weak from fasting, Satan may oppress him with illness. What then should he do? Why, respond to the devil just as Paul did, saying, "When I am weak, then am I strong," and "Power is made perfect in weakness."[64]

On the other hand, in a letter to the lady Paula, whose twenty-year-old daughter, Blaesilla, had recently died, Jerome chides her for fasting. He imagines Christ saying to her that such fasting, which simply gratifies her grief, is displeasing to him. "Such fasts are my enemies. I receive no soul which forsakes the body against my will." It would be suicide for her to die in this way. Interestingly, Blaesilla's death had likely been hastened by her severe self-abasement, which Jerome had then most heartily encouraged; he still approved of it when he wrote to Paula. Toward the end of the letter, he rebukes her for her public display of grief during the funeral procession. Not only is it a bad witness, since Christians are supposed to rejoice in the "homegoing" of loved ones, but also he knows what the Roman crowd viewing the procession were probably saying: The girl was "killed with fasting." "How long must we refrain from driving these detestable monks out of Rome?" "They have misled this unhappy lady." Apparently the fasting in which the already sick Blaesilla had engaged, which almost certainly contributed to her death, was, in Jerome's opinion, pleasing to Christ. But Paula's fasting was displeasing to Christ because her motivations were wrong. And if she had died because of it, it would have been sinful; consequently Christ would not have received her soul, since it would have forsaken her body against his will.[65]

There are some very fine lines to draw here. And we can rest assured that Jerome drew them very close to those extremes of asceticism that earned for the rigorist Messalians, as an example, the status of heretics by official proclamation of the orthodox community. Most of the church fathers would not have gone as far as Jerome did in exhorting others to persevere in subduing and denying the flesh. But all shared the view that the soul was of infinitely greater value than the body. They did, however, as we have seen, espouse an obligation to care for the body. Hence the tension between these two obligations as perceived by the Christian community at that time and for a long time thereafter.

Leaving persecution, martyrdom, and asceticism, we turn to those forms of suffering that are the common lot of mankind. Even a cursory and random reading of the church fathers reveals that they regarded suffering as an essential aspect of God's sanctifying of his people. This belief, combined with a firm assurance that God is sovereign, and an equally firm trust that he does all thing for their ultimate good, engendered in them an imperative to preach and practice endurance in the face of all afflictions. Cyprian and Tertullian, who wrote in Latin, and Clement of Alexandria, who wrote in Greek, lived when Christians were subject to persecution and possible martyrdom. They differ from each other significantly in their backgrounds, personalities, and emphases, and hence they reflect the diversity of theology that then prevailed within the realm of orthodoxy. Yet, in the most foundational and essential areas of Christian values, they display a profound unity: Christians are subject to the whole range of afflictions that beset fallen humanity in a fallen world. Indeed, Christians must face even greater sufferings than pagans, because both God and Satan will buffet them. Satan does so in order to discourage them and hence to tempt them to sin; God does so as paternal chastening (including both training and discipline) that leads to sanctification. Accordingly, the Christian must practice patient endurance in defiance of Satan and in resignation to the salutary and salubrious providence of God. It should be noted that both the Greek and the Latin words typically translated as "patience" have the underlying meaning of "patient endurance."

Cyprian was the most pastoral of these three church fathers. He also most clearly represents the mainstream of orthodoxy. Two of his most pastoral writings are *Mortality,* written during a time of plague, and *The Good of Patience.* In the latter he asserts that "a crown for sorrow and suffering cannot be obtained unless patience in sorrow and suffering precede."[66] For with patience

we may endure all afflictions. . . . It is a salutary precept of our Lord and Master: "He who has endured even to the end will be saved. . . ." We must endure and persevere . . . so that, having been admitted to the hope of truth and liberty, we can finally attain that same truth and liberty, because the very fact that we are Christians is a source of faith and hope. However, in order that hope and faith may reach their fruition, there is need of patience.

After quoting Romans 8:24–25, he says, "Patient waiting is necessary that we may fulfill what we have begun to be, and through God's help, that we may obtain what we hope for and believe." He quotes Galatians 6:9–10 and comments that Paul here "warns lest anyone, through lack of patience grow tired in his good work; lest anyone either diverted or overcome by temptations, should stop in the middle of his course of praise and glory and his past works be lost." After quoting Ezekiel 33:12 and Revelation 3:11, he says that "these words urge patient and resolute perseverance, so that he who strives for a crown, now with praise already near, may be crowned because his patience endures." He immediately asserts that patience "not only preserves what is good, but also repels what is evil," for "it struggles . . . against the acts of the flesh and the body whereby the soul is stormed and captured." He then enumerates various sins against which patience is the only efficacious defense and states that if patience is strong "the hand that has held the Eucharist will not be sullied by the blood-stained sword."[67] Later he maintains that patience is

necessary in respect to various hardships of the flesh and frequent and cruel torments of the body by which the human race is daily wearied and oppressed. . . . It is necessary to keep struggling and contending in this state of bodily weakness and infirmity; and this struggle and strife can not be endured without the strength of patience. But different kinds of sufferings are imposed on us to test and prove us, and many forms of temptations are inflicted upon us by loss of wealth, burning fevers, torments of wounds, by the death of dear ones. . . . The just man is proved by patience, as it is written, "In thy sorrow endure and in thy humiliation keep patience, for gold and silver are tried in the fire."[68]

He then gives the example of Job: "Thus Job was examined and proved and raised to the pinnacle of praise because of the virtue of patience." He describes Job's various afflictions and says that

lest anything at all might remain which Job had not experienced in his trials, the devil even armed his wife against him. . . . Nevertheless, Job was not broken by these heavy and continuous assaults, and in spite of these trials and afflictions he extolled the praise of God by his victorious patience.[69]

A little later he exclaims:

Let us . . . maintain the patience through which we abide in Christ and with Christ are able to come to God. . . . It is patience that both commends us to God and saves us for God. . . . It vanquishes temptations, sustains persecutions, endures sufferings and martyrdoms to the end. It is this patience which strongly fortifies the foundations of our faith. It is this patience which sublimely promotes the growth of hope.[70]

As the climax of his argument, he exhorts, "Let us . . . persevere and let us labor . . . watchful with all our heart and steadfast even to total resignation."[71]

In his treatise entitled *Mortality*, Cyprian comments on the phenomenon that some Christians were troubled because this

disease carries off our people equally with the pagans, as if a Christian believes to this end, that, free from contact with evils, he may happily enjoy the world and this life, and, without having endured all adversities here, may be preserved for future happiness. . . . But what in this world do we not have in common with others as long as this flesh . . . still remains common to us?

He gives as examples famine, the ravages of war, drought, shipwreck; "and eye trouble and attacks of fever and every ailment of the members we have in common with others as long as this common flesh is borne in the world."[72]

After giving Job and Tobias as examples of endurance, he reminds his readers that this

endurance the just have always had; this discipline the apostles maintained from the law of the Lord, not to murmur in adversity, but to accept bravely and patiently whatever happens in the world. . . . We must not murmur in adversity, beloved brethren, but must patiently and bravely bear with whatever happens, since it is written: "A contrite and humble heart God does not despise."[73]

Hence, "the fear of God and faith ought to make you ready for all things," such as loss of property, diseases, loss of wife and children and other dear ones. So

let not such things be stumbling blocks for you but battles; nor let them weaken or crush the faith of the Christian, but rather let them reveal his valor in the contest, since every injury arising from present evils should be made light of through confidence in the blessings to come. . . . Conflict in adversity is the trial of truth.[74]

Note further Cyprian's emphasis on the activity of God and the passivity of the Christian in death. Cyprian writes that Christians who died of the current pestilence "have been freed from the world by the summons of the Lord."[75] Later he asserts that "those who please God are taken from here earlier and more quickly set free, lest, while they are tarrying too long in this world, they be defiled by contacts with the world." He then suggests that "when the day of our own summons comes, without hesitation but with gladness we may come to the Lord at His call." For "rescued by an earlier departure, you are being freed from ruin and shipwrecks and threatening disasters!" Therefore, "Let us embrace the day which assigns each of us to his dwelling, which on our being rescued from here and released from the snares of the world, restores us to paradise and the kingdom." Consider the loved ones already in heaven and the joys that await us there. "To these, beloved brethren, let us hasten with eager longing! Let us pray that it may befall us speedily to be with them, speedily to come to Christ."[76]

We see that in Cyprian's thought it is God who calls; it is he who issues the summons. God takes the Christian from the world; God frees him; God rescues him; God releases him; God restores him to heaven. The Christian is passive—he *is being* freed; he *is being* rescued; he *is being* released; he *is being* restored. This is God's activity. The Christian's activity is to yearn for heaven. Hence he should pray for an early departure from life. Yearning for death and praying to die are categorically different from taking one's own life. There is no room here for suicide. Patient endurance of all afflictions, perseverance to the end, final resignation to the will of God in the midst of those very situations that God is using to test and to refine the Christian: such thought is antithetical to the taking of one's own life.

Tertullian's message is similar:

Let us strive, then, to bear the injuries that are inflicted by the Evil One, that the struggle to maintain our self-control may put to shame the enemy's efforts. If, however, through imprudence or even of our own free will we draw down upon ourselves some misfortune, we should submit with equal patience to that. . . . But if we believe some blow of misfortune is struck by God, to whom would it be better that we manifest patience than to our Lord? In fact, more than this, it befits us to rejoice at being deemed worthy of divine chastisement. . . . Blessed is that servant upon whose amendment the Lord insists, at whom He deigns to be angry, whom He does not deceive by omitting His admonition. From every angle, then, we are obliged to practice patience, because we meet up with our own mistakes or the wiles of the Evil One or the warnings of the Lord alike.[77]

Later he gives Job as the most significant example of patient endurance:

Far from being turned away by so many misfortunes from the reverence which he owed to God, he set for us an example and proof of how we must practice patience in the spirit as well as in the flesh, in soul as well as in the body, that we may not succumb under the loss of worldly goods, the death of our dear ones, or any bodily afflictions. What a trophy over the Devil God erected in the case of that man! What a banner of His glory He raised above His enemy . . . when [Job] severely rebuked his wife who, weary by now of misfortunes, was urging him to improper remedies. . . . Thus did that hero who brought about a victory for his God beat back all the darts of temptation and with the breastplate and shield of patience soon after recover from God complete health of body and the possession of twice as much as he had lost.[78]

Here also there is no room for suicide. The most basic principles of patient endurance for the Christian militate against the very thought of suicide. Cyprian never mentions suicide. Tertullian, however, after mentioning that Christ "tells us to give to the one who asks," remarks that "if you take His command generally, you would be giving not only wine to a man with a fever, but also poison or a sword to one who wanted to die."[79] Giving wine to the febrile was thought to be very harmful. He includes assisting in suicide in the same category. The thought is that one simply will not supply the means if asked. Elsewhere he classifies anyone who "cuts his own throat" as demented or insane, and the context suggests that such a one is possessed by a demon.[80] There is absolutely no suggestion in the writings of Cyprian and Tertullian that for contemporary Christians suicide either was an attraction or posed a theoretical, much less a practical, problem. Indeed, all the evidence points in the opposite direction.

Of all the church fathers, none was more significantly influenced by Greek philosophy than Clement of Alexandria. To him, Greek philosophy was a *praeparatio evangelica* that contained more truth than falsehood. He eagerly drank from the springs of the pagan past, rejoicing in the plethora of wisdom that he felt God had revealed to the Greeks, partially through a supposed early acquaintance with Hebrew Scripture. Nevertheless, he did not accept all that these philosophers offered. How could he? Not only did they frequently contradict each other but they were often at variance with Scripture. Clement's style, however, was not to draw attention to points of disagreement but, as a means of apologetics, to emphasize primarily matters of consonance. Sometimes he is obscure; at other times he can be easily misunderstood, especially when he draws the reader's attention to certain philosophical tenets, not to endorse them but rather to illustrate a particular Christian truth. Here is a pertinent example:

the philosophers also allow the good man an exit from life in accordance with reason, in the case of one depriving him of active exertion, so that the hope of action is no longer left him. And the judge who compels us to deny Him whom we love, I regard as showing who is and who is not the friend of God. In that case there is not left ground for even examining what one prefers—the menaces of man or the love of God.[81]

An "exit from life in accordance with reason" is, of course, the suicides permitted by certain philosophical schools. The Christian also has an "exit from life in accordance with reason," says Clement, and that is martyrdom. But we must remind ourselves that Clement, as we saw above, unequivocally condemns seeking martyrdom and strongly encourages flight in the face of persecution. Hence this cannot be taken as an endorsement of suicide, as is made even more clear by the discussions of suffering and sanctification that are scattered throughout Clement's *Stromateis*.

Even when addressing suffering and sanctification, Clement's terminology is so philosophical, his vocabulary so peppered with jargon, especially with Stoic jargon, that he can be easily misunderstood, especially if sentences, even paragraphs, are taken out of context. The concept of *apatheia* (insensibility to suffering) is central to Stoic thought. It is also of vital importance to Clement. But in Clement it is significantly informed by those essential scriptural principles that are basic to other church fathers' values. So also for Clement suffering is an essential aspect of Christian growth, and he frequently stresses God's paternal, sovereign care of his people. He says, for example, that the true Christian

will never . . . have the chief end placed in life, but in being always happy and blessed, and a kingly friend of God. Although visited with ignominy and exile, and confiscation, and above all, death, he will never be wrenched from his freedom, and signal love to God. The charity which "bears all things, endures all things" is assured that Divine Providence orders all things well.[82]

Clement enlarges on these themes later:

Though disease, and accident, and what is most terrible of all, death, come upon [the true Christian], he remains inflexible in soul,—knowing that all such things are a necessity of creation, and that, also by the power of God, they become the medicine of salvation, benefiting by discipline those who are difficult to reform; allotted according to dessert, by Providence, which is truly good. . . . He undergoes toils, and trials, and afflictions, not as those among the philosophers who are endowed with manliness, in the hope of present troubles ceasing, and of sharing again in what is pleasant, but knowledge has inspired him with the firmest persuasion of receiving the hopes of the future. [He] withstands all fear of everything terrible, not only of death, but also poverty and disease, and ignominy, and things akin to these.[83]

Penury and disease, and such trials, are often sent for admonition, for the correction of the past, and for care for the future. Such a one prays for relief from them, in virtue of possessing the prerogative of knowledge, not out of vainglory . . . having become the instrument of the goodness of God. . . . He is not disturbed by anything which happens; nor does he suspect those things, which, through divine arrangement, take place for good. Nor is he ashamed to die, having a good conscience, and being fit to be seen by the Powers. Cleansed, so to speak, from all the stains of the soul, he knows right well that it will be better with him after his departure.[84]

The apatheia that Clement lauds as a Christian ideal can never logically lead to suicide:

[By] going away to the Lord . . . *he does not withdraw himself from life. For that is not permitted to him.* But he has withdrawn his soul from the passions. For that is granted to him. And on the other hand he lives, having put to death his lusts, and no longer makes use of the body, *but allows it the use of necessaries, that he may not give cause for dissolution [of the body]* [my emphases].[85]

This is a magnificent blending of certain Stoic principles that are compatible with Clement's Christianity. But it is a Stoicism that has been Christianized to such a degree that suicide is permitted neither in the active sense of withdrawing from life nor in the passive sense of causing the dissolution of the body by failing to provide it with "necessaries."

Just as for Cyprian and Tertullian, so also for Clement, Job is the outstanding example of endurance. The Christian "will bless when under trial, like the noble Job. . . . He will give his testimony by night; he will testify by day; by word; by life, by conduct, he will testify."[86] Later he mentions Job once more, here prefacing his praise with a commendation of the Stoics for the good qualities of their teaching:

Fit objects for admiration are the Stoics, who say that the soul is not affected by the body, either to vice by disease, or to virtue by health; but both these things, they say, are indifferent. And indeed Job, through exceeding continence, and excellence of faith, when from rich to become poor, from being held in honour dishonoured, from being comely unsightly, and sick from being healthy, is depicted as a good example for us, putting the Tempter to shame, blessing his Creator.[87]

George Fisher succinctly describes the salient and essential differences between Stoicism and early Christianity:

Stoicism exhibits no rational ground for the passive virtues, which are so prominent in the Stoic morals. There is no rational end of the cosmos; no grand and worthy consummation towards which the course of the world is tending. Evil is not overruled to subserve a higher good to emerge at the last. There is no inspiring future on which the eye of the sufferer can be fixed. The goal that bounds his vision is the conflagration of all things. Hence there is no basis for reconciliation to sorrow and evil. Christianity in the doctrine of the kingdom of God, furnishes the element which Stoicism lacked, and provides thus a ground for resignation under all the ills of life, and amid the confusion and wickedness of the world. For the same reason, the character of Christian resignation is different from the Stoic composure. It is submission to a wise and merciful Father, who sees the end from the beginning. Hence, there is no repression of natural emotions, as of grief in case of bereavement; but these are tempered, and prevented from overmastering the spirit, by trust in the Heavenly Father. In the room of an impassable serenity, an apathy secured by stifling natural sensibility, there is the peace which flows from filial confidence.[88]

Fisher's assessment can be applied to Clement, whose agenda was not to denigrate any philosophical school, including Stoicism, but to appropriate the schools' best features. Although he was influenced more than any other church father by Greek philosophy (much more by Platonism than by Stoicism), nevertheless, Clement's most basic values were thoroughly Christian. Stoic *apatheia* was for him a means to godliness, a tool for sanctification through perseverance and patient endurance of all afflictions sent or permitted by the sovereign, omniscient, and paternally benevolent Deity. If any church father could have endorsed suicide under any circumstances, it would have been Clement. And in numerous places, especially in his *Stromateis,* it would have been very natural, indeed nearly inevitable, to have done so, *if* he had harbored even the remotest sympathy for it. But it was so far from his mind, so discordant with his values, and so remote from his concerns as an ethical or practical problem, that even his condemnation of it is only made in passing. This is the case also with Tertullian and, as we shall see in the next section, with the other condemnations of suicide in patristic literature before the fourth century.

Discussion of Suicide in Patristic Sources

Justin Martyr (ca. 100–165) imagines a pagan suggesting, "All of you, go kill yourselves and thus go immediately to God, and save us the trouble." Justin replies, "If . . . we should kill ourselves we would be the cause, as far as it is up to us, why no one would be born and be instructed in the divine doctrines, or even why the human race might cease to exist; if we do act thus, we ourselves will be opposing the will of God."[89] L. W. Barnard, in his insightful study of Justin, says, on the basis of this passage, that Justin "shows us men and women . . . who thought it a duty to preserve life so long as God delayed to take it."[90] There is, of course, a difference between a duty not to take one's life and a duty to preserve it, a distinction made by Justin in the context surrounding the passage quoted, when he juxtaposes the Christian's refusal to kill himself and his willingness to die for his faith. Although this passage is a direct condemnation of suicide for Christians, it is simply an explanation, to pagans, of why Christians do not kill themselves. Nor is it bolstered by any moral reasoning or defense. Rather, it simply maintains that it is wrong for Christians to kill themselves because God wants them in the world and the human race needs them, for without Christians there would be no one to instruct humanity in the truth. Since God sustains the human race for the sake of his people, if Christians were all removed from the world, the human race would cease to exist. His position resembles some earlier pagan and later Christian condemnations of suicide based on the premise that since God has stationed each one in this life, no one has a right to desert that post to which God has assigned him.

The *Epistle to Diognetus*, an anonymous piece probably written in the late second century, contains a somewhat similar passage:

The soul is locked up in the body, yet is the very thing that holds the body together; so, too, Christians are shut up in the world as in a prison, yet are the very ones that hold the world together. Immortal, the soul is lodged in a mortal tenement; so, too, Christians, though residing as strangers among corruptible things, look forward to the incorruptibility that awaits them in heaven. The soul, when stinting itself in food and drink, is the better for it; so, too, Christians, when penalized, increase daily more and more. Such is the important post to which God has assigned them, and it is not lawful for them to desert it.[91]

There is no suggestion in either passage that suicide posed a moral problem for the Christian community. Rather, the question is why Christians do not kill themselves, and the answer is that God has assigned them for an important purpose to a post that they must not abandon.

The Clementine *Homilies*, falsely attributed to Clement of Rome, who lived in the late first century and early second century, but written in their present form probably in the mid–fourth century, were based on an original composed in the late second or early third century. Although the *Homilies* display a marked Ebionite or Elkesaite orientation, in many ways their theology is not inconsistent with contemporary orthodoxy. In *Homilies* 12 Peter encounters a pagan woman who, because of a variety of afflictions, is considering committing suicide. He admonishes her, "Do you suppose, O woman, that those who destroy themselves are freed from punishment? Are not the souls of those who thus die punished with a worse punishment in Hades for their suicide?"[92] This is a novel position, that suicide will compound one's future punishment; hence it is unfortunate that we cannot know whether this incident was in the original or added by a fourth-century redactor.

Tertullian remarks that some pagans, "led by the impulses of their own mind, put an end to their lives." Under this rubric he includes the Roman matron Lucretia; the legendary Carthaginian queen Dido; the wife of Hasdrubal, the Carthaginian general who surrendered to Scipio; Cleopatra; and the philosophers Heraclitus, Empedocles, and Peregrinus, the last of whom, after a brief stint as a Christian, became a Cynic and ended his life by self-immolation during the Olympic Games in 165.[93] Tertullian's assessment of these suicides and of those who sacrificed their lives or bravely endured horrible sufferings is that "if earthly glory accruing from strength of body and soul is valued so highly" that pagans would undergo such things "for the reward of human praise," then the sufferings that Christian martyrs endure "are but trifling in comparison with the heavenly glory and divine reward."[94]

In his *Apology* he compared Lycurgus, who had "hoped to starve himself to death because the Spartans had amended his laws," with the Christian, who, "even when condemned, gives thanks."[95] Later he mentions Empedocles' and Dido's self-immolation. Here he becomes sarcastic: "Oh, what strength of mind!" he exclaims about the former; and, about the latter, "Oh, what a glorious mark of chastity!" He says that he will "pass over those who by their own sword or by some other gentler manner of death made sure of their fame after death." On these suicides and on certain examples of bravery and fortitude, he comments that "such recklessness and depravity, for the sake of glory and renown, raise aloft among you the banner of courage." But, in the opinion of pagans, the man who "suffers for God, is a madman."[96]

Tertullian does not condemn these pagan suicides, at least not directly. His sole purpose, as Timothy Barnes expresses it in his study of Tertullian, is contrast: "If glass is so precious, how valuable must be a genuine pearl! Why should Christians hesitate to die for the truth, when others die for false ideals such as their own glory?"[97] "These are all pagans with false ideals. How much more should the Christian endure for the sake of truth and for celestial glory!"[98] Tertullian's sarcasm shows his readers what he thinks of these suicides. If pagans are willing to kill themselves for such unworthy reasons, how much more understandable it is that Christians willingly die for their faith. It would require some hermeneutical gymnastics to find a support of suicide here.

Lactantius (ca. 240–320) was a Latin rhetorician whose accomplishments attracted the attention of the emperor Diocletian, who appointed him professor of oratory in Nicomedia. He was converted to Christianity, and when the Great Persecution began (303), he felt compelled to resign his position. He turned to writing Christian apologetics directed, on the one hand, to educated pagans, and, on the other, to Christians who were troubled by philosophical attacks against their faith. The major argument of his *Divine Institutes* is that "pagan religion and philosophy are absurdly inadequate. Truth lies in God's revelation, and the ethical change which the teaching of Christ brings points conclusively to its accuracy."[99] The first two books, "Concerning False Religion" and "Concerning the Origin of Error," attempt to refute polytheism. Book 3, "Concerning False Wisdom," tries "to prove the falsity of pagan philosophy, its contradictions, and its uselessness in practice."[100] The remainder of the work is devoted to demonstrating the truth of Christianity. Lactantius' major statement on suicide appears in book 3. Discussing the Pythagoreans and Stoics, both of whom believed in the immortality of the soul (although the latter regarded it as right to take one's own life under some circumstances), he says that many of them, "because they suspected that the soul is immortal, laid violent hands upon themselves, as though they were about to depart to heaven." He then gives as examples Cleanthes, Chrysippus, Zeno, Empedocles, Cato, and Democritus. He asserts that

nothing can be more wicked than this. For if a homicide is guilty because he is a destroyer of man, he who puts himself to death is under the same guilt, because he puts to death a man. Yea, that crime may be considered to be greater, the punishment of which belongs to God alone. For as we did not come into this life of our own accord; so, on the other hand, we can only withdraw from this habitation of the body which has been appointed for us to keep, by the command of Him who placed us in this body that we may inhabit it, until He orders us to depart from it. . . . All these philosophers, therefore, were homicides.[101]

Some years after completing his *Divine Institutes,* Lactantius was asked to produce an epitome of it. It is interesting to note that the space he devotes to suicide in this much shorter abridgement is more than in the original. In the *Epitome* he asks whether we should approve those

who, that they might be said to have despised death, died by their own hands? Zeno, Empedocles, Chrysippus, Cleanthes, Democritus, and Cato, imitating these, did not know that he who put himself to death is guilty of murder, according to the divine right and law. For it was God who placed us in this abode of flesh: it was He who gave us the temporary habitation of the body, that we should inhabit it as long as He pleased. Therefore it is to be considered impious, to wish to depart from it without the command of God. Therefore violence must not be applied to nature. He knows how to destroy His own work. And if any one shall apply impious hands to that work, and shall tear asunder the bonds of the divine workmanship, he endeavours to flee from God, whose sentence no one will be able to escape, whether alive or dead. Therefore they are accursed and impious, whom I have mentioned above, who even taught what are the befitting reasons for voluntary death; so that it was not enough of guilt that they were self-murderers, unless they instructed others also to this wickedness.[102]

We should note that in the earlier passage suicides are condemned as worse than homicides, for suicides desert the place to which God has appointed them. In the *Epitome* the argument is essentially the same, although Lactantius adds the offenses of attempting to flee from God by committing violence against nature, and encouraging others to do the same. His tone in the *Epitome* is even more outraged and vitriolic than in the *Institutes.* Suicides are not only homicides but are impious as well.

In passing we may observe that a contemporary of Lactantius, the historian Eusebius (ca. 265–ca. 339), writes that "tradition relates" that Pilate, the Roman official who had sentenced Jesus to death by crucifixion, "fell into such great calamity that he was forced to become his own slayer and to punish himself with his own hand, for the penalty of God, as it seems, followed hard after him."[103] In a case such as Pilate's, suicide from despair is seen as God's penalty, a condemnation for sin, hardly setting a precedent for Christian suicide.

John Chrysostom (349–407) was a fervent and eloquent preacher whose concerns were primarily pastoral. In his *Commentary on Galatians,* when dealing with Galatians 1:4 (Jesus "gave himself for our sins to deliver us from the present evil world, according to the will of our God and Father"), he criticizes those heretics who regard the material world as evil. He takes the words *evil world* to mean evil actions, and a depraved moral principle. . . . Christ came not to put us to death and deliver us from the present life in that sense, but to leave us in the world, and prepare us for a worthy participation of our heavenly abode. Wherefore He saith to the Father, "And these are in the world, and I come to Thee; I pray not that Thou shouldest take them from the world, but that Thou shouldest keep them from the evil," i.e., from sin. Further, those who will not allow this, but insist that the present life is evil, should not blame those who destroy themselves; for as he who withdraws himself from evil is not blamed, but deemed worthy of a crown, so he who by a violent death, by hanging or otherwise, puts an end to his life, ought not to be condemned. *Whereas God punishes such men more than murderers, and we all regard them with horror, and justly; for if it is base to destroy others, much more is it to destroy one's self* [my emphasis].[104]

Chrysostom here maintains that encouragement to suicide is a reasonable consequence of dualistic heresy. But as far as he is concerned, true Christians—"we all" would be the orthodox—regard suicides with horror, and justly so. This would be a preposterous statement if there had been even a strong minority sentiment in the orthodox Christian community that would justify suicide to escape "the present evil world."

Ambrose (ca. 339–97), Augustine's mentor, was much influenced by both Neoplatonism and Stoicism.[105] His position on suicide, however, seems to have been no more affected by Stoicism than was that of Clement of Alexandria. In his treatise *Death as a Good*, he comments on Paul's statement "For to me to live is Christ and to die is gain" (Phil. 1:21):

For Christ is our king; therefore we cannot abandon and disregard His royal command. How many men the emperor of this earth orders to live abroad in the splendor of office or perform some function! Do they abandon their posts without the emperor's consent? Yet what a greater thing it is to please the divine than the human! Thus for the saint "to live is Christ and to die is gain." He does not flee the servitude of life like a slave, and yet like a wise man he does embrace the gain of death.[106]

Here once more we see the familiar assertion that one is to stay at the post to which God has assigned him until God chooses to remove him.

Elsewhere Ambrose writes to his sister Marcellina, "You make a good suggestion that I should touch upon what we ought to think of the merits of those who have cast themselves down from a height, or have drowned themselves in a river, lest they should fall in the hands of persecutors, seeing that holy Scripture forbids a Christian to lay hands on himself."[107] Then, after giving an example of a virgin's committing suicide to preserve her chastity, he describes an instance of a woman's endurance under torture leading to death, implying, in answer to the question raised above, that suicide to avoid persecution is wrong, but suicide to preserve virginity is laudable. It is noteworthy that Ambrose simply asserts that Scripture forbids suicide and appears to assume that his addressee would share this opinion. This, incidentally, appears to be the earliest extant blanket appeal to Scripture for a condemnation of suicide.

Very similar are the views of Jerome. In a letter written to the lady Paula, who was distraught over the death of her daughter Blaesilla, he says,

Have you no fear, then lest the Savior may say to you: "Are you angry, Paula, that your daughter has become my daughter? Are you vexed at my decree, and do you, with rebellious tears, grudge me the possession of Blaesilla? You ought to know what my purpose is both for you and for yours. You deny yourself food, not to fast but to gratify your grief, and such abstinence is displeasing to me. Such fasts are my enemies. I receive no soul which forsakes the body against my will. A foolish philosophy may boast of martyrs of this kind; it may boast of a Zeno, a Cleombrotus, or a Cato. My spirit rests only upon him 'that is poor and of a contrite spirit and that trembleth at my word' [Is. 66:2]."[108]

Elsewhere, Jerome qualifies this otherwise unlimited condemnation of suicide: "It is not ours to lay hold of death, but we freely accept it when it is inflicted by others. Hence, even in persecutions it is not right for us to die by our own hands, except when chastity is threatened, but to submit our necks to the one who threatens."[109]

We should note that both Ambrose and Jerome make one exception to their condemnation of suicide: they sanction suicide when committed to preserve one's chastity. However, they do condemn suicide to escape persecution. The latter was pretty much academic for the orthodox community by this time, since persecution leading to martyrdom had generally ceased to be a threat with the legalization of Christianity in 313. The only specific example of Christians committing suicide to avoid martyrdom is given by Eusebius in his *Ecclesiastical History*, where he expresses neither approval nor disapproval:

Why need one rekindle the memory of those in Antioch, who were roasted on heated gridirons, not unto death, but with a view to lengthy torture; and of others who put their right hand into the very fire sooner than touch the accursed sacrifice? Some of them, to escape such trials, before they were caught and fell into the hands of those that plotted against them, threw themselves down from the tops of lofty houses, regarding death as a prize snatched from the wickedness of evil men.[110]

This passage ought to be interpreted in light of the implied condemnation of this type of suicide by Ambrose,[111] and the very specific condemnation of it by Jerome.[112]

Both Ambrose and Jerome assume, however, the probity of suicide to preserve chastity. Here we enter into an anomaly in early Christian thought: the approbation of suicide to preserve chastity, especially to preserve virginity. Only a minority of the sources surveyed mention it; the few that do, approve it.[113] The earliest of these is Eusebius. He tells of a virtuous woman and her two virgin daughters at Antioch who threw themselves into a river to escape the salacious designs of the Roman soldiers.[114] Later, after describing the endurance of martyrs under the most severe tortures, he writes:

And the women, on the other hand, showed themselves no less manly than the men, inspired by the teaching of the divine Word: some, undergoing the same contests as the men, won equal rewards for their valour; and others, when they were being dragged away to dishonour, yielded up their souls to death rather than their bodies to seduction [*phthora*, "moral corruption"].[115]

Then he gives an example of a "most noble and chaste" married lady in Rome who, when faced with imminent threat of sexual violation, "transfixed herself with a sword. And straightway dying she left her corpse to her procurers; but by deeds that themselves were more eloquent than any words she made it known to all men, both those present and those to come hereafter, that a Christian's virtue is the only possession that cannot be conquered or destroyed."[116] Eusebius' approval of these cases is obvious.

We have already noted that Ambrose appears to approve such suicide. The remarks of the leading twentieth-century authority on Ambrose, F. Homes Dudden, are worthy of inclusion here:

On one occasion Ambrose was requested by his sister Marcellina to state his opinion concerning virgins who committed suicide to avoid violation. He did not, however, express himself very clearly. On the one hand, he told the story of the suicide of St. Pelagia of Antioch and of her mother and sisters in a manner which suggests that, if he did not actually commend, he certainly did not condemn their act. On the other hand, he spoke with unqualified admiration of another Antiochene virgin, who, being sentenced to violation in a brothel, on account of her refusal to sacrifice, prepared to undergo the penalty, without anticipating it by suicide. In relating the incident, he said, "A virgin of Christ may be dishonoured, but she cannot be polluted. Everywhere she is the virgin of God and the temple of God. Places of infamy do not stain chastity; on the contrary chastity abolishes the infamy of the place."[117]

Ambrose's reasoning, as expressed in the last three sentences quoted here from his treatise *Concerning Virgins*, corresponds very closely to Augustine's, who, as we shall see, on these very grounds condemns suicide even to preserve chastity.

Jerome, as has already been observed, is unequivocal in his approbation of these acts of suicide. For him, they are the only exception to his firm conviction that suicide is illicit for Christians. To appreciate why such an exception was made by these church fathers, one must be aware of the extent to which the early Christian community recoiled from what they regarded as the gross immorality of pagan culture. Early Christian sources condemned nearly all aspects of pagan immorality as related features of a society that they regarded as rotten to its very core because of sin. With sweeping strokes of moral indignation, early Christian apologists condemned gladiatorial shows and cruel executions, along with abortion, infanticide, homicide generally, and a broad variety of sexual practices ranging from homosexuality to adultery, from fornication to perversions within the marriage bond. The range of imagination employed in sexual activities by the pagans, and the open display of it, appears to have caused the early Christian community to react more strongly against sexual sins than against any other realm of contemporary immorality. And the numerous injunctions in the New Testament to refrain from sexual sins supported their moral indignation.

These factors alone, however, were not sufficient to produce a climate conducive to regarding the preserving of one's chastity as a higher moral obligation than refraining from suicide. Sexual abstinence is occasionally praised or recommended in the New Testament, and as early as the late first or early second century Ignatius calls Christian women who voluntarily remain virgins Christ's brides and jewels. But it is not until the mid- to late second century that some sources begin to suggest that celibacy is a higher good than marriage and an essential quality for the true ascetic. That virginal celibacy was continuing to grow in esteem, gradually becoming nearly the highest virtue, is illustrated by the fact that instances of Christian women committing suicide to preserve their chastity are not found before the fourth century. It is this one motivation for suicide (which was by then approved) that first caught Augustine's attention and caused him to address the subject of suicide.

All the implicit and explicit condemnations of suicide in Christian literature prior to or contemporary with Augustine are encapsulated and elaborated by Augustine. There is no figure in the early centuries of

Christianity who had a more significant influence on later western Christian thought than he. So similar was he to his eastern contemporaries, Basil of Caesarea, Gregory Nazianzen, and Gregory of Nyssa (the Cappadocian fathers), and to John Chrysostom that to see him as a spokesman for western (as opposed to eastern) Christianity would be simplistic. Yet there is in Augustine's works a melody that is hauntingly "medieval" in many of its nuances. The end of his long life marks a watershed in Western history. When he died in 430, Rome had already been sacked (twenty years earlier) by the Goths, and Roman North Africa was falling to the Vandals. The unity of the Mediterranean world was beginning to disintegrate as its western half was increasingly affected by forces from the north, some already Christianized, and was slowly being drawn into an emerging European, rather than a strictly Mediterranean, ethos.

Hence we need to approach Augustine as something of a Janus figure. His influence on medieval Christianity is enormous. Much more important, for the present study, is a consideration of the extent to which he shares and transmits the values of his antecedents and contemporaries as they pertain to suicide. As early as Rousseau, some have claimed that Augustine took his arguments against suicide from Plato's *Phaedo* and not from the Bible. It is common to find modern scholars making such amazing claims as "There is little reason to think that Augustine's position is authentically Christian."[118] It should be obvious to the attentive reader that a survey of the patristic literature demonstrates that it is simply wrong to suggest that Augustine formulated what then became the "Christian position" on suicide. Rather, by removing certain ambiguities, he clarified and provided a theologically cogent explanation of and justification for the position typically held by earlier and contemporary Christian sources.

Augustine's best-known discussion of suicide is found in book 1 of the *City of God*. This is a digression that he could not have intended to be a systematic and comprehensive treatment of the moral issues involved in a consideration of suicide, regardless of the extent to which portions of this digression on suicide were used as authoritative by later generations. His discussion of suicide must be appreciated within the context of his immediate purposes in formulating a position to which a consideration of suicide is only incidental.

In his introductory letter to the first installment of this work, published in 414, Augustine says that he had undertaken the writing of the work in order to defend the City of God, that is, the community of those "predestined to reign with God from all eternity" (as he eventually defines it),[119] against the pagans. Just four years earlier (410), Rome had been captured and ravaged by Alaric and his Goths. This had sent a shockwave throughout the empire. Even though pagan temples had been closed by imperial decree about two decades earlier and public worship of the traditional deities forbidden, the city of Rome had remained largely pagan, especially its upper classes, who clung tenaciously and defiantly to their ancient religious practices, refined by the increasingly popular Neoplatonism, which had become nearly a religion itself. The sack of Rome was, in the pagans' opinion, the final proof of the gods' displeasure with the official neglect of their worship. It was in response to such sentiments that Augustine began, essentially as an encouragement to his fellow Christians in the face of troubling accusations by pagans, what was, over the next thirteen years, to evolve into the *City of God*.

Shortly after finishing this massive work, Augustine wrote his *Retractations*, in which he describes the schema of the *City of God*. Here he says that the first five books were designed to refute those who tie the prosperity of the empire to the favor of the gods and adversity to their disfavor.[120] Book 1 begins with the assertion that Christianity had mitigated rather than aggravated the violence of the recent sack of Rome in particular, and of war in general. Christians show a clemency antithetical to the typical savagery of the pagans (1.1–7). He argues that prosperity and adversity affect both the good and the bad alike (1.8–9). Christians lose nothing when deprived of temporal goods, even of life itself, since all must die sooner or later (1.10–11). Furthermore, it is not a matter of great concern whether the dead bodies of Christians are abused and left unburied, as happened in several instances during the recent sack of Rome. Nevertheless, if possible, Christians pay respect to the bodies of their dead (1.12–13). He then describes the consolations that Christians experience when in captivity and reminds the pagans of their own Regulus, who, centuries before, had endured captivity in an exemplary manner for the sake of his religion, albeit a false religion (1.14–15). Some pagans took great delight in pointing out that even Christian women were sexually violated by the barbarian Goths during their ravaging of Rome. Augustine replies that the virtue of one thus violated is not polluted (1.16). It is here that Augustine detours into a discussion of suicide by women to preserve their chastity.[121]

Who is so lacking in human compassion, he asks, as to refuse to excuse them for doing this? But other women did not kill themselves under the same circumstances, because they did not want to escape "another's criminal act by a crime of their own." Anyone who faults the latter lays himself open to a charge of folly. At this point Augustine turns from a consideration of this specific type of suicide to make his *first general condemnation of suicide,* which rests on two grounds:

1. If no one on his own authority has a right to kill even a guilty man, then certainly one who kills himself is a homicide. The more innocent he is in respect to that for which he puts himself to death, the more guilty he is for killing himself.

2. We rightly execrate Judas' deed, and truth declares that when he hanged himself he increased rather than atoned for his detestable betrayal. Truth declares this to be so because by killing himself, Judas, in despairing of God's mercy, while displaying a self-destructive sorrow, left no room for a saving repentance. How much more, then, ought one who has no fault in himself worthy of such a punishment refrain from self-slaughter. When Judas killed himself, he killed a criminal. He died guilty not only of Christ's death, but of his own as well.

Augustine returns to the initial question: What of those who commit suicide to preserve their chastity? "Why then should a person who has done no evil do evil to himself, thus killing an innocent person lest he have to submit to another's wrongdoing and in so doing perpetrate his own sin upon himself, lest another's sin be perpetrated upon him?" Here ends book 1, section 17.

Augustine devotes book 1, section 18, to the question of whether the fear of being morally polluted by another's lust is legitimate. Augustine's answer is a resounding "no." If the lust is another's, there is no moral pollution for the one victimized, since purity is a virtue of the mind. We need not consider his arguments here. His conclusion to this section is that a woman who has been violated by another's sin has in herself no fault worthy of being punished by voluntary death. How much less, then, is she right in killing herself to ensure that she not be violated. He then expresses a strong admonition: Let there be no certain murder when the offense itself, although another's, still is only pending and uncertain.

Having established that guilt attaches only to the ravisher if the will of the victim does not consent to the act, he considers in book 1, section 19, the case of the legendary Roman matron Lucretia, who killed herself because she had been violated and was unable to endure living with the horror of the indignity that she had suffered. The Romans venerated her as a paragon of virtue, but, says Augustine, in killing herself she received the greater punishment, since the ravisher was only exiled. What kind of justice is this? And, after all, her suicide was not due to any great value that she placed on chastity but rather was due to the weakness of shame. Her sense of honor could not tolerate the thought that some might think that she had willingly submitted to an adulterous sexual act. But this is not the way Christian women acted who were violated but still survived. Not only did they not avenge another's crime, but they would not compound the wrong by adding crimes of their own by committing murders against themselves. They have within themselves the glory of chastity, the witness of their conscience. This they have in the sight of God and they do not ask for anything more. There is, indeed, nothing more for them to do that they could rightly do, "lest they deviate from the authority of divine law while doing wrong to avoid people's suspicion."

In book 1, section 20, Augustine makes his *second general condemnation of suicide* on the following grounds:

1. It is significant, he says, that in the sacred canonical books no divinely given command or permission can be found for us to kill ourselves either to attain immortality or to avoid or escape any evil.

2. Quite to the contrary, the killing of oneself must be understood to be forbidden when the law says, "You shall not kill," especially because it does not add "your neighbor" as it does when it forbids bearing false witness. Even though the commandment against bearing false witness against one's neighbor also should be understood to include the prohibition against bearing false witness against oneself, the absence of the addition of "your neighbor" to the commandment not to kill shows that there is no exception, not even the very individual to whom the command is addressed.

He maintains in book 1, section 21, that not all killings of men are acts of homicide: for example, he exempts obeying legitimate orders to execute a criminal or to kill in war. He then gives some extraordinary examples of legitimate killings. Abraham was prepared to kill Isaac at God's command and would rightly have done so if God had not intervened. Samson destroyed himself along with his enemies. God's Spirit, who had previously worked miracles through him, must certainly have ordered him to do this. He concludes this section by saying that other than these two exceptions (i.e., killing prescribed by a just law or directly by God), whoever kills a human being, either himself or anyone at all, is entwined in the crime of homicide.

He next poses the question of whether suicide is ever a sign of greatness of soul. Those who have killed themselves are perhaps to be admired for their greatness of soul but not praised for the soundness of their wisdom. But if one considers the matter carefully, greatness of soul may not properly be attributed to one who has killed himself because he lacked the strength to endure hardship or another's wrongs. An inability to bear physical oppression or the stupid opinion of the rabble is rather the sign of weakness of character. If suicide can be taken as a sign of greatness of soul, then Theombrotus should be an outstanding example: When he read Plato's dialogue that discusses the immortality of the soul, he went right out and killed himself so that he could go immediately to a better life. And Theombrotus had not been suffering under any hardship whatsoever. Would not Plato himself have done the same thing if that intellect by which he perceived the soul's immortality had not also shown him that such an act must be forbidden?

Many, of course, have killed themselves rather than fall into the hands of the enemy. But the patriarchs, prophets, and apostles did not do so. Indeed, Christ advised the latter that when they were persecuted in one town they should flee to another. He could have advised them to kill themselves to avoid falling into the hands of their persecutors. Instead, he promised to prepare eternal mansions for them. Augustine ends book 1, section 22, by asserting that regardless of what kinds of examples many pagans give of their ancestors thus ending their own lives, "it is obvious that this is not right for those who worship the true God."[122]

In the next two sections he contrasts two examples from Rome's past. Cato, whom the Romans regarded as a man of learning and integrity, committed suicide to avoid falling into Caesar's hands. Why did he commit suicide? Augustine suggests that he apparently did not want to allow Caesar to receive the praise he would win by pardoning him. Augustine begins book 1, section 24, by asserting that Job, who chose to continue to suffer horrible physical distress rather than kill himself, is to be preferred over Cato. So also are other saints mentioned in the sacred writings who chose to endure captivity and slavery rather than to end their own lives. Now he brings up a virtuous pagan to contrast with Cato; that is Regulus, whom Augustine had already given as an example of patient endurance (1.15). Since Regulus chose to stay alive under the most trying of circumstances, there can be no doubt that he judged it to be a great crime for a person to kill himself. Augustine says that he could give other examples of pagans who had no fear of death but chose to endure domination by the enemy rather than to inflict death on themselves. "How much more will Christians, who worship the true God and long for a heavenly country, abstain from this crime." For Christians assume, under such circumstances, that Divine Providence has subjected them to enemies either to try or to correct them. For God does not abandon them in their state of humiliation. Furthermore, since they are under no obligation to kill a conquered enemy *(hostis)*, "what, then, is the source of this evil error that a person should kill himself, either because his enemy [*inimicus*] has sinned against him or may sin against him, although he would not dare to kill even an enemy [*inimicus*] who had sinned or may sin against him?" With this question Augustine ends book 1, section 24, and is obviously working his way back to the question that precipitated his digression on suicide.

In book 1, section 25, he deals with the proposition that one sin should not be avoided by the commission of another sin. There is always the possibility that when subjected to another's lust one may be enticed to consent to the sin. Accordingly, some say that one so threatened ought to kill himself, not on the ground of another's sin, but rather on the ground of the potential for one's own sin. But, replies Augustine, a mind that is subject to God and his wisdom rather than to the body and its lusts will never consent to the physical desire aroused by another's lust. "In any event, if the killing of oneself is a detestable crime and a damnable sin just as obvious truth proclaims, who is so stupid as to say, 'Let us now sin immediately, lest perhaps we sin later; let us now commit homicide immediately lest perhaps we fall into adultery later'?" Surely it is better to take a chance on an uncertain adultery in the future than on a certain homicide now. Is it not better to commit a crime that repentance may heal than an act of wickedness that affords no opportunity for repentance? Augustine says that he included these comments "for the sake of those men or women who think that they must do mortal violence to themselves in order to avoid, not another's sin, but a sin of their own." He proceeds to assure them that the mind of a Christian who trusts in his own God, hoping in him and relying on his help, will not consent to participate in another's sin. Augustine will resume discussion of the subject in book 1, section 27, the final section of this digression on suicide.

Augustine has clearly condemned as sinful, but understandable, the suicides of Christian women who considered death preferable to being ravished by barbarians during the recent sack of Rome. But what of those women of the past who, in the face of persecution, chose to commit suicide to preserve their chastity and have not only become heroines of the faith but also are venerated as martyrs in the Catholic Church by throngs of people who visit their shrines? It is with this difficult question that he introduces book 1, section 26, a section that addresses the broader question, "What explanation should be given for those unlawful acts committed by saints?" Regarding those women who killed themselves during times of persecution in the past and are now venerated as martyrs, he does not "dare to give a rash judgment." Perhaps divine authority instructed the church by some trustworthy evidence that their memory should be honored. Maybe these women acted not under human misconception but by divine command. In this case, they were not erring but obeying. But this he also has no way of knowing. If the latter is true, then the case is comparable to Samson's. There must be absolutely no doubt about the certainty of the divine command. He concludes this section with the assertion that

no one should inflict a voluntary death on himself by fleeing temporal troubles, lest he fall into eternal troubles; that no one ought to do so on account of another's sins, lest by this very act he create his own very serious sin, when he would not have been polluted by another's sin; that no one ought to do so because of past sins, because he needs his present life all the more so that his sins may be healed by repentance; that no one ought to do so from a desire for the better life for which we hope after death, because this better life, which comes after death, does not receive those responsible for their own death.

This could have been a quite appropriate concluding statement of this digression, which deals with a variety of hypothetical exceptions to the prohibition of suicide. It is noteworthy that the hypothetical exception not included here is the one to which the immediately preceding section was devoted, to which Augustine feels he must devote more attention.

In book 1, section 27, Augustine resumes his examination of the question of whether one may commit suicide to escape being lured into sin by enticing pleasure or impelled into sin by raging pain. If we ever consent to this, there is no drawing the line: then why not kill oneself immediately after being baptized? For what reason would anyone chose to endure the pressures of life, with its temptations? Why waste our time exhorting to holiness and to the avoiding of sin when we could persuade people to take a shortcut that would avoid all risks of sin? That would not be foolishness but madness. Because it is wicked even to suggest this, it is certainly wicked to kill oneself. "For if any just cause were possible for suicide, I am sure that there could not be one more just than that. But since not even this one is just, therefore there is no just cause for suicide." Here ends the digression on suicide, and Augustine resumes the subject that had precipitated this digression with a word of encouragement: "So, faithful Christians, don't regard your life as a burden because your enemies mock your chastity" (1.28).

Augustine has covered the bases very well in condemning different motivations for suicide: (1) a desire to escape from or avoid temporal troubles; (2) a desire to escape from or avoid another's sinful actions (suicide to protect one's chastity would be included here); (3) guilt over past sins; (4) a desire for the better (i.e., eternal) life; and (5) a wish to avoid sinning. He emphatically maintains that if there were any just cause for suicide, it would be the last. He makes only passing mention of martyrdom in this digression on suicide, and that is in his refutation of the pagans' approval of suicide to avoid captivity. He says that the patriarchs, prophets, and apostles certainly did not commit suicide to avoid persecution, and in reference to the apostles quotes Jesus' admonition that when persecuted in one city, they should flee to another (1.22). He will shortly be devoting much attention to the subject, but it will not be to the martyrdom of fellow Catholics; rather, it will be to the courting of martyrdom by, and the "heroic" suicides of, members of a schismatic, heretical group, the Donatists.[123]

The Donatist movement was named after its leader, Donatus, who was bishop in Carthage from 313 to about 355. The movement had actually been formed two years earlier by rigorists who condemned what they regarded as the laxness of the church in accepting back into fellowship those who had apostatized during the Great Persecution under Diocletian. It was essentially a protest movement that regarded itself as the one true and holy church. The Catholics, they maintained, because of their toleration of low standards of holiness, were apostates. The Donatists saw themselves as upholders of purity of discipline in the face of Catholic compromise with the "world" and its system, including the ostensibly Christian emperors. From its inception, the sect was both on the offensive and on the defensive; they were the church of the righteous who alone were pure.

The schismatic basis for the Donatist movement evoked a negative response both from the Catholic Church and from the emperor Constantine, who, beginning in 317, attempted to coerce the Donatists back into the fold. Persecution encouraged rather than discouraged these rigorists and merely confirmed them in their convictions. They appear to have been only spasmodically persecuted until early in the fifth century, when a series of repressive measures were promulgated by imperial edict. In 415 the death penalty was specified for those Donatists who continued to assemble.

Augustine greeted these draconian measures with enthusiasm, except for the death penalty, which he consistently opposed in principle: it, like suicide, removed any possibility of repentance.[124] Furthermore, it provided the Donatists with the martyrdom that so many of them seem to have wanted. Augustine's position on coercion had changed over the years, along with his evolving ecclesiology. Earlier he had maintained that only spiritual measures should be used against heretics. Now he advocated force to bring them into the Catholic Church, for outside the Catholic Church there could be no salvation. He applied the *cogite intrare* ("compel them to enter") of Luke 14:23 to the treatment of heretics by civil authorities, hoping that by these measures they could be saved when reason and instruction failed.

Undoubtedly Augustine's change of heart on the question of religious coercion was catalyzed by those aspects of the Donatist movement that he found exceptionally objectionable: their provoking persecution through acts of violence and obnoxious defiance, and their "heroic" suicides. The most noteworthy practitioners of these tactics that Augustine so loathed were the Circumcellions, a fringe group of Donatists who were generally an embarrassment to the more moderate members of the sect. The Circumcellions often roamed the countryside, inciting peasants and slaves to rebellion, engaging in indiscriminate as well as systematic acts of violence, destroying Catholic churches, and harassing, sometimes maiming, and occasionally even killing Catholic clerics. They once attempted to kill Augustine by an ambush that he escaped only because he had accidentally taken the wrong road on a journey.[125] It is impossible to determine with accuracy whether it is fair to saddle the entire Donatist movement with complicity in the actions of the Circumcellions, or to know when the fanatical actions of the latter were simply an extension of the ideology of the former, especially in their provoking of martyrdom and in their "heroic" suicides.

Augustine, perhaps unfairly, attributes both of these acts quite indiscriminately to the Donatists generally. In one of his earliest anti-Donatist works, the *Contra litteras Petiliani,* written between 401 and 405, he asks, "If you are suffering persecution, why do you not retire from the cities in which you are, that you may fulfill the instructions" of Christ to flee when persecuted? Why are you always "eager to annoy the Catholic Churches by the most violent disturbances, whenever it is in your power, as is proved by innumerable instances?"[126] But what disturbed him far more was their practice of "heroic" and very dramatic suicide. Just before committing suicide, they would shout *Deo laudes:* "You are so furious, that you cause more terror than a war trumpet with your cry of 'Praise to God'; so full of calumny, that even when you throw yourselves over precipices without any provocation, you impute it to our persecutions."[127] This was written before the death penalty had been imposed against Donatists who persisted in assembling, and apparently Augustine's point is that their propensity to suicide was so ingrained that their acts of self-destruction could not be mitigated by the claim that they were acting to avoid being put to death by their persecutors.[128]

Several years later (416), after the promulgation of several decrees against the Donatists, one of which imposed the death penalty for those who continued to assemble, Augustine wrote to Donatus, a priest of the Donatist sect, who had been arrested. Augustine writes:

You are angry because you are being drawn to salvation, although you have drawn so many of our fellow Christians to destruction. For what did we order beyond this, that you should be arrested, brought before the authorities, and guarded, in order to prevent you from perishing? As to your having sustained bodily injury, you have yourself to blame for this, as you would not use the horse which was immediately brought to you, and then dashed yourself violently to the ground; for, as you well know, your companion, who was brought along with you, arrived uninjured, not having done any harm to himself as you did.[129]

Augustine then argues that it is "fitting that you should be drawn forcibly away from a pernicious error, in which you are enemies to your own souls."[130] The "pernicious error" to which he refers is twofold: in the broadest sense it is the heretical teaching of the Donatist sect that would lead to spiritual death; in a narrower sense it is the act of suicide, from which Donatus was forcibly restrained, which would have caused physical as well as spiritual death. Augustine maintains that if

mere bodily safety behooves to be so guarded that it is the duty of those who love their neighbour to preserve him even against his own will from harm, how much more is this duty binding in regard to that spiritual health in the loss of which the consequence to be dreaded is eternal death! At the same time let me remark, that in that death which you wished to bring upon yourself you would have died not for time only but for eternity, because even though force had been used to compel you—not to accept salvation, not to enter into the peace of the Church, the unity of Christ's body, the holy indivisible charity, but—to suffer some evil things, it would not have been lawful for you to take away your own life.[131]

He next argues that the Scriptures give no precedents for such self-destruction and seeks to refute the Donatist claim that 1 Corinthians 13:3 does:

I have heard that you say that the Apostle Paul intimated the lawfulness of suicide, when he said, "Though I give my body to be burned," supposing that because he was there enumerating all the good things which are of no avail without charity, such as the tongues of men and of angels, and all mysteries, and all knowledge, and all prophecy, and the distribution of one's goods to the poor, he intended to include among these good things the act of bringing death upon oneself. But observe carefully and learn in what sense Scripture says that any man may give his body to be burned. Certainly not that any man may throw himself into the fire when he is harassed by a pursuing enemy, but that, when he is compelled to choose between doing wrong and suffering wrong, he should refuse to do wrong rather than to suffer wrong, and so give his body into the power of the executioner, as those three men did who are being compelled to worship the golden image, while he who was compelling them threatened them with the burning fiery furnace if they did not obey. They refused to worship the image: they did not cast themselves into the fire, and yet of them it is written that they "yielded their bodies, that they might not serve nor worship any god except their own God." This is the sense in which the apostle said, "If I give my body to be burned."[132]

Augustine then argues that the Donatists' interpretation of 1 Corinthians 13:3 is incorrect since they are devoid of charity both in their actions and in their state, and ends with an appeal to the *cogite intrare* of Luke 14:23 as justification for employing coercion against recalcitrant Donatists.

A year later, Augustine wrote a treatise entitled *Concerning the Correction of the Donatists* in the form of a letter. The Donatists can be easily distinguished from true martyrs, Augustine maintains, for "true martyrs are such as those of whom the Lord says, 'Blessed are they which are persecuted for righteousness sake.' It is not, therefore, those who suffer persecution for their unrighteousness, and for the divisions which they impiously introduce into Christian unity, but those who suffer for righteousness' sake, that are truly martyrs."[133] Some, however, may think that the Donatists have been driven to suicide by the persecutions. That is not so, says Augustine, because when they were not being persecuted and the pagan temples were still permitted to be open, they would come to the temples and provoke the pagans to kill them. Others

went so far as to offer themselves for slaughter to any travellers whom they met with arms, using violent threats that they would murder them if they failed to meet with death at their hands. Sometimes, too, they extorted with violence from any passing judge that they should be put to death by executioners, or by the officer of his court. . . . It was their daily sport to kill themselves by throwing themselves over precipices, or into the water, or into the fire. For the devil taught them these three modes of suicide, so that, when they wished to die, and could not find any one whom they could terrify into slaying them with the sword, they threw themselves over the rocks, or committed themselves to the fire or the eddying pool.[134]

That the devil is the cause of the Donatists' acts of self-destruction by no means exculpates them. Rather, for Augustine it is evidence of the extent to which these acts of "heroic" suicide are profoundly execrable.

In a letter written in 420, Augustine makes the interesting argument that he who thinks that it is "advantageous and allowable" to kill himself should also kill his neighbor

since the Scripture says: "Thou shalt love thy neighbor as thyself." But when no laws or lawful authorities give comment, it is not lawful to kill another, even if he wishes and asks for it and has no longer the strength to live, as is clearly proved by the Scripture in the Book of Kings, where King David ordered the slayer of King Saul to be put to death, although he said that he had been importuned by the wounded and half-dead king to kill him with one blow and to free his soul struggling with the fetters of the body and longing to be released from those torments. Therefore, since everyone who kills a man without any authorization of lawful power is a murderer, anyone who kills himself will not be a murderer if he is not a man. I have said all this in many ways in many other sermons and letters of mine.[135]

This point, however—that it is a sin to aid in the suicide of one who strongly desires to die but does not have the strength to kill himself—does not appear elsewhere in any of his discussions of suicide.

Now Augustine brings up a matter that he says he does not recall ever having addressed before. The Donatists, "embarrassed by the extreme scarcity of examples" that would set "a precedent for the crime of self-destruction," claim that they have found one in 2 Maccabees 14:37–46, specifically in the person of Razias, who had taken his own life rather than submit to captivity by the enemy. Augustine says of him:

Since he was in high esteem among his own, and was most zealous in the Jewish religion . . . and since for this reason this same Razias was called the father of the

Jews, what wonder if an overweening pride found its way, so to speak, into the man so that he chose to die by his own hand rather than suffer the indignity of slavery at the hands of an enemy after having enjoyed such eminence in the sight of his countrymen? Deeds like that are usually praised in pagan literature. But although the man himself is praised in these Books of the Maccabees, his deed is merely related, not praised, and it is set before our eyes as something to be judged rather than imitated. . . . Obviously, Razias was far from those words which we read: "Take all that shall be brought upon thee, and in thy sorrow endure, and in thy humiliation have patience" [Ecclus. 2:4]. Therefore, he was not a man of wisdom for choosing death, but of impatience in not bearing humiliation.[136]

Patience—that is, patient endurance—was just as fundamental a principle for Augustine as it was for earlier and contemporary church fathers. Patient endurance was to Augustine a distinct quality of God's people, whether of the Old Covenant or of the New. In 415 he had written a treatise entitled *De patientia*, which begins with the statement that patience is a virtue of the soul that is not only a gift of God but is predicated of God himself. In much of its emphasis this treatise is similar to earlier works on patience that we have already considered. The major difference is that the earlier discussions, written as they were while Christianity was an illicit cult, devoted much attention to patient endurance of persecution. Like earlier authors, Augustine presents Job as the supreme example of patience:

At him let those men look who bring death upon themselves when they are being sought out to be given life, and who, by taking away their present life, reject also the life to come. For, if they were being forced to deny Christ or to do anything contrary to justice, they ought, as true martyrs, to bear all things patiently rather than to inflict death upon themselves in their impatience. If he could have done it righteously to escape evil, holy Job would have destroyed himself so that he might have escaped such diabolic cruelty in his own possessions, in his own sons, in his own limbs. But he did not do it. Far be it that a wise man commit against himself what not even his foolish wife suggested. Because, if she had suggested it, she would deservedly have had the reply which she heard on suggesting blasphemy: "Thou hast spoken like one of the foolish women: if we have received good things at the hand of God, why should we not receive evil?" And, had he lost his patience either by blaspheming, as she had wished, or by killing himself, which she had not dared to suggest, he would have died and would be among those about whom it has been said: "Woe to them that have lost patience." And he would have increased rather than escaped punishment, for, after the death of his body, he would be hurried away to the penalties of blasphemers or homicides or the more grievous ones of parricides. For, if parricide is more heinous than any homicide in that one slays not merely a man, but one's neighbor, and in that type of murder one's guilt is more serious the closer the person one has destroyed, then without doubt he is a worse sinner who commits suicide, for no one is closer to a man than himself. What now are those wretched men doing, who suffer self-inflicted punishments here and afterwards pay the penalty due, not only for their impiety toward God but also for their cruelty toward themselves? And then they look for the glory of martyrdom! Even if they were suffering persecution in order to bear witness to Christ, and killed themselves so as not to suffer anything from their persecutors, it would rightly be said of them: "Woe to those who have lost patience." For, how could the reward of patience be given to them justly if it was impatient suffering that was to be crowned? Or if he murders himself, a crime which he is forbidden to commit against a neighbor, how will he, to whom it has been said: "Thou shalt love thy neighbor as thyself," be judged innocent?[137]

It is interesting to note that Augustine now introduces the argument that the degree of heinousness of murder depends on the degree of propinquity of the murdered to the murderer. Hence suicide is the most reprehensible type of murder. More significant overall, however, is that suicide, for Augustine, is the fruit of the lack of patient endurance. At the beginning of this treatise, he had told his readers that patience is a gift of God, and the treatise ends on that extended note. Patience will also prove to be the climax of Augustine's second digression on suicide in the *City of God,* which is his final statement on the subject.

In 426 or 427 Augustine published book 19 of the *City of God,* along with the remainder of the work. This, the last section of Augustine's *magnum opus,* opens with a discussion of three pagan treatments of life's *summum bonum* and *summum malum.* Augustine then presents a fourth that is opposed to these pagan perspectives, all of which maintain that the summum bonum for oneself resides in oneself. For the Christian, the summum bonum is eternal life and the summum malum is eternal death. "Truth" laughs at those who place the summum bonum in such things as the body or soul, pleasure or virtue, or in anything that they think they can achieve by their own efforts. What pain and turbulence may not strike the wise man's body? What if the mind is affected by the senses, that is, if one becomes deaf or blind, or if one is rendered insane by some disease? The insane say or do many senseless things, mostly alien or even opposed to their own purpose and character. And what of those who suffer the assaults of demons? Where is their intellect when the evil spirit is using their souls and bodies according to its own will? And who is confident that this evil cannot happen to the wise man in this life? As to the virtues (temperance, prudence, justice, fortitude, and patience), there can be nothing but perpetual warfare with internal vices.

How, then, Augustine asks, can the Stoics claim that all these ills that beset the body, the mind, and the will are not ills at all, since they admit that if the wise man cannot or ought not endure them, he is compelled to inflict death on himself and depart from this life? So great is their stupidity that they call their wise man "happy," even if he becomes blind and deaf and dumb, loses the use of his limbs, is racked with pain and afflicted with every other imaginable evil, and finally is driven by these things to kill himself. What a "happy" life it is that seeks to end itself! If it is "happy," let him remain in it. But these things must be evil that conquer that good that is called fortitude and compel it to give up and escape a life that they crazily call "happy." The very word *escape* admits how weak their position is, as evidenced by the example of the well-known suicide of Cato.

Augustine next tackles the Peripatetics and the Old Academics, who, he alleges, call this life happy because if things become too miserable, they say they have the freedom to escape from it. But this position, he maintains, is absurd, because the happiness of this life then depends upon one's freedom to leave it, thus making its happiness congruent with the brevity of its wretchedness. Great is the power in these evils that force even the wise man to rob himself of his existence as a man, since they say that the first and greatest command of nature is that a man should be reconciled to himself and, as a consequence, naturally shun death; and that, as a living creature, he should be such a friend to himself and so wish to live in this union of body and soul that he would make continued existence his aim. The power in these evils must be great, since it overcomes this natural feeling that causes us to use all our strength in our efforts to avoid death. It so thoroughly defeats nature that what was avoided is now desired and sought, and if it is not achieved in some other way, is inflicted on a person by himself. Great, indeed, Augustine exclaims, is the power in these evils that make the virtue of fortitude a homicide, if it is proper to call fortitude that which is so thoroughly overcome by these evils that it cannot safeguard one from killing himself but rather drives him to it. The wise man ought to endure death patiently, death, that is, which he does not inflict upon himself. If, indeed, a man is compelled by these evils to kill himself, surely these philosophers must admit that they are not only evils but, in fact, intolerable evils.

Such a life, weighed down by such evils, should by no means be called happy. The men who call it that, when they are defeated by the increasing burden of ills and then surrender to adversity by killing themselves, should instead surrender to truth and believe that enjoyment of the supreme good is not a goal to be attained in our moral state. For our virtues bear witness to life's miseries most eloquently when they support us in the midst of life's dangers, toils, and griefs. If our virtues are true, they do not claim to possess the power to ensure that we will not experience any miseries. True virtues are not guilty of such mendacity. But true virtues do say that our human life, although it must be miserable owing to the many evils of this age, *is* happy in expectation of the future age, but only if it is grounded on salvation. Hence the apostle Paul, speaking about men who live in accord with true piety, says, "Now we are saved by hope. But hope that is seen is not hope. For how would one hope for that which he sees? But if we hope for that which we do not see, we wait for it with patience" (Rom. 8:24–25). Augustine concludes this, his final discussion of suicide, by asserting that just as Christians have been saved by hope, so also have they been made happy by hope. Just as Christians do not already possess a present salvation but look forward to a future salvation, so also it is with their happiness. All must be *per patientiam*. Christians are afflicted with various evils but they must patiently endure them until they come to heaven, where they will be made ineffably happy.

Such is the salvation that will be in the future age, which will itself also be the ultimate happiness. Philosophers, since they do not see this happiness and, accordingly, are not willing to believe in it, try in this life to counterfeit for themselves the falsest kind of happiness by a virtue that is as much more arrogant as it is more fraudulent.

Conclusion

Augustine's most frequently cited discussion of suicide, which is also his earliest thorough treatment of it,[138] is his digression on suicide in book 1 of the *City of God*, which he could not have intended to be a systematic theological, much less philosophical, analysis of the subject. Augustine entered the discussion convinced that suicide was a reprehensible sin and a crime. He was speaking to his fellow Christians, who would not have been particularly surprised by anything that he was saying because they held the same basic values as Augustine and his older contemporaries who had already penned condemnations of suicide. The very fact that, in his discussion of suicide, his general condemnations of the act are almost incidental to his main line of argument is in itself compelling evidence for the stability of a tradition of condemnation of suicide. Indeed, if it were not for the exception that a few church fathers had made of some virgins "martyred" by their own hand to preserve their chastity in the face of persecution, the subject of suicide would almost certainly never have come up in book 1 of the *City of God*, and the only discussion of it in this work would then be that which appears in book 19.

It is also unlikely that Augustine would have used the terms that he did to describe the immorality of suicide if his Christian audience would have found his emphatic and unequivocal condemnation of the act at all remarkable. His first reference to suicide is to the suicide of Christian women in Rome who chose death in lieu of possible sexual violation by the conquering Goths. He calls their act a *facinus*. He also refers to suicide as a *scelus*, in fact a *detestabile facinus et damnabile scelus*, a *peccatum*, indeed a *peccatum gravissimum*, a *crimen homicidii*. Augustine refers to one who commits it as a *homicida*. The deed is *non licet;* it is *nefas*, a deviation *ab auctoritate legis divinae*, for which *nulla causa iusta* is possible. It is, in Augustine's mind, so obvious that the immorality of suicide would be self-evident to Christians that he can say that *veritas manifesta* itself proclaims that suicide is a *detestabile facinus et damnabile scelus*. So certain is he of the agreement of the Christian reader that he declares that to believe otherwise than that Samson's self-destruction was in response to a direct command from God's Spirit *fas non est*.

Augustine based his condemnation of suicide most fundamentally on the same presuppositions and values that caused the earlier church fathers to condemn the act. His position is more developed than theirs. Earlier sources simply *assumed* that suicide was a sin. Recall the words with which they describe it: it is opposed to the will of God (Justin); suicides are punished more severely than others (Clementine *Homilies*); it is not permitted (Clement); we all justly regard suicides with horror because God punishes the murderer of self more than he does the murderer of another (John Chrysostom); nothing can be more wicked than suicide (Lactantius); Christ will not receive the soul of a suicide (Jerome); Scripture forbids a Christian to lay hands on himself (Ambrose). These are all simply assertions with which the earlier authors who made them were so confident that their Christian readers would be in agreement that they felt no need to defend them. The last example given, that Scripture forbids a Christian to lay hands on himself, was from Augustine's mentor, Ambrose, who does give the suicide of a woman to preserve her chastity as the only exception to this ostensibly "scriptural" prohibition. It is, of course, the question of this exception that precipitates Augustine's digression on suicide in book 1 of the *City of God.*

The only difference between Augustine and his predecessors who deal with suicide is that in book 1 of the *City of God* Augustine attempts to answer possible objections to the traditional Christian condemnation of suicide. His defense of the traditional position is fourfold:

1. Scripture neither commands suicide nor expressly permits it, either as a means of attaining immortality or as a way to avoid or escape any evil.

2. It must be understood to be forbidden by the sixth commandment.

3. If no one on his own authority has a right to kill even a guilty man, then one who kills himself is a homicide.

4. The act of suicide allows no opportunity for repentance.

There are three major themes in Augustine's anti-Donatist writings that do not appear in his digression on suicide in book 1 of the *City of God:*

1. Provoking martyrdom is a form of suicide and hence a sin. Persecution by pagans was a moot point by this time. Consequently, Augustine's treatment of voluntary martyrdom, since it involves those outside the orthodox community who were responding to efforts by the Catholic Church to compel them to enter the orthodox fold, differs somewhat in force and emphases from earlier condemnations of voluntary martyrdom by members of the orthodox community.

2. "Heroic" suicides by these same folk, when they were unable to provoke others to martyr them, have no known parallel in earlier Christian experience. While the act and circumstances are novel, Augustine's condemnation of such suicides is entirely consistent with the position that he had already articulated in book 1 of the *City of God.*

3. In one of his last anti-Donatist treatises (*Letters* 204, written in 420), Augustine argues that the Donatists' suicides violate the foundational Christian principle of patient endurance. Already, in his treatise on patience, written five years earlier, he had condemned suicide precisely on these grounds. In his final discussion of suicide in book 19 of the *City of God,* written about a decade later, he uses patient endurance as the central principle for a condemnation of suicide as encouraged by various pagan philosophical schools.

Did Augustine formulate the Christian position on suicide? No; but he is the first Christian to discuss it thoroughly. Did he contribute anything new to the Christian position? Here again the answer is "no," except for his unequivocal condemnation of suicide to preserve chastity. It is unlikely that any of the earlier sources that I have cited would have disagreed with any of his arguments, except regarding suicide to preserve chastity, especially virginity. These authors were intelligent men who based their conclusions on their own understanding of Scripture, which they regarded as providing fundamental truth and the only basis for establishing their values and ethics. That none of the extant sources prior to Augustine had recourse to the sixth commandment as forbidding suicide is not remarkable, since earlier sources did not so much argue against suicide as assume its essential sinfulness. Granted, it is interesting historically, as a matter of record, to identify the earliest use of the sixth commandment for this purpose. But it would be significant in a discussion of the development of the Christian position on suicide only (1) if sources prior to Augustine had directly or indirectly approved of suicide generally, thus making him the earliest surviving Christian source to condemn the act; or (2) if earlier Christian authors who did condemn suicide had attempted to justify their position from Scripture (which they did not) but had failed to base any part of their argument on the sixth commandment. Neither of these, of course, is true.

There is no evidence that, at any time during the centuries under consideration, suicide was a debated issue in the Christian community. The church fathers were anything but shy about condemning moral laxity and the diverse sins of their Christian audiences. Indeed, many of them warmed to that task with an enthusiasm of moral vigor, and they dealt not only with matters specifically prohibited by Scripture but with *adiaphora* (grey areas) as well. Nevertheless, one never finds an exhortation to refrain from suicide even in the writings of those authors who condemn the act in no uncertain terms, owing simply to the fact that it was not an option for Christians.[139] The absence of a debate over suicide in the literature of early Christianity is an indication not that the Christian community was indifferent to suicide as an ethical issue but rather that its condemnation as a sinful act was generally assumed throughout the period under consideration.

NOTES

Abbreviations

AF.   *Apostolic Fathers,* trans. K. Lake (Cambridge: Harvard University Press, 1912–13)

ANF.   *Ante-Nicene Fathers,* [various translators] ([various dates]; reprint, Grand Rapids: Eerdmans, 1951)

FC.   *Fathers of the Church,* [various editors and translators] (Washington, D.C.: Catholic University of America, 1948–)

NPNF-1.   *Select Library of Nicene and Post-Nicene Fathers of the Christian Church,* [various translators], 1st ser. ([various dates]; reprint, Grand Rapids: Eerdmans, 1976–79)

NPNF-2.   *Select Library of Nicene and Post-Nicene Fathers of the Christian Church,* [various translators], 2d ser. ([various dates]; reprint, Grand Rapids: Eerdmans, 1976–79)

1. Exod. 21:22–25, the one possible exception, is patient of two different interpretations: the "serious injury" applies (1) to the mother or (2) to the baby. Regardless, the passage does not involve intentional, induced abortion.

2. We now recognize, however, that they often confused abortion and contraception owing to their rudimentary knowledge of obstetrics and embryology.

3. For a thorough discussion, see David Daube, "The Linguistics of Suicide," *Philos. Public Affairs* 1 (1972): 387–437.

4. C. A. Mounteer, "Guilt, Martyrdom, and Monasticism," *J. Psychohist.* 9 (1981): 145.

5. Ibid., 146–53.

6. Glanville Williams, *The Sanctity of Life and the Criminal Law* (1957; reprint, New York: Alfred A. Knopf, 1970), 254–55.

7. A. Alvarez, "The Historical Background," in *Suicide: The Philosophical Issues,* ed. M. P. Battin and D. J. May (New York: St. Martin's, 1980), 25.

8. M. P. Battin, *Ethical Issues in Suicide* (Englewood Cliffs, N.J.: Prentice Hall, 1982), 29 and 72–73.

9. Ibid., 89.

10. Ibid., 71.

11. L. I. Dublin, *Suicide: A Sociological and Statistical Study* (New York: Ronald, 1963), 119.

12. George P. Fisher, *The Beginnings of Christianity* (New York: Scribner's, 1911), 174–75.

13. Ibid., 175.

14. Ambrose, *Death as a Good* 1.1, in *FC* 65:70.

15. Ibid., 2.3, in *FC* 65:71.

16. Ibid., 8.31, in *FC* 65:93.

17. Ibid. 12.57, in *FC* 65:112.

18. Peter Brown, *The Cult of the Saints: Its Rise and Function in Latin Christianity* (Chicago: University of Chicago Press, 1981), 69–70.

19. John Chrysostom, *Homily 8 on Philippians*, in *NPNF*-1, 13:233.

20. Tertullian, *Patience* 9, in *FC* 40:209.

21. "Similitude" 10.4.3, in *Shepherd of Hermas*, in *AF* 2:305.

22. Adolf Harnack, *The Expansion of Christianity in the First Three Centuries*, trans. J. Moffat (1905; reprint, New York: Books for Libraries, 1972), 69–70.

23. E.g., pseudo-Justin, *Letters* 17; Hippolytus, *Apostolic Tradition* 20; Polycarp, *Letters* 6; pseudo-Clement, *De virginitate;* Tertullian, *Ad uxorem* 2.4; Justin, *1 Apology* 67; Jerome, *Letters* 52.15 and 16.

24. Clement of Alexandria, *Stromateis* 4.26, in *ANF* 2:439.

25. Ibid., 4.4, in *ANF* 2:412.

26. Tertullian, *Apology* 42.4, in *FC* 10:107.

27. Cyprian, *Mortality* 5, 18, 24, in *FC* 36:202–3, 214, 219.

28. Basil of Caesarea, *The Long Rules* 55, in *FC* 9:331.

29. John Chrysostom, *Homily 8 on Colossians*.

30. Augustine, *Sermons* 345.2

31. Ibid., 84.1, in M. M. Getty, *The Life of the North Africans as Revealed in the Sermons of Saint Augustine* (Washington, D.C.: Catholic University of America, 1931), 24–25.

32. Ibid., 344.5, in Getty, *Life of the North Africans* (n. 31), 25.

33. There is an enormous literature on the subject of martyrdom and persecution in early Christianity. The most authoritative and reliable treatment is W.H.C. Frend, *Martyrdom and Persecution in the Early Church* (Oxford: Blackwell, 1965).

34. Clement, *Stromateis* 4.4, in *ANF* 2:412.

35. Ibid., 4.4, in *ANF* 2:412.

36. Ibid., 4.10, in *ANF* 2:423.

37. Ibid., 4.4, in *ANF* 2:411.

38. Tertullian, *Scorpiace* 1.11.

39. Tertullian, *Patience* 13.6.

40. Tertullian, *Ad uxorem* 1.3

41. Tertullian, *Flight in Time of Persecution* 6.3, in *FC* 40:287.

42. For a discussion of this case, see Timothy D. Barnes, *Tertullian: A Historical and Literary Study* (Oxford: Clarendon, 1971), 168–71.

43. Frend, *Martyrdom* (n. 33), 197.

44. Ignatius, *To the Romans* 4, in *AF* 1:231.

45. Eusebius, *Ecclesiastical History* 4.15.

46. *Martyrdom of Polycarp* 4, in *AF* 2:317.

47. Tertullian, *To Scapula* 5, in *FC* 10:160.

48. See, e.g., Tertullian, *Apology* 5.

49. What may have been more common were Christians provoking persecution and potential martyrdom by symbolic acts such as the destruction of pagan idols. Canon 60 of the Synod of Elvira, held around 305, condemned such acts on the grounds that the gospel does not suggest deeds of this kind and the apostles did not act in this fashion. The synod decreed that people who die as a result of doing so should not be regarded as martyrs. See C. J. Hefele, *A History of the Christian Councils* (Edinburgh: T. and T. Clark, 1871), 163.

50. Lucian, *The Death of Peregrinus* 13, in *Selected Satires of Lucian*, trans. L. Casson (New York: Norton, 1968), 369.

51. Marcus Aurelius, *Meditations* 11.3.

52. Clement, *Stromateis* 4.4, in *ANF* 2:411.

53. Boniface Ramsay, *Beginning to Read the Fathers* (New York: Paulist, 1985), 126.

54. Clement, *Stromateis* 7.11, in *ANF* 2:541–42.

55. Cyprian, *Mortality* 17, in *FC* 36:213.

56. See, as a beginning point, E. R. Dodds, *Pagan and Christian in an Age of Anxiety* (1965; reprint, New York: Norton, 1970), especially 26–36.

57. E.g., Clement, *Stromateis* 3.7; Lactantius, *The Divine Institutes* 5:22; Ambrose, *Letters* 63:91.

58. Augustine *City of God* 14.3, trans. Henry Bettenson (London: Penguin, 1972), 550–52. See R. M. Miles, *Augustine on the Body* (Missoula, Mont.: Scholars, 1979).

59. Jerome, *Letters* 10.

60. Ibid., 39.2, in *NPNF*-2, 6:50.

61. Ibid., 38.2.

62. Ambrose, *Letters* 79.

63. Ambrose, *Concerning Repentance* 1.13.63.

64. Jerome, *Letters* 3.5.

65. Ibid., 39, in *NPNF*-2, 6:53. The cynical reader might suggest that Jerome condemned Paula's fasting and public grief from fear that her actions might draw attention to his own role in Blaesilla's death. Jerome appears, however, to be making a theologically categorical distinction between the asceticism of the daughter and the austerities of her mother.

66. Cyprian, *The Good of Patience* 10, in *FC* 36:273.

67. Ibid., 12–14, in *FC* 36:275–77.

68. Quoting Ecclus. 2:4–5.

69. Cyprian, *The Good of Patience* 17–18, in *FC* 36:279–81.

70. Ibid., 20, in *FC* 36:282–83.

71. Ibid., 24, in *FC* 36:287.

72. Cyprian, *Mortality* 8, in *FC* 36:204–5.

73. Ibid., 11, in *FC* 36:207, quoting Ps. 50:19.

74. Ibid., 12, in *FC* 36:208.

75. Ibid., 20, in *FC* 36:215.

76. Ibid., 26, in *FC* 36:220–21.

77. Tertullian, *Patience* 11.2–5, in *FC* 40:212.

78. Ibid., 14.2–6, in *FC* 40:218–19.

79. Tertullian, *Flight in Time of Persecution* 13.2, in *FC* 40:304.

80. Tertullian, *Apology* 23.3, in *FC* 10:71–72.

81. Clement, *Stromateis* 4.6, in *ANF* 2:414.

82. Ibid., 4.7, in *ANF* 2:418.

83. Ibid., 7.11, in *ANF* 2:540–41.

84. Ibid., 7.13, in *ANF* 2:547.

85. Ibid., 6.9, in *ANF* 2:497.

86. Ibid., 2.20, in *ANF* 2:374.

87. Ibid., 4.5, in *ANF* 2:412.

88. Fisher, *Beginnings* (n. 12), 175.

89. Justin Martyr, 2 *Apology* 4, in *FC* 6:123.

90. L. W. Barnard, *Justin Martyr: His Life and Thought* (Cambridge: Cambridge University Press, 1967), 154.

91. *Epistle to Diognetus*, in J. Quasten, *Patrology*, vol. 1, *The Beginnings of Patristic Literature* (1950; reprint, Westminster: Christian Classics, 1983), 251.

92. *Clementine Homilies* 12.14, in *ANF* 8:295.

93. Tertullian, *To the Martyrs* 4.9, in *FC* 40:24.

94. Ibid., 9, in *FC* 40:27–28.

95. Tertullian, *Apology* 46.14, in *FC* 10:113.

96. Ibid., 50.4–11, in *FC* 10:123–25.

97. Barnes, *Tertullian* (n. 42), 218–19.

98. Ibid., 227.

99. C. P. Williams, "Lactantius," in *The New International Dictionary of the Christian Church*, ed. J. D. Douglas, 2d ed. (Grand Rapids: Zondervan, 1974), 575.

100. P. de Labriolle, *History and Literature of Christianity from Tertullian to Boethius* (1924; reprint, New York: Barnes and Noble, 1968), 205.

101. Lactantius, *Divine Institutes* 3.18, in *ANF* 7:88–89.

102. Lactantius, *Epitome* 39, in *ANF* 7:237.

103. Eusebius, *Ecclesiastical History* 2.7.1, trans. K. Lake and J. Oulton (Cambridge: Harvard University Press, 1926–32), 1:125–27.

104. John Chrysostom, *Commentary on Galatians* 1.4, in *NPNF*-1, 13:5. The translation of Gal. 1:4 preceding the quotation is my own.

105. F. Homes Dudden, *The Life and Times of St. Ambrose* (Oxford: Clarendon, 1935), 502 ff.

106. Ambrose, *Death as a Good* 3.7, in *FC* 65:73–74.

107. Ambrose, *Concerning Virgins* 3.7.32, in *NPNF*-2, 10:386.

108. Jerome, *Letters* 39.3, in *NPNF*-2, 6:51.

109. Jerome, *Commentarius in Ionam prophetam* 1.6, in *Patrologia cursus completus, Series Latina*, ed. Jacques Paul Migne (Paris: J. P. Migne, 1844–65), 1.12:390–91, my translation.

110. Eusebius, *Ecclesiastical History* 8.12.2, vol. 2, p. 298, in the edition cited in n. 103.

111. Ambrose, *Concerning Virgins* 3.7.32.

112. Jerome, *Commentarius in Ionam prophetam* 1.6.

113. Chrysostom, in his *Homilia encomastica* on the most famous of these virgin suicides, Pelagia (who died about 313), enthusiastically approved her act. John Chrysostom, *Homilia encomastica*, in *Patrologia cursus completus, Series Graeco-Latina*, ed. Jacques Paul Migne (Paris: J. P. Migne, 1857–66), 49:579–84.

114. Eusebius, *Ecclesiastical History* 8.12.3–4.

115. Ibid., 8.14.14, vol. 2, p. 309, in the edition cited in n. 103.

116. Ibid., 8.14.17, vol. 2, p. 311, in the edition cited in n. 103.

117. Dudden, *Life and Times* (n. 105), 157.

118. Battin, *Ethical Issues* (n. 8), 71.

119. Augustine, *City of God* 15.1, p. 595 in the edition cited in n. 58.

120. Augustine, *Retractations* 2.69.

121. All subsequent quotations from the *City of God* in the present paper are my own translations.

122. The only examples of Christians committing suicide to avoid torture are those during the Great Persecution mentioned by Eusebius (*Ecclesiastical History* 8.12.2). Eusebius expresses neither approval nor disapproval. This type of suicide must have been very uncommon, since it attracted so little attention by the sources. It is likely that it was so rare that Augustine was unaware of specific examples. He was so thorough in his various discussions of suicide that it is most improbable that he would have missed such incidents if they were well known. And if he had been aware of them, it would be totally uncharacteristic of him to have shied away from wrestling with the possible problems posed by such cases. He will later address the subject when considering the Donatists, a schismatic, heretical sect.

123. For a thorough, scholarly treatment of the Donatist movement, see W.H.C. Frend, *The Donatist Church* (Oxford: Clarendon, 1952).

124. Augustine, *Letters* 153.18.

125. Possidius, *Vita Augustini* 12.

126. Augustine, *Contra litteras Petiliani* 2.19.43, in *NPNF*-1, 4:539–40.

127. Ibid., 2.85.186, in *NPNF*-1, 4:574.

128. Ibid., 2.20.46, in *NPNF*-1, 4:541.

129. Augustine, *Letters* 173.1, in *NPNF*-1, 1:544.

130. Ibid., 173.2, in *NPNF*-1, 1:544.

131. Ibid., 173.3–4, in *NPNF*-1, 1:545.

132. Ibid., 173.5, in *NPNF*-1, 1:545.

133. Augustine, *Letters* 185.2.9, in *NPNF*-1, 4:636.

134. Ibid., 185.3.12, in *NPNF*-1, 4:637–38.

135. Augustine, *Letters* 204, in *FC* 32:6.

136. Ibid.

137. Augustine, *Letters* 13.10, *FC* 16:246–48.

138. The earliest mention of suicide in Augustine's writings is in his *De libero arbitrio*, begun shortly after his conversion and published in three books between 388 and 395. For an analysis of Augustine's quite incidental comments on suicide there, see n. 46 in the original version of the present paper in *Suicide and Euthanasia: Historical and Contemporary Themes*, ed. Baruch A. Brody (Dordrecht: Kluwer Academic, 1989), 149–51.

139. The only hint that there might be even a minor problem can be read into the *City of God* 1.25, where Augustine says that he included the discussion of the question of suicide committed in order to avoid sinning, "for the sake of these men or women who think that they must do mortal violence to themselves in order to avoid, not another's sin, but a sin of their own." When he returns to the subject in 1.27, he concedes that "if any just cause were possible for suicide, I am sure that there could not be one more just than that." But we should not take this as anything more than an acknowledgment of the realities of the spiritual warfare that caused even Paul, in his yearning to be entirely free from sin, finally

to cry out, "Wretched man that I am! Who will deliver me from this body of death?" (Rom. 7:24). The scenario of the discouraged Christian, who, vitally concerned about his propensity to sin, asks his spiritual counselor why he can't just end the battle by going to heaven immediately, is more likely than one in which a person who wants to kill himself argues that this might be a justifiable cause.

This is not to say that there are no cases of newly converted Christians committing suicide with the intention of going directly to heaven. But the earliest examples that I have been able to locate come from the British Isles and survive in documents written centuries after Augustine's time. See J. J. O'Dea, *Suicide: Studies on its Philosophy, Causes, and Prevention* (New York: Putnam, 1882), 75–76.

FIVE

Medicine and Faith in
Early Christianity

The attitudes toward medicine and healing found in early Christianity are as varied and contrasting as those of classical pagan
society.[1] Some classical sources display a high regard for medicine as
administered by physicians, or for popular folk medicine. Others show a
fascination with medical theory, if not with medical practice, as an off-
shoot of philosophical speculation. Many thinkers saw medicine as part
of the natural order and, correlatively, accepted a natural causality of
disease and thus employed the services of physicians—if not always for
prophylaxis, at least for cure. Some of those who believed that diseases
had natural causes saw these only as proximate and the supernatural
as the ultimate cause, and therefore sought direct divine intervention.
Others, however, viewed illness as entirely supernatural in its causation,
not distinguishing between proximate and ultimate causality, and thus
also sought supernatural means of healing. Many of the educated, at
various times, were adherents of philosophical systems in which a body-
soul dichotomy was central, but still paid considerable attention to the
care of the body, while a small minority vilified the body, heaping abuse
upon it, and glorified disease.

   All of these attitudes are also seen in early Christianity, and many of
them are to be found even today, for they seem to be universal. Attitudes
that involve or recognize the supernatural as a causal agent and, even
peripherally, as a force in healing are, of course, present only among
those who have an active belief in the supernatural. While among pagans

and Christians the same range of attitudes toward medicine and healing existed, there was one essential difference between pagans and at least those Christians who had actively embraced the gospel. This vital difference not only impinged upon, but affected in the most fundamental way, all of these attitudes, making them, when held by Christians, inherently and qualitatively different from the corresponding attitudes held by pagans. This pervasive difference between pagans and Christians resulted from the highly personal relationship existing between the individual Christian and an omnipotent God who was typically viewed as having a direct concern with and involvement in the life of the believer. This is not to deny that there are some remarkable similarities between Christianity and certain pagan cults, especially the mystery religions with a Near Eastern origin. In some of these, devotion to a deity may have been quite pronounced, but even then it was, in the mind of the initiate, devotion to *a* deity, not to *the* Deity. It was henotheism, perhaps, but not monotheism; devotion to one god among many whose favor was sought, not devotion to the omnipotent God whose favor had already been gained through entering into a covenant relationship with him. The predominant undergirding principle in the relationship between a Christian and his God was that of a reciprocal love supporting a dependent trust by the Christian in his God. This cannot be said of any other religion in the ancient world, with the obvious exception of Judaism.

The importance of Judaism for the most basic Christian understanding of the nature of God and his relationship with his covenant—in this case, new covenant—people did not depend merely on the acceptance of the Old Testament by individual theologians, since the God of the New Testament is essentially the God of the Old in orthodox Christian thought. Regardless of the varied attitudes of early Christians toward Jews and Judaism, and irrespective of the contradictory opinions of church fathers concerning the applicability and importance of the Old Testament (including the Jewish apocryphal books) to the Christian and the place of Israel in the present and in the eschatological future, it is undeniable that the God of Judaism was viewed by orthodox Christians as the God of Christianity, and pre-Christian Judaism as a *praeparatio evangelica*. It was a praeparatio evangelica that was accepted by all the early orthodox Christian sources and, directly or indirectly, had a profound effect on the question of the relationship of medicine and faith, an effect that we shall consider later in this paper.

The Influence of Greek and Roman Philosophy

There was a second *praeparatio evangelica*, regarded as built upon the special revelation of the Old Testament and anticipatory of the special revelation of the New, and that was the secular learning to which many early Christian thinkers felt themselves to be the heirs, specifically those aspects of Greek philosophy held to be compatible with Christianity. It is reasonable to suppose that the attitudes of church fathers toward medical theory were affected, at least in part, by their relationship with the prevailing philosophical systems of which contemporary medical theory was an intricately involved but subsidiary part.

After its initial Jewish beginnings, the gospel took root in a syncretistic, gentile, and thoroughly pagan society made up of diverse cultures. The Greek tongue, in which the New Testament was written and in which the gospel was preached, was a unifying factor in the Mediterranean world of the early centuries of our era. Greek thought had penetrated the whole Roman Empire deeply, and evangelists made use of those ideas in pagan thought and tradition that were compatible with Judeo-Christian teaching.[2] To exploit the useful in secular learning was not to compromise the gospel but was simply cultural accommodation as well as "spoiling the Egyptians," an endeavor to which some second-century apologists devoted themselves with great enthusiasm. This was an especially congenial task for some apologists, given the philosophical climate of that time. Of the four major philosophical schools,[3] Stoicism and Middle Platonism (as influenced by Stoicism) were oriented to religious questions,[4] as part of a general movement of the educated classes toward monotheism or a belief in a doctrine of providence.[5] By the second century A.D. the "idea of a philosopher as a man interested in God was taken for granted."[6] This was also a time marked by philosophical eclecticism. Seneca's famous comment "Whatever has been well said by anyone is mine" was quoted with approbation by both Justin Martyr and Clement of Alexandria.[7] Christian apologists took "great pains to argue that the revelation was in harmony with philosophy at its best because philosophers had in part been inspired by the Logos."[8] As Stanley Jaki writes, "Christian belief in a personal, rational Creator pictured Him as being the weight, measure, and number of the universe. . . . Such a firm conviction could only rejoice at the presence of genuine fragments of truth in antique learning."[9] Jaki is speaking of Clement of

Alexandria. But Clement was by no means the first of the church fathers to have had such an attitude.

Justin Martyr (died ca. 165) had apparently been a Platonist but discovered in Christianity what he had failed to find in Greek philosophy. When he was converted, there was no need for him to take off the mantle of the Greek philosopher because he believed that Christianity was the absolute philosophy, the only philosophy that was "safe and profitable."[10] Robert Grant writes, "What Justin had done when he moved from philosophy to Christianity was to discover a new religious sanction for his inherited and acquired culture."[11] This overstates the position a little. Justin could indeed look back on his philosophical quest as a personal *praeparatio evangelica*. But he was a *converted* man who saw in Greek philosophy much that appeared quite incompatible with scriptural teaching. He also saw in it much that reinforced scriptural revelation. It is one thing to accept certain pagan philosophical premises as consonant with and anticipatory of the gospel. It is quite another simply to use the language of Greek philosophy in one's apologetics. All the extant apologists of the second century, intentionally or not, did the latter. Justin did both. But it was in Alexandria that the first systematic attempt was made to elaborate Christian dogma by employing the methods of Greek philosophy. And it was Clement who was "the first to take proper cognisance of what this use involves."[12]

In Clement (ca. 150–ca. 220) and Origen (ca. 184–ca. 253), the great Alexandrian fathers, "the Christian faith and Greek philosophical tradition became embodied in one and the same individual. . . . [thus producing] a highly complex synthesis of Greek and Christian thought."[13] This synthesis, however, was by no means a wholesale adoption of Greek philosophy, but a borrowing of what appeared to the synthesizer to be compatible with scriptural truth as he perceived it. Both Clement and Origen were motivated by a firm conviction that a faith corroborated by philosophical reasoning was preferable to a simple faith. This opinion, of course, was not shared by all. Even those who agreed with it varied in determining how far one might safely go in such an endeavor. Origen attempted to do with the Bible what earlier Alexandrian scholars had done with Homer. He saw in Scripture a literal meaning and a spiritual sense that was either allegorical or typological. Combining his theology, which was strongly tempered by Greek philosophy, with a minute philological scrutiny of many of the books of the Bible, he produced monuments of allegorical hermeneutics built upon a tradition in Alexandria going back as far as Philo, which brought Greek philosophy into the service of scriptural explication. In addition, Origen was fascinated with the Greek doctrine of cosmic cycles and flirted with metempsychosis. While he ultimately rejected the latter, he adapted the former to his Christian cosmology, with dangerous implications, in the opinion of many in subsequent generations. Origen was the most influential and distinguished of all the theologians of the early church, with the possible exception of Augustine. He was also probably the most prolific author in the ancient church, truly the philosopher's theologian and the theologian's philosopher. Origen's methods and conclusions had a lasting effect, particularly on the Cappadocian fathers, Basil (ca. 329–79), Gregory Nazianzen (ca. 330–ca. 390), and Gregory of Nyssa (ca. 335–94).

The Cappadocian fathers were great admirers and avid readers of Origen. Basil and Gregory Nazianzen collaborated in compiling the famous anthology of Origen's writings, the *Philocalia.* They were trained in philosophy, although much more in classical Greek philosophy (as part of a liberal education) than in the Neoplatonism of their own day. It is unlikely that they even recognized the extent to which their Christian heritage had by then been tempered by classical ideas, the philosophical tradition having been so naturalized into, and made nearly inseparable from, Christianity. While they often spoke of individual pagan philosophers and philosophical schools with contempt or ridicule, they evinced a profound respect for everything in Greek learning that was close to or compatible with their Christianity, which was expressed in highly philosophical terms.

John Chrysostom (ca. 349–407), a younger contemporary of the Cappadocian fathers, received his secular education under the famous sophist Libanius, who nurtured in him a love for classical culture. He studied theology under Diodorus, bishop of Tarsus, from whom he imbibed Antiochine hermeneutics, which explicated Scripture through grammatical analysis. While never hostile to Origen, Chrysostom rejected his and the Alexandrian school's allegorical interpretations. Best known for his eloquent and fervent preaching, he was the least philosophical of the fathers considered thus far, although thoroughly steeped in classical learning.

The Latin West also had Augustine (354–430), an intellectual giant who had been deeply influenced by Neoplatonism before his conversion. At nineteen he had read Cicero's *Hortensius,* and it had inspired him to study philosophy.[14] His pursuit of philosophy gave him no more satisfaction than had Justin's; nor did his detour into Manicheism. For Augustine, as for Justin, the study of pagan philosophy, particularly Neoplatonism (which he regarded as closer to Christianity than any of the other pagan philosophies),[15] was something that helped to bring him to Christianity. And Christianity was true philosophy. But Augustine's thinking had been significantly influenced by his immersion in Neoplatonism. Peter Brown writes that "Plotinus and Porphyry are grafted almost imperceptibly into his writings as the ever present basis of his thought."[16] His epistemology allowed no dichotomy between his faith and his reason, although he held firmly to the conviction that, after conversion, the latter depended upon the former. To quote Brown again: "He felt himself intimately bound to the vast prestige of the Christian scholarship of the Greek world, above all to the great Origen of Alexandria . . . [and] to a firm belief that a mind trained on philosophical methods could think creatively within the traditional orthodoxy of the church."[17]

Augustine's erstwhile mentor, Ambrose of Milan (ca. 339–97), was also influenced by Neoplatonism. Scholars have long remarked on "how deeply imbued with Platonism Ambrose was."[18] He drew upon the pagan philosophers extensively in his sermons, in which one can find literal borrowings from Plotinus. Ambrose's major modern biographer writes that he endeavored to combine much of Stoicism with Christianity.[19] While pagan philosophy permeated Ambrose's writings, providing him with convenient literary flourishes and oratorical thrusts, it did not permeate his thought, his epistemology, or his theology. With some qualifying cautions, the reverse may be maintained for Augustine. In this matter, Augustine was much closer to the spirit of both the Alexandrian and the Cappadocian fathers than was Ambrose or the latter's contemporary, Jerome. Jerome (ca. 345–ca. 419) had studied in Rome, where his education had included law and philosophy. Although he had little or no firsthand intimacy with the Greek classics, his love for the pagan Latin luminaries is well known. He was a scholar with a scholar's tastes, one of the most cultured and learned of the fathers, who had drunk deeply from the well of his pagan heritage.

Attitudes of Christians toward Health, Illness, Suffering, and Medicine

What might such church fathers, who were ostensibly sympathetic to much in their classical heritage, have found in pagan tradition—particularly in pagan philosophy—that had a bearing on their attitudes toward medicine in the broadest sense? In the first place, they inherited and exploited to the fullest the positive metaphorical value of the idea of the physician as one who unselfishly succors the ill, enduring unpleasant tasks in caring for the unhealthy, often administering necessarily painful means for effecting a cure, or helping people maintain health through regimen. Ludwig Edelstein suggests that the greatest debt that ancient philosophy had to medicine was the use of medical analogies, giving "a prominent place to the analogy of body and soul, to the similarity between the training of the body and the discipline of the soul, to the consideration of medicine as a counterpart of ethics."[20] Just as pagan philosophers delighted in medical analogies drawn from the physician-patient relationship, calling themselves "physicians of the soul," so also did church fathers. They saw their spiritual office as that of *medici animarum,* following the example of the ultimate *medicus,* Christ, who is described as the Great Physician, the *verus medicus, solus medicus, verus archiater, ipse et medicus et medicamentum*—himself both the physician and the medication. Much has been written by modern scholars on the use of such physician-patient analogies by church fathers. Included in these discussions is usually a treatment of their use of medical analogies in which medical theory, particularly rudimentary anatomy and physiology, theories of natural causality, and descriptions of specific medical or surgical techniques that were employed in the treatment of particular medical problems provide homiletically rich comparisons.[21] Some modern scholarship dealing with this was at least partially motivated by a desire to disprove assertions (which were common especially in the nineteenth and early twentieth centuries) that the church fathers were virulently hostile to science as well as ignorant of it.

In pagan philosophy there were, however, some very substantial areas that Christian thinkers had to reject. Greek philosophy had been traditionally concerned with cosmology and cosmogony. The foundational principle of Christian cosmogony and cosmology was, "In the beginning God created the heavens and the earth." Christian cosmogony was creation, and Christian cosmology was predicated upon a belief in a Creator who transcended but was very involved in his creation. Religion was, in Greek philosophy, only an ennobled form of naturalism, and for all intents, nature was the supreme being, distinct from which nothing was able to exist. Even the gods, or whatever there is that transcends man, are subordinate to nature, are limited by it, and thus must work within it.

Man is the product of nature, and is not created by anything or anyone who transcends nature. In contrast, for the Christian, man's understanding of his place in the world depended on his "grasp of his own and of the material world's fundamental contingency, as everything rested on a sovereign, creative act of God."[22]

At the end of each of the six days of creation the Genesis account says, "And God saw that it was good." That the material world was not rendered essentially evil by the Fall is demonstrated by the Incarnation. Herbert Butterfield observes, "It has always been realised in the main tradition of Christianity that if the Word was made flesh, matter can never be regarded as evil in itself."[23] Individuals or groups (e.g., Gnostics, Manicheans, Marcionites) on the periphery of Christianity who conceived of matter as inherently evil also balked at the doctrine of the Incarnation. In early Christianity a less radical dualism appeared frequently that did not classify matter as inherently evil but strained the bounds of orthodoxy by exaggerating the Pauline σάρξ-πνεῦμα dichotomy into a severe asceticism. A moderate dualism was central to Platonism too, which, like Cynicism, fostered a rigid asceticism, particularly during the early centuries of our era. Radical dualism, as it appeared in classical culture, whether identified with Christianity or not, was based on a variety of premises, assumed various forms, and had both Greek and Near Eastern (particularly Persian) roots. Some Greek philosophical schools such as Stoicism, Platonism, and Pythagoreanism, however, which held to a doctrine of eternal returns or endless recurring cycles, also held to a principle of the "conservation of evil in nature," which stated that throughout eternity the total quantity of matter was to remain the same. Orthodox sources from the early church which addressed the philosophical doctrine of eternal returns or endless recurring cycles and the principle of the "conservation of evil in nature" categorically and unequivocally rejected both. Even Origen, who received such censure for his doctrine of goal-directed cosmic cycles guided by the omnipotent and benevolent Creator, rejected the idea that matter was evil and stressed the inherent goodness of matter as it existed and was regulated by God's laws.[24]

Generally, the educated pagan of the early Christian centuries, unless he had adopted a rigid and severe asceticism based on a radical dualism, did not excessively vilify the body. Although he might possibly disparage his material side as worth little in comparison with his spiritual, he sought healing when ill. Most typically he would regard his illness as due to natural causes and would seek the help of a physician. There were also healing cults available, especially that of Asclepius, which attracted the sick either by offering an alternative or a complement to strictly human medical care, or by providing a last resort when such care had failed. The various attitudes toward medicine described in the opening paragraph of the present paper would have governed, or at least affected, the choice of action a pagan took when ill. How then, did the cultivated church fathers, steeped in classical culture, view the role of medicine?

A fundamental principle that was shared, if not always specifically articulated, by all the fathers mentioned above is that the material world was created by God for man's use. Justin, whose cosmology is biblically based and nonspeculative, believed simply that God, in his goodness, created all things in the material world for man's sake,[25] that is, that the purpose of creation was the benefit of the human race,[26] and that all earthly things were made subject to man.[27] Clement held that, within God's created order, understanding is from God, and many things in life arise from the exercise of human reason, although its kindling spark comes from God. Health obtained through medicine is one of these things that has its origin and existence as a consequence of divine Providence as well as human cooperation.[28] Consistently enough, Clement elsewhere writes that the art of healing, which he describes as the relief of the ills of the body, is an art learned by man's wisdom.[29] Origen, in a homily on Numbers, quotes Ecclesiasticus 19:19—"All wisdom is from God"—and a little later asks, if all knowledge is from God, what knowledge could have a greater claim to such an origin than medicine, the knowledge of health?[30] Just as God causes herbs to grow, so also did he give medical knowledge to men.[31] God did this in his kindness, knowing the frailty of our bodies and not wishing for us to be without succor when illness strikes.[32] Thus Origen can call medicine "beneficial and essential to mankind."[33] Basil also regarded all the arts as God's gift, given to remedy nature's deficiencies. Accordingly, the medical art was given to relieve the sick, "in some degree at least."[34] Gregory of Nyssa records that, when his sister was ill, their mother had begged her to let a physician treat her, arguing that God gave the art of medicine to men for their preservation.[35] John Chrysostom also writes that God gave us physicians and medicine,[36] and Augustine attributes the healing properties of medicine to God.[37]

If God is acknowledged as the source of both healing substances and the knowledge of how to apply them, and if he gave them to men to succor their ills, then it might well be maintained that health is itself a good. Augustine regarded health as a blessing from God,[38] a God-given good to be sought for its own sake, like wisdom and friendship.[39] But health, although a desirable thing, was a relative good and could at times be an evil, depending on its role in the life of the healthy man. Jerome, for instance, in writing to a remarkably healthy centenarian, asserts that while the health of the unrighteous is a gift of the devil to lead them to sin, the health of the righteous is a gift of God to make them rejoice.[40] Accordingly, Jerome can urge another correspondent not only to rejoice in health but also to rejoice in sickness.[41]

It is here that we enter into a major paradox of Christianity, one that is frequently misunderstood and that makes the Christian attitude to both health and illness, as evidenced in the majority of early Christian sources, significantly different from that of the pagan. Some Greeks and Romans regarded suffering as having value, in that it might contribute to the sufferer's growth, maturity, and sense of values. Among the pagans, a few severe ascetics sought suffering for its supposed expiatory, propitiatory, or purificatory ends. Some Christians also sought suffering, particularly the suffering involved in persecution leading to martyrdom. A few rigidly ascetic Christians inflicted suffering on themselves for reasons similar to those of their pagan counterparts, a phenomenon that, in its extreme and bizarre forms, was by no means approved of by the fathers whose works we are now considering, even though most of these fathers had been ascetics for part or most of their lives.

The attitudes of the fathers under consideration toward suffering, particularly the suffering associated with illness, are a curious mixture of popular Stoicism, with which it was possible to agree or disagree without reference to Christianity; and spiritual explanations derived from or built upon biblical teaching. Clement expresses admiration for the Stoics who say that the soul is not influenced by the body, either to vice by disease or to virtue by health. He then discusses the debilitating and distracting force of pain and observes that one who is suffering from disease will be distraught unless he has achieved the habit of self-command and is "high-souled."[42] Such observations would be acceptable to many pagans. Later he comes closer to Christian principles when he asserts that pain, disease, and other such trials often are sent for admonition, for correction of the past, and to make one mindful of the future. Since the Gnostic (i.e., the true and instructed Christian) has the advantage of his knowledge *(gnosis)*, he prays for relief from them.[43] Origen, in his reply to Celsus, says that Christians endure the appointed evils, that is, troubles that occur among men, as trials of the soul; for by them their souls are tested, either being convicted of failure or being shown to be reliable. So prepared are Christians for evils that they say, "Prove me, O Lord, and try me; test my kidneys and my heart by fire" (Ps. 26:2; 25:2 LXX).[44]

Basil, as we saw above, writes that medicine was given by God to succor us.[45] That, however, was in his opinion the secondary reason, the primary being to provide a model, a parallel, or an example of the cure of the soul. One of the reasons that Christians are permitted to fall ill is so that, through the suffering involved in the disease and in the cure, they may draw valuable instruction to apply to the cure of the soul in need of spiritual medicine, cautery, or surgery. While God will not allow the Christian to be tried more than he can bear, some are left to struggle against their afflictions, and are rendered more worthy of reward because of these trials. Illness often is a punishment for sin that is imposed for repentance. Sometimes it is to keep the Christian from pride. Thus, when suffering calamity at God's hand the Christian is admonished to ask two things of God: first, understanding of the reason he has inflicted these blows; and second, deliverance from these pains, or the capacity to endure them patiently.

Gregory Nazianen, in a way that would have given no offense to the pagan, stresses the power of the mind to rise above physical ills, maintaining that illness should be used to strengthen one's character by the practice of patience,[46] and he laconically remarks that a lingering illness from which he suffered was for his own benefit.[47] When his father became seriously ill and expressed surprise that God would allow him to suffer from sickness and bodily pain, Gregory replied that it was not at all remarkable, since even the great saints of the past were afflicted with suffering. He gave three reasons why they were permitted to suffer: (1) for the cleansing of their clay (i.e., earthen vessels, bodies); (2) as a touchstone of virtue and a test of philosophy; and (3) for the education of the weaker who learn from the example of the stronger.[48] John Chrysostom, in a sermon on 1 Timothy 5:23,[49] addresses the same question, broadening it, in some instances, to include Christians in general. He gives twelve explanations for suffering: (1) so that Christians may not too easily be exalted into presumption by the greatness of their good works and miracles; (2) so that others may not have a greater opinion of them than is appropriate for mere men; (3) so that the power of God may be made obvious in advancing the word preached through the efficacy of men who are infirm; (4) so that their endurance may be a more striking evidence that they are serving God not for a present reward; (5) to demonstrate their belief in a resurrection and an eternal life; (6) so that others who suffer will find consolation in their example; (7) so that when exhorted to imitate them, others will be aware that they possessed a similar nature; (8) so that Christians may learn whom they ought to consider as happy and whom wretched, for "Whom the Lord loves He chastens, and scourges every son whom He receives" (Heb. 12:6); (9) because tribulation makes those who are troubled more approved, for "tribulation produces patience" (Rom. 5:3); (10) so that if Christians have any blemishes, they may put them away; (11) because the Christians' crowns and rewards are thus increased; and (12) because, if Christians give thanks to God in the midst of their suffering, they deliver a blow to the devil.[50]

Elsewhere Chrysostom stresses that when Christians give thanks in circumstances under which others curse and complain, they see "how great a philosophy is here."[51] This "philosophy" is then far superior to the philosophies of the pagans because the Christian can rejoice and give thanks in suffering, for God would not permit Christians to suffer were it not for their good.[52] God alone knows what is good for his children; thus they should bear all things, whether poverty or disease.[53] If Christians were always healthy, they would grow self-confident; God allows affliction to remind Christians of the weakness of their nature.[54] Sometimes God punishes his children's bodies to bring their spiritual needs to their attention.[55] A good example of this is Hezekiah, who grew proud when he had received many blessings. When he fell sick, he was humbled and drew near to God.[56]

Jerome writes, "Am I in good health? I thank my Creator. Am I sick? In this case also I praise God's will. For 'When I am weak, then am I strong,' and the strength of the spirit is made perfect in the weakness of the flesh."[57] He describes the lady Paula as having the same attitude. In her frequent sicknesses she also used to say, "When I am weak, then am I strong."[58] Sicknesses, according to Jerome, can cause a man to adjust his priorities. He describes a young lady who had suffered from a burning fever for nearly thirty days. This fever, he maintains, had been sent to teach her to renounce her excessive attention to her body and to draw her to more serious pursuits.[59] In a somewhat similar vein, Ambrose writes that while luxury ignites the sins of the flesh, sickness of the body restrains one from sin.[60] He tells a correspondent that God had sent the latter's recent sickness for his health and admonition, bringing him more pain than peril, and finally healing him with faith.[61]

We have seen above that Augustine regarded health as a good to be sought, but he reminds his readers that although God has not promised Christians health he has promised eternal life, a heaven where there will be no fear and trouble.[62] When Christians suffer affliction, because it is hard and painful and against natural inclinations, they pray for its removal. But since they do not know why God permits the particular tribulation, they do not know for what they should pray. Augustine says that God allows Christians to endure physical ills because such ills heal the swelling of pride, test and prove patience, and punish and eradicate sins.[63] Further, infirmities remind Christians of their mortality and cause them to rely on God.[64] In one letter Augustine brings this to a personal level. He says that he is confined to bed, and can neither walk, stand, nor sit because of the pain and swelling of a boil or tumor. "Even so, since it pleases the Lord, what else is to be said but that I am well?" He then asks for prayer that he may have self-control and patience and that the Lord would be so present with him that he would fear no evil.[65]

We have seen that the fathers whom we have considered thus far regarded the created world as good insofar as it is the product of God's benevolent plan and his beneficent provision for man's sustenance. Medicine is part of that plan and provision, given by God to help to succor man's ills in this fallen world. Yet suffering, which includes that caused by illness and infirmity, is good in that it is used by God in the lives of his children, just as he ultimately uses all things, for their spiritual good. In view of these fathers' belief that manifold spiritually edificatory benefits of physical suffering accrue to the sufferer who is receptive to God's instruction, what, in their opinion, is the proper perspective for Christians to have on secular medicine?

Origen discusses God's condemnation of the Jewish king Asa, who, when he was ill, "did not seek the Lord but the physicians" (2 Chron. 16:12). He sees two possible explanations. Either Asa called on physicians who used charms and trickery, or he had faith in the physicians alone and did not place his hope in God. "For those who are adorned with religion use physicians as servants of God, knowing that He Himself gave medical knowledge to men, just as He Himself assigned both herbs and other things to grow on the earth. They also know that the physician's art has no strength if God is not willing, but it is able to do as much as God wills."[66] Both explanations of God's reaction to Asa's reliance upon physicians are pertinent to Christians. The fathers all stressed the diabolical nature of magic and, as we shall see more fully, the importance of recognizing the role of the physician as subordinate to the place of God in the healing of Christians.

Were all Christians to use medical means for the healing of their bodies? To this question Origen gives an answer that distinguishes between two classes of Christians. A little earlier in his text he had said, "God has allowed us to marry wives, because not everybody is capable of the superior condition which is to be absolutely pure."[67] When discussing the Christian's use of medicine he writes, "A man ought to use medical means to heal his body if he aims to live in the simple and ordinary way. If he wishes to live in a way superior to that of the multitude, he should do this by devotion to the supreme God and by praying to Him."[68] This attitude, that the more spiritual or devout Christians should refrain from the use of medicine and rely strictly upon God for healing, is an opinion not held, or at least not expressed, by many church fathers. It is, however, a stand taken by numerous Christians of different theological persuasions throughout the history of Christianity. It does not indicate dualism and should never be used as a criterion for determining whether a Christian was orthodox or heretical.

In his *Long Rules,* Basil dealt with the question of "whether recourse to the medical art is in keeping with the practice of piety." He writes,

We must take great care to employ this medical art, if it should be necessary, not as making it wholly accountable for our state of health or illness, but as redounding to the glory of God. . . . In the event that medicine should fail to help, we should not place all hope for the relief of our distress in this art. . . . To place the hope of one's health in the hands of the doctor is the act of an irrational animal. This, nevertheless, is what we observe in the case of certain unhappy persons who do not hesitate to call doctors their saviors. Yet, to reject entirely the benefits to be derived from this art is the sign of pettish nature. . . . We should neither repudiate this art altogether nor does it behoove us to repose all our confidence in it. . . . When reason allows, we call in the doctor, but we do not leave off hoping in God.[69]

Under what circumstances would "reason allow" one to use the medical art? Basil writes that there is great danger of falling "into the error of thinking that every kind of suffering requires medical relief. Not all sicknesses for whose treatment we observe medicine to be occasionally beneficial arise from natural causes, whether from faulty diet or from any other physical origin." Those who are ill because of living improperly should make use of the medical art. But there are other causes of illness. It is often a punishment for sin; sometimes it is at Satan's request (e.g., the suffering of Job); at other times an illness that even leads to death is inflicted on one (e.g., Lazarus) who can bear it as a model of patience; and sometimes it is imposed on a great man of God so that he will be seen to be of the same nature as the rest of mankind. Of these Basil exclaims, "What profit would there be for such men in having recourse to medicine? Would there not rather be danger that in their solicitude for the body they would be led astray from right reason?"

How does Basil's position, thus far expressed, compare with Origen's division between Christians of the common sort, who resort to medicine, and those of a superior order, who rely entirely upon God? In the first place, we must be aware that Basil's *Long Rules* was written as a standard for monks and, as Eric Osborn observes, Basil did not allow for a double standard for monk and layman; instead "there was a single standard but only the monk could achieve it."[70] Thus, for all practical purposes, the standards expressed in *The Long Rules* are those for "superior Christians," and for them medicine is of significantly less importance than reliance upon God for healing, and is, after all, to be used only in one of the five cases described.

Basil, in the same work, stresses that when a man employs the medical art and a cure is obtained, he should receive it with thanksgiving. He mentions the case of Hezekiah and the poultice of figs prepared by Isaiah and applied to the boil (carbuncle) from which he suffered. Hezekiah "did not regard the lump of figs as a primary cause of his regaining his health . . . but gave glory to God and added thanksgiving for the creation of the figs."[71] Medicines and physicians' skill are both from God. This is a common theme in the literature surveyed. In Augustine's mind it is by no means inconsistent for a Christian to go to a physician, and indeed a sick man acts wisely in availing himself of a physician's skill.[72] In his regulations for his sister's convent he stipulates that physicians should be consulted in times of illness and their orders obeyed.[73] He writes that regardless of who assists in the restoration of health, the cure ultimately comes from God,[74] for medicines have no power unless God supplies it; yet God can cure without medicines.[75] Hence, when the Christian is scourged in the body, he should pray to God for relief.[76] Likewise, Jerome urges medical care for sick monks,[77] but he maintains that physicians labor in vain without the aid of the

Lord.[78] Ambrose also advises that physicians should be sent for in time of sickness,[79] but castigates those who, when ill, call the physician and, only if his efforts fail, pray to God for healing.[80]

When John Chrysostom was exiled and moved from place to place under the most adverse circumstances, which culminated ultimately in his death, he lamented in a letter to the lady Olympias that he was deprived of the services of physicians, which he sorely needed. Olympias was sick herself, and John beseeched her "to employ various and skilled physicians and to take medicines that are effective in correcting these conditions." He lauds patience under suffering and then says that no suffering experienced in life is worse than bodily infirmities—not loss of goods, loss of honors, exile, imprisonment, bondage, abuse, scoffings, the loss of one's children, not even death itself. He cites the case of Job, who only when he was delivered over to sickness and sores longed for death.[81] In discussing 1 Corinthians 6:20—"glorify God in your body"— he writes that he glorifies God in the body, which, among other things, makes such provision for itself as is sufficient for health.[82] In explicating Romans 13:14—"make no provision for the flesh in regard to its lusts"— he says that we owe the body many things, food, warmth, rest, medicine when ill, clothing, and a thousand other things. But he cautions us not to make it the mistress of our life.[83]

This was a theme dear to some pagan thinkers as well: do not have such concern with your body that you are distracted from the pursuit of virtue. Balance and right priorities: these were values lauded especially by Clement of Alexandria, of whom Eric Osborn says, "During the first five centuries Christian theology never became more Greek, never merged more fully with classical philosophy than it did in Clement."[84] Clement writes that those who die of disease depart in a state of weakness while they still desire to live. Hence their souls are impure and bear their lusts like weights of lead, except for those who have been conspicuous in virtue.[85] The latter are, of course, those who have a Stoical endurance under suffering and do not cling to life desperately. Basil, in his discussion of medicine in *The Long Rules,* urges that "whatever requires an undue amount of thought or trouble or involves a large expenditure of effort and causes our whole life to resolve, as it were, around solicitude for the flesh must be avoided by Christians."[86] While Clement addresses an élite circle of Christians possessed of sophisticated, philosophical *gnosis,* and Basil speaks to his monastic community, John Chrysostom exhorts Christian society at large. Preaching about a mother who had refused to resort to magical means urged upon her by ostensibly Christian friends for the cure of her critically ill child, John commends her and bemoans to his audience how little concerned Christians are with heaven, although they will undergo anything for the sake of this life. "Be ready for death," he urged his audience, and asks, "Why do you cling to the present life? Why do you not look to the future?"[87]

Augustine contrasts the "ultimate bliss" of heaven with the evils of this world,[88] and points out that even if health is restored to one who is ill, his death is only delayed.[89] He notes the irony that so many when faced with troubles cry out, "O God, send me death; hasten my days!" But when sickness comes, they rush to the physician, promising him money and rewards.[90] He laments what men will do just to live a few more days. If they fall ill and all the physicians who examine them despair of their life, and then if some physician capable of curing them frees them from their desperate state, how much do they promise him? They will give up the sustenance of life just to live a little longer.[91]

What, then, is the essence of the attitudes of these fathers to the use of medicine? Medicines and the skill of physicians are blessings from God. It is not *eo ipso* wrong for a Christian to employ them, but it is sinful to put one's faith in them entirely since, when they are effective, it is only because their efficacy comes from God, who can heal without them. Hence, to resort to physicians without first placing one's trust in God is both foolish and sinful. Likewise, to reject medicine and the medical art entirely not only is not recommended but is disparaged. Origen may seem an exception to this position, but he is not. He does acknowledge the appropriateness of the medical art for Christians generally, but suggests that those of a superior spiritual nature should seek healing through devotion and prayer alone, without recourse to medicine. For his monks Basil recommends the use of medicine only when the cause of the illness is obviously natural; otherwise, if the infirmity is thought to have been allowed or sent by God for an edificatory end, medicines and physicians are to be avoided. The other fathers do not, so far as I have been able to determine, place any similar restrictions on the use of medicine. All agree that suffering, even from disease, when it afflicts the Christian, is sent or permitted for his ultimate good by a God who loves him and will cause all things to work together for his good. Since one's spiritual welfare is infinitely more important than one's bodily state, and since the Christian is but a pilgrim in this world, an alien with heaven as his home, an undue concern for the body—to the point where one's mind revolves around its needs—and a desperate clinging to life are a tragic contradiction of Christian values.

The fathers surveyed thus far were chosen because they all acknowledged their debt to, or were obviously in various respects deeply influenced by and dependent upon, their classical heritage and did not express a strong antipathy or hostility to it. The effect of their classical leanings and learning on their attitudes toward medicine seems to have been limited to the productive use of analogies drawn from the physician-patient relationship and from medical theories and practices. Their attitudes toward the use of medicines and physicians by Christians, however, are thoroughly tempered by spiritual principles for the most part quite foreign to pagan sympathies, but explicitly congenial to those of late pre-Christian Judaism.

Jewish Antecedents

In the Old Testament, God is the physician of his people,[92] and they are not to have recourse to magic[93] or to pagan healing means.[94] The use of natural means of healing, however, is not precluded, and these are employed even in ostensibly miraculous healings.[95] But medical knowledge was probably limited to folk remedies.[96] By the second century B.C., Jewish medical practitioners seem to have been common both in Palestine and abroad, and they appear to have adopted Greek rational-speculative medicine insofar as it was not antithetical to Jewish religious principles. The apocryphal book known variously as Ecclesiasticus or the Wisdom of Jesus ben Sira, written in Hebrew in Jerusalem during the early second century B.C. and translated into Greek in Alexandria by ben Sira's grandson roughly a half century later, contains much information on the Judaism of Palestine at that time. Ben Sira lauds health and urges his readers to take care of their own (18:19). He acknowledges that God grants healing, life, and blessing (34:17). In chapter 38:1–15 there is a discussion of the role of physicians.[97] The passage opens with a command to "honor the physician with the honor due him, according to your need of him, for the Lord created him" (38:1). Ben Sira's argument proceeds along these lines: Healing comes from God, and the physician's art is admirable. God created medicines from the earth; thus "a sensible man will not despise them." God is glorified through the skill he gave to men to compound medicines (38:2–8). At this point ben Sira's emphasis changes: "My son, if you are sick do not be negligent, but pray to the Lord, and He will heal you. Give up your faults and direct your hands aright, and cleanse your heart from all sin. Bring a sweet-smelling offering." However, "give the physician his place, for the Lord created him. . . . There may be a time when your recovery lies in the hands of physicians, for they too will pray to the Lord to give them success in diagnosis and healing to save their patient's life" (38:9–14).[98]

The position of the church fathers whom we have considered thus far is essentially compatible with that of ben Sira. There is, however, no evidence of a direct dependence.[99] Such a dependence would only have been literary, since the similarity of thought goes much deeper; indeed, it feeds upon the very roots of a religious tradition in which a covenant relationship based upon love, trust, and the dependence of man upon his omnipotent Creator was central. It is this special quality of Judaism and Christianity that is little affected by classical thought in general or pagan philosophy in particular. There was probably no Jew more Hellenized than Philo, who lived in Alexandria in the first century A.D. He writes that God gives medicines and the medical art through himself alone but can heal without them. And Philo criticizes those who resort to the physician and turn to God only after medical care has failed.[100] Such sentiments are consonant with those of ben Sira. They are also harmonious with the attitudes of the church fathers we have discussed, men who had drunk deeply from the wells of classical culture. But they are remote from attitudes typical of the church fathers' classical heritage.

The Attitudes of Some Christian "Extremists" toward Medicine

But what of those patristic sources that rejected classical culture? Tertullian (ca. 160–after 220) is one of the best known and most influential in this category. "Quid Athenae Hierosolymis?" he exclaimed; "What concord is there between the Academy and the Church?"[101] He goes on to say that the Gnostics derived their idea of the eons from the Platonists, the Stoics supplied the Marcionites with their deity, Zeno identified God with matter, Heraclitus identified him with fire, Epicurus taught the annihilation of the soul, and all of them denied the possibility of resurrection.[102] Philosophical speculation spawns heresy; so Tertullian emphatically insisted that there must be an absolute breach between "science" and "faith." "For him the breach was absolute, and it involved an irreconcilable opposition between the claims of Christ and those of the world."[103] Faith, in his opinion, was superior to reason because of its suprarational characteristics.[104] Although his rejection of philosophy was vitriolic and unequivocal, and probably absolutely sincere, his knowledge of it was extensive, since he needed to know it thoroughly to be able to refute heretics on what he considered to be their own ground. It was inevitable, though, that he was deeply influenced by it. Timothy Barnes writes that "Tertullian would have deplored the attempts of Justin, Clement and Origen to reconcile Christianity and pagan philosophy. He explicitly rejected a Stoic, Platonic or dialectical Christianity. But in a wider sense, he had himself reconciled Christianity and classical culture. For he used the benefits of a traditional education and the fruits of his pagan erudition to defend and to propagate what he considered to be the truth."[105]

Tertullian, probably motivated simply by interest or curiosity, had studied medicine.[106] He too was fond of using physician-patient and medical analogies in his writings, as were classical philosophers and many other church fathers. He refers to medicine as "the sister of philosophy."[107] Although philosophers "indulge a stupid curiosity on natural objects, which they ought rather intelligently to direct to their Creator and Governor,"[108] the Christian knows that medicines and the medical art were given by God. "Let Aesculapius have been the first who sought and discovered cures. Isaiah mentions that he ordered Hezekiah medicine when he was sick. Paul, too, knows that a little wine does the stomach good."[109] Thus medicine is appropriate for the Christian. Tertullian saw in suffering a warning for Christians,[110] and held that pride was checked in the apostle Paul by earaches or headaches.[111] His position on the use of suffering in the Christian's life and the suitability of the uses of the medical art for Christians appears quite consistent with the views of the other fathers surveyed.[112] His becoming a Montanist, a member of a group declared heretical that was similar in some respects to modern evangelical charismatics, seems not to have affected his attitude toward medicine except to reinforce the absolute necessity of recognizing God's hand in the healing process.

The Syrian Tatian (ca. 120–?), who was a student of Justin Martyr, is sometimes compared with Tertullian. After Justin's death, Tatian broke with the Roman church and returned to Syria, where he founded his own school. He rejected all pagan culture with vehement contempt, sarcasm, and bitterness. His *Oration to the Greeks* was a fierce diatribe against Greco-Roman culture and society. He enjoined a strict asceticism. Irenaeus maintained that he was the founder of the Encratites. We find that term, however, applied indiscriminately to all ascetic sects of the Gnostics. Irenaeus also accused Tatian of Gnosticism, identifying him with the Gnostic Valentine and with Marcion, the founder of a heresy that bore his name and had much in common with Gnosticism. Although Tatian resembled both the gnostics and the Marcionites in his severe asceticism, his affinity with Gnosticism has been convincingly challenged by some prominent scholars, including Jean Daniélou. Daniélou writes that "Tatian's theology derives fundamentally from his teacher Justin and from the mainstream of Christian tradition, and the deviations are peripheral only. The system . . . of the Gnostics is radically different."[113] He goes on to point out that Tatian's age was characterized "by a general dualist spirit." He identifies three systems current at that time: "The Pauline dualism of σάρξ-πνεῦμα; the Platonist dualism of the sensible and intelligent orders of reality; and the Gnostic dualism of the Pleroma, the transcendent world of the Supreme God, and the Kenoma, the material universe made by the Demiurge and dominated by the evil powers."[114] Tatian stressed creation by the Logos, and his dualism was basically Pauline, tempered by a Platonist pessimism about matter. But it was not his dualism that produced his attitude toward medicine, although it did condition it.

In his *Oration to the Greeks,* Tatian asserts that when diseases arise within anyone, demons ascribe the cause to themselves. Sometimes they cause disturbances within men, but if they are countered by the word of God, they depart and the sick man is healed.[115] He goes on to say that a πάθος is not destroyed by an ἀντιπάθεια, just as a madman is not cured by hanging amulets on himself. Both are demonic practices, in the same way as using material means thought to effect love in someone desired or to do harm to someone hated. When men resort to such things they become the slaves of demons. These material substances have no power in themselves—whether amulets, roots, or herbs—but, if one places one's faith in them, demons then work through them. If God had produced these things in order to bring about men's wishes, he would then be a creator of evil things. But it is the depravity of demons that makes use of natural substances for evil ends.[116] He then focuses specifically on medicine, saying that it, and everything included in it, is an invention of the same kind. Anyone who is healed by trusting in matter (which has efficacy only because demons are using it) would have been healed better by having recourse to the power of God. He asks why one who trusts in matter is unwilling to trust in God. The demons do not really cure, but by their craft make men their prisoners. He compares them to robbers who hold a person for ransom and free him when paid.[117]

Tatian's position on demons was entirely orthodox, although it was extreme. It differed only in degree from the position of the fathers we have considered above. Justin and Clement shared with Tatian the belief that the pagan gods were demons, fallen angels, who were cruel and intent on the destruction of mankind. Tertullian was of the same persuasion, as was Origen, in whose writings demonology occupies a considerable place. Generally, pagans believed not only in their gods but in demons as well. It was, in Michael Green's words, "an age which was hagridden with the fear of demonic forces dominating every aspect of life and death."[118] Belief in demons usually included their involvement in disease. Tatian held that demons caused disease and thus could cure it. Origen believed that demons could cause disease but expressed some doubt about whether they could cure. One exception was Asclepius, the Greek healing god, whose healing miracles few if any Christians denied. That he was a demon was frequently asserted in early Christian sources. We are on the periphery of a quagmire as we look into early Christian demonology, particularly possession manifested in disease and madness, which was treated by exorcism. Suffice it to say that during the period under consideration a distinction, if not always precise, was usually made between possession and illnesses, which were dealt with (as we have seen) in various ways by the church fathers who addressed their attention to them. A notable exception is Tatian, whose attitude toward medicine seems to have been the product of an extreme demonology conditioned by an orthodox Pauline dualism accentuated and rendered pessimistic by Platonism. It was this, not his rejection of pagan culture per se, that caused him to repudiate medicine. While it was his overall extremism that led him to separate from the Roman church and to become a heretic, the views expressed in the *Oration to the Greeks* were still within the bounds of orthodoxy, and there is a good possibility that this work was written fairly shortly after his conversion.

If my assessment is correct, Tatian's rejection of medicine was not a product of anything similar to the radical heretical dualism of Marcion (died ca. 160). Marcion's quasi-Gnosticism, which led to a severe asceticism predicated upon the conviction that the body is inherently evil, provided a framework productive of such hostility to medicine that he even eliminated the "beloved physician" from Paul's description of Luke in Colossians.[119] Fridolf Kudlien groups together, as "people whose hostility against physicians and medicine is almost outrageous," Tertullian, Marcion, Tatian, and Macarius.[120] Tertullian hardly seems to fit in this category. Marcion and Tatian do, but each for quite different reasons. Kudlien further asserts that "Tatian and Makarios argued that one is not allowed to cure diseases since they are sent from God, so that to take medicine would make you an atheist."[121] We have seen that this was by no means the reason why Tatian rejected the use of medicine. Let us see whether it is an accurate description of Macarius' position.

Classical attitudes extolling frugality and simplicity, the Neoplatonic ideal of the "flight of the alone to the alone," and many other factors in pagan society fostered a climate conducive to asceticism. This was so especially when the Christian demand for sacrifice and a perhaps exaggerated emphasis on the Pauline σάρξ-πνεῦμα dichotomy stirred in the hearts of Christians a desire to demonstrate a maximum commitment to Christ by denial of self and withdrawal from the world. Macarius the Egyptian, whose life spanned most of the fourth century, was a famous figure in the Christian ascetic movement. Of him we know very little.[122] Under his name circulated a collection of spiritual homilies in which there is one passage that is sometimes cited as inimical to medicine and physicians.[123] The anonymous author, writing for cenobitic (rather than anchoritic) monks, quotes Matthew 6:31–32 and then reminds his readers that they believe that their souls have received spiritual healing from Christ. That being the case, should not their bodily sicknesses likewise lead them to him rather than to earthly physicians? "See how you deceive yourself, because you acknowledge that you believe, yet not truly believing as you should." He considers the possible objection that God gave herbs and drugs and provided physicians for the diseases of the body. He agrees that this is true. God, because of his boundless philanthropy and kindness, gave these things to succor man after the Fall, since he did not wish entirely to destroy mankind. These were his gifts to the men of the world, for those "who are not yet able to entrust themselves entirely to God. . . . But you, who live in solitude, having drawn near to God" should entrust yourself to God alone.

We should note that he does not condemn the use of medicine by the average Christian. He is speaking to his monks. His is a position entirely compatible with that of Origen, only expressed in more exclusive terms since it is addressed only to those "superior Christians" who, instead of relying on medicine as the multitude does, should seek healing, in Origen's words, "by devotion to the supreme God and by praying to him."[124]

Pseudo-Macarius' position,[125] however, is more extreme than that of Basil, who allowed his monks the use of medicine under some conditions. Although the spiritual homilies attributed to Macarius may well have arisen in a Messalian community, the attitude toward medicine seen here need not be attributed to Messalianism, since it is an attitude that, although not common, is shared by Christians ranging from Origen to some modern charismatic sects and was probably present, to some degree, during every period in church history.

A rejection or criticism of medicine somewhat different from that made by Tatian, Marcion, or (with obvious qualifications) Macarius is that expressed by Arnobius, in the early fourth century. Converted late in life, he apparently knew very little about the Bible but soon wrote his *Adversus gentes* "with the enthusiasm of a recent convert [who] is better equipped to denounce idolatry than to set forth positive Christian themes."[126] His work was less Christian apologetics than an attack on paganism. In it he repudiated the Old Testament and did not use the New. He criticizes Asclepius' lack of success in working through the hands of fallible physicians, who waver in their diagnoses and often fail in their treatments. A physician is merely "a creature earth-born and not relying on true science," in that physicians do not depend on the power of God, who can heal without medicines.[127] His emphasis on the errors of physicians shows a side to his bias that transcends religious and other barriers. In classical, medieval, and modern societies there always were and there still are those who abuse medical practitioners for their failings. Arnobius' hostility seems to have been born of such a prejudice combined with a rejection of paganism, from which he had just fled, and an entirely orthodox concern with God as the ultimate healer, a basic principle of the religion to which he had just been converted.

Conclusions

With the exception of Tatian and Arnobius (who reject medicine while remaining within the bounds of orthodoxy) and Marcion (whose radical dualism was not, by any stretch of the imagination, Christian), the sources discussed in this paper display an attitude toward medicine which recognizes God as the source of all salubrious aspects of the created order, and the bestower of the wisdom to use them to man's advantage. God as the source of healing can also heal without the use of means. The Christian, as one who loves, trusts in, and depends upon this omnipotent God who loves and cares for his children, must rely upon God when ill, recognizing that illness itself (as well as any other form of suffering), can be a good when the Christian is receptive to edification by it. This attitude is much more consistent with the spirit of Judaism, particularly late pre-Christian Judaism, than it is with any strains of classical culture. However sympathetic it may be to medicine, it is an attitude that rejoices in God's display of power in miraculous healings in cases when physicians have failed, or simply in lieu of their care. For instance, Gregory Nazianzen, who was entirely supportive of secular medicine, enthusiastically recounts the healing of his father when all the physicians' efforts had failed.[128] Gregory of Nyssa describes how his sister was healed by God when she refused to see a physician because of her modesty.[129] Jerome, although supportive of secular medicine, delights in recounting the miracles wrought by Hilarion on those whom physicians could not cure.[130] And Augustine, in the *City of God*, describes a series of miraculous healings not only of those of whom physicians had despaired, but also of those who were saved from the agony of surgery, and of a physician cured of a condition for which his own skill did no good.[131] Augustine was by no means belittling physicians or medicine. His perspective on secular medicine was positive, as positive as that of the many other fathers whom our sources show as vigorous and enthusiastic in their efforts to succor the sick, as an act of Christian charity, through the employment of medicine and its practitioners as a material manifestation of God's love. And this was often done in early versions of "hospitals," institutions of medical care such as that founded near Caesarea by Basil, who, we may recall, allowed his monks to use medical means only on a quite circumscribed basis.

Modern scholarly appraisals of the attitudes of the early church to the use of secular medicine vary in their explanations of instances of apparent resistance to medicine's appropriateness or validity for Christians.[132] Some assert that a negative attitude toward human medicine can be best explained by seeing it as an outgrowth of, or as ancilliary to, various heretical tendencies. There is some truth in this, if the idea is not taken too far. Hostility to medicine by heretics such as Marcion was a product of a radical dualism quite inconsistent with Christian beliefs. That of Tatian, however, was not the result of his heretical inclinations but of his quite orthodox, though extreme, demonology. But his attitude was tempered by his dualism, which was not heretical, except insofar as it was made radical by a Platonic dualism that is qualitatively different from

Pauline dualism. Tatian's rejection of medicine, although extreme and bizarre, is still within the scope of orthodoxy. Other scholars find the roots of a rejection of medicine by early Christians in the severe asceticism that is itself born of a non-Christian dualism or a Pauline dualism pushed to its limits. The orthodox limits of Pauline dualism, as brought to bear on the question of the suitability of human medicine for the Christian, have led to positions such as that of pseudo-Macarius, who urges those who would be most devout to seek their bodily healing from the same source from which their spiritual healing came. This position is fundamentally the same as Origen's and is not *radically* different from that of Basil. Although extreme, it is orthodox in its basic principles, even if held by individuals, such as Messalians, who were declared heretical for some of their ascetic excesses. Lastly, some scholars argue that a negative attitude toward medicine may have been a widely held position in the very early church, gradually overcome, in the next three to four centuries, by common sense, reason, and very importantly, an ameliorating Hellenistic influence, with later resistance being the manifestation of the two tendencies discussed in the preceding sentences. This position is untenable in light of the essentially spiritual component central to the question of the Christian's use of medicine, a spiritual component similar to that of pre-Christian Judaism but alien to all strains of classical culture and predicated upon the relationship of the believer to his omnipotent and loving Creator. This relational principle tempered and provided the framework for the entire range of attitudes toward secular medicine, a range of attitudes that has been, and to a degree still is, present within Christianity.

NOTES

Abbreviations

ANF.   *Ante-Nicene Fathers,* [various translators] ([various dates]; reprint, Grand Rapids: Eerdmans, 1951)

FC.   *Fathers of the Church,* [various editors and translators] (Washington, D.C.: Catholic University of America, 1948–)

NPNF-1.   *Select Library of Nicene and Post-Nicene Fathers of the Christian Church,* [various translators], 1st ser. ([various dates]; reprint, Grand Rapids: Eerdmans, 1976–79)

NPNF-2.   *Select Library of Nicene and Post-Nicene Fathers of the Christian Church,* [various translators], 2d ser. ([various dates]; reprint, Grand Rapids: Eerdmans, 1976–79)

1. There is a fairly extensive literature on medicine in the early church, particularly studies of the extent of individual church fathers' medical knowledge, and their literary use of that knowledge. Mention should be made of the following in the former category: A. Harnack, "Medicinisches aus der ältesten Kirchengeschichte," *Texte Untersuchungen zur Geschichte der altchristlichen Literatur* 8, no. 4 (1892): 37–152; Stephen d'Irsay, "Patristic Medicine," *Ann. Med. Hist.* 9 (1927): 364–78; idem, "Christian Medicine and Science in the Third Century," *J. Relig.* 10 (1930): 515–44; H. J. Frings, "Medizin und Arzt bei den griechischen Kirchenvätern bis Chrysostomos" (Ph.D. diss., Rheinische Friedrich-Wilhelms-Universität zu Bonn, 1959); and H. Schadewaldt, "Die Apologie der Heilkunst bei den Kirchenvatern," *Veröffentlichungen der Internationalen Gesellschaft für Geschichte der Pharmazie* 26 (1965): 115–30.

2. A notable and very early example is Paul's Areopagus address in Acts 17.

3. Stoicism, Middle Platonism, Epicureanism, and Aristotelianism (i.e., the Peripatetic school).

4. Robert M. Grant, *Augustus to Constantine: The Thrust of the Christian Movement into the Roman World* (New York: Harper and Row, 1970), 106–8; Werner Jaeger, *Early Christianity and Greek Paideia* (Cambridge, Mass.: Belknap, 1961), 43–44.

5. Michael Green, *Evangelism in the Early Church* (Grand Rapids: Eerdmans, 1970); 19, Grant, *Augustus to Constantine* (n. 4), 107.

6. Jaeger, *Early Christianity* (n. 4), 31.

7. See Grant, *Augustus to Constantine* (n. 4), 109.

8. Ibid., 142.

9. Stanley L. Jaki, *Science and Creation: From Eternal Cycles to an Oscillating Universe* (Edinburgh: Scottish Academic, 1974), 168.

10. Justin Martyr, *Dialogue with Trypho* 8, in *ANF* 1:198.

11. Grant, *Augustus to Constantine* (n. 4), 112.

12. Jean Daniélou, *Gospel Message and Hellenistic Culture*, trans. J. A. Baker (Philadelphia: Westminster, 1973), 303.

13. Jaeger, *Early Christianity* (n. 4), 38.

14. Augustine, *Confessions* 8.7.

15. See, e.g., ibid., 8.2; idem, *City of God* 8.5.

16. Peter Brown, *Augustine of Hippo* (Berkeley: University of California Press, 1967), 95.

17. Ibid., 113.

18. Pierre Courcelle, "Anti-Christian Arguments and Christian Platonism: From Arnobius to St. Ambrose," in *The Conflict between Paganism and Christianity in the Fourth Century*, ed. Arnaldo Momigliano (Oxford: Clarendon, 1963).

19. F. Homes Dudden, *The Life and Times of St. Ambrose* (Oxford: Clarendon, 1935), 502 ff.

20. Ludwig Edelstein, "The Relation of Ancient Philosophy to Medicine," in *Ancient Medicine: Selected Papers of Ludwig Edelstein*, ed. Owsei Temkin and C. Lilian Temkin (Baltimore: Johns Hopkins Press, 1967), 360.

21. All works mentioned in n. 1 are concerned, at least in part, with these matters. In addition, see Rudolph Arbesmann, "The Concept of 'Christus Med-

icus' in St. Augustine," *Traditio* 10 (1954): 1–28; A. S. Pease, "Medical Allusions in the Works of St. Jerome," *Harvard Stud. Class. Philol.* 25 (1914): 73–86; and H. Schipperges, "Zur Tradition des 'Christus Medicus' im frühen Christentum und in der älteren Heilkunde," *Arzt und Christ* 11 (1965): 12–20.

22. Jaki, *Science and Creation* (n. 9), 183.

23. Herbert Butterfield, *Christianity and History* (New York: Scribner's, 1949) 121.

24. Origen, *Contra Celsum* 4.65–68.

25. Justin Martyr, *1 Apology* 10.2.

26. Justin Martyr, *2 Apology* 4.2.

27. Ibid., 5.2.

28. Clement of Alexandria, *Stromateis* 6.17.

29. Clement, *Christ the Educator* 1.2.6.

30. Origen, *Homily 18 on Numbers 3*.

31. Origen, *Annotations on III Kings* 15:13.

32. Origen, *Homily 1 on Psalm 37* 1.

33. Origen, *Contra Celsum* 3.12, trans. Henry Chadwick (Cambridge: Cambridge University Press, 1953), 135.

34. Basil of Caesarea, *The Long Rules* 55, in *FC* 9:331.

35. Gregory of Nyssa, *Life of St. Macrina*.

36. John Chrysostom, *Homily 8 on Colossians*.

37. Augustine, *On Christian Doctrine* 4.16.33.

38. Augustine, *Tractate 30 on John* 1; idem, *Tractate 32 on John* 9.

39. Augustine, *On the Good of Marriage* 9.

40. Jerome, *Letters* 10.

41. Ibid., 39.2.

42. Clement, *Stromateis* 4.5.

43. Ibid., 7.14.

44. Origen, *Contra Celsum* 8.56.

45. Basil, *The Long Rules* 55.

46. Gregory Nazianzen, *Letters* 31.

47. Gregory Nazianzen, *Panegyric on Basil* 26.

48. Gregory Nazianzen, *On the Death of His Father* 28.

49. 1 Tim. 5:23 reads: "Use a little wine for the sake of your stomach and your frequent infirmities."

50. John Chrysostom, *Homily 1 on the Statues*, for which his text was 1 Tim. 5:23; in *NPNF*-1, 9:331–44.

51. John Chrysostom, *Homily 8 on Colossians*, in *NPNF*-1, 13:297.

52. John Chrysostom, *Homily 1 on the Statues*.

53. John Chrysostom, *Homily 33 on Hebrews* 8.

54. John Chrysostom, *Homily 10 on 2 Timothy*.

55. John Chrysostom, *Homily 38 on John* 2.

56. John Chrysostom, *Homily 33 on Hebrews* 8.

57. Jerome, *Letters* 39.2, in *NPNF*-2, 6:50.

58. Ibid., 108.19, in *NPNF*-2, 6:205.

59. Ibid., 38.2.

60. Ambrose, *Concerning Repentance* 1.13.63.

61. Ambrose, *Letters* 79.

62. Augustine, *Tractate 32 on John 9.*

63. Augustine, *Letters* 130.

64. Augustine, *On Psalm 39* 18.

65. Augustine, *Letters* 38, in *FC* 12:169.

66. Origen, *Adnotationes in Librum III Regum* 15:23, in *Patrologia cursus completus, Series Graeco-Latina,* ed. Jacques Paul Migne (Paris: J. P. Migne, 1857–66), 17:53–55; my translation.

67. Origen, *Contra Celsum* 8.55, trans. by Chadwick (n. 33), 494.

68. Ibid., 8.60, trans. by Chadwick (n. 33), 498.

69. Basil, *The Long Rules* 55, in *FC* 9:331–36.

70. Eric Osborn, *Ethical Patterns in Early Christian Thought* (Cambridge: Cambridge University Press, 1976), 110; cf. 96: For Basil, "the discipline of the monk is simply a continuation of the discipline which is imposed on every baptised Christian."

71. Eusebius, discussing the same incident, maintains that it teaches that "by no means should those things designed for men for the treatment of the body be discarded as worthless; moreover, that these are to be used since the prophet advised their use" (*Commentaria in Isaiam* 38.21, in *Patrologia . . . Graeco-Latina* [n. 66], 24:359; my translation).

72. Augustine, *Sermons* 87.10–11.

73. Augustine, *Letters* 211.13.

74. Augustine, *Tractate 30 on John 3.*

75. Augustine, *On Christian Doctrine* 4.16.33.

76. Augustine, *Tractate 7 on John* 12.

77. Jerome, *Letters* 125.16.

78. Jerome, *On Isaiah* 8.

79. Ambrose, *Exposition of Psalm 118* 19.

80. Ambrose, *On Cain* 1.40.

81. John Chrysostom, *Letters to Olympias,* in *NPNF*-1, 9:293–94.

82. John Chrysostom, *Homily 4 on Timothy.*

83. John Chrysostom, *Homily 14 on Romans.*

84. Osborn, *Ethical Patterns* (n. 70), 51.

85. Clement, *Stromateis* 4.4.

86. Basil, *The Long Rules* 55, in *FC* 9:331.

87. John Chrysostom, *Homily 8 on Colossians,* in *NPNF*-1, 13:298–99.

88. Augustine, *City of God* 19.4, trans. Henry Battenson (London: Penguin, 1972), 857.

89. Augustine, *Tractate 30 on John 3.*

90. Augustine, *Sermons* 84.1, in M. M. Getty, *The Life of the North Africans as Revealed in the Sermons of Saint Augustine* (Washington, D.C.: Catholic University of America, 1931), 24–25.

91. Ibid., 344.5, in Getty, *Life of the North Africans* (n. 31), 25.

92. Cf. Exod. 15:26; Deut. 32:39.

93. Exod. 22:18; Deut. 18:10; Isa. 3:2–3, 28:15, 47:9, 47:12; Jer. 27:9; Ezek. 13:17–23; Mic. 5:12.

94. Perhaps 2 Chron. 16:12–13.

95. Isa. 38; 1 Kings 17:17–24; 2 Kings 4:18–37, 5:1–14.

96. Of more value for rabbinic than for biblical medical history are Julius Preuss, *Biblical and Talmudic Medicine,* trans. Fred Rosner (New York: Sanhedrin, 1978); and Fred Rosner, *Medicine in the Bible and Talmud* (New York: Ktav, 1977).

97. For a discussion of the passage, see A. Stöger, "Der Arzt nach Jesus ben Sirach (38:1–15)," *Arzt und Christ* 11 (1965): 3–11; S. Noorda, "Illness and Sin, Forgiving and Healing: The Connection of Medical Treatment and Religious Beliefs in Ben Sira 38:1–15," in *Studies in Hellenistic Religions,* ed. M. J. Vermaseren (Leiden: E. J. Brill, 1979), 215–24.

98. Verse 15 in LXX differs from the Hebrew. In the former the thought is, "Let the one who sins before his Maker fall into the hands of a physician"; in the latter, "A man who sins before his Maker will be strong before [i.e., resist] the physician." For a discussion, see Noorda, "Illness and Sin" (n. 97), 220–21, especially n. 18.

99. The only instance that I have seen of a direct quotation of any part of the passage in question by an early church father is by Clement (*Christ the Educator* 2.8). He quotes verses 1, 2, and 8 in the context of an argument in which he is attempting to demonstrate that unguents were given for use, not for voluptuousness.

100. See Noorda, "Illness and Sin" (n. 97), 220 n. 17, for Greek text and references.

101. Tertullian, *On Prescription against Heretics* 7, in *ANF* 3:246.

102. Ibid.

103. Charles N. Cochrane, *Christianity and Classical Culture: A Study of Thought and Action from Augustus to Augustine* (London: Oxford University Press, 1957), 227.

104. Jaeger, *Early Christianity* (n. 4), 33.

105. Timothy David Barnes, *Tertullian: A Historical and Literary Study* (Oxford: Clarendon, 1971), 210.

106. Ibid., 205.

107. Tertullian, *De anima* 2.

108. Tertullian, *Ad nationes* 2.4, in *ANF* 3:133.

109. Tertullian, *De corona* 8, in *ANF* 3:97.

110. Tertullian, *On Flight in Persecution* 1–2.

111. Tertullian, *On Purity* 13.

112. He is sometimes criticized as antagonistic to medicine because of his outspoken deprecation of techniques employed in abortion (Tertullian, *De anima* 25; idem, *Ad nationes* 1; idem *Apology* 9). This, in an early Christian author, tells us nothing about his attitude toward a "proper" use of the medical art, a misunderstanding demonstrated by Kudlien, who includes Tertullian among those early Christians who rejected medicine. Fridolf Kudlien, "Cynicism and Medicine," *Bull. Hist. Med* 43 [1974]: 317. Schadewaldt, "Apologie der Heilkunst" (n. 1), 126, shares Kudlien's misapprehensions.

113. Daniélou, *Gospel Message* (n. 12), 395.

114. Ibid., 396.

115. Tatian, *Oration to the Greeks* 16.

116. Ibid., 17.

117. Ibid., 18.

118. Green, *Evangelism* (n. 5), 190.

119. Schadewaldt, "Apologie der Heilkunst" (n. 1), 127.

120. Kudlien, "Cynicism and Medicine" (n. 112), 317–18.

121. Ibid., 318.

122. Palladius includes a brief description of him in his *Lausiac History* 17, written around 420.

123. Pseudo-Macarius, *Homily* 48.3–6, in *Patrologia . . . Graeco-Latina* (n. 66), 34:809–11; my translation.

124. Origen, *Contra Celsum* 8.60, trans. Chadwick (n. 33), 498.

125. In practice these Egyptian monks did employ physicians. Palladius, who was one of them for some years, relates that he was sent to Alexandria by his brotherhood to be cured of hydropsy by the physicians there (Palladius, *Lausiac History* 35.12). He tells of one monk who had the gift of healing and had cured many who had come to him. He became afflicted with an "ulcerous condition known as cancer [φαγέδαινον]" and was under the care of a physician. So great was his "spiritual preparation" that he carried on a conversation and wove palm leaves while the physician performed what is described as quite extensive surgery (Palladius, *Lausiac History* 24.1, trans. Robert T. Meyer [London: Longmans, Green, 1965], 83). Other instances of the use of physicians and medicine in these monastic communities are sufficient to indicate that exclusive reliance on healing by divine intervention was not the strict practice.

126. Grant, *Augustus to Constantine* (n. 4), 196–97.

127. Arnobius, *Against the Heathen* 1.48; cf. 3.23 in *ANF* 6:426, 470.

128. Gregory Nazianzen, *On the Death of His Father* 28–29.

129. Gregory of Nyssa, *The Life of St. Macrina*.

130. Jerome, *Life of St. Hilarion* 14, 15.

131. Augustine, *City of God* 22.8.

132. E.g., those cited in nn. 1 and 112, above.

SIX

Tatian's "Rejection" of Medicine
in the Second Century

Tatian, a second-century Syrian convert to Christianity, was an apologist best known for vitriolically denouncing pagan culture, who was himself denounced as a heretic.[1] The dates of his birth and death are unknown. His *floruit* is generally given as 160–80. It is certain that he spent some time in Rome as a student of Justin Martyr. Around 172 he returned to Syria, where he is supposed to have founded an ascetic sect known as the Encratites, who later were declared heretical for their rejection of marriage, and of the eating of meat and the drinking of wine, and for aspects of their theology that bordered on Gnosticism. Because of his later association with Encratism and his rigorous denunciation of virtually all features of pagan culture while still within the orthodox community, he remains a controversial figure.[2]

Tatian appears to have been a prolific writer. Only two of his works, however, are extant, one of which is the *Oratio ad Graecos*.[3] The *Oratio* belongs to the genre of Christian apologetics. A feature that was common to the genre was an attack on pagan teachings, morals, and religion, and an attempt to show that the teachings of Christianity, especially its monotheism and its promise of judgment for sin, were older and more venerable than pagan religion and philosophy. Most of the second-century apologists were, if not thoroughly conciliatory, at least irenic, and sought to emphasize those aspects of paganism that were least in conflict with divine revelation. Tatian, by contrast, was vehemently polemical and uncompromising, taking obvious delight in ridiculing and denouncing all aspects of classical culture.[4]

Scholars continue to debate whether Tatian wrote the *Oratio* before or after he left the pale of orthodoxy for Encratism. Some see signs of a developed Gnosticism in the *Oratio;* others deny that a close and unbiased scrutiny of the evidence can support this interpretation. Jean Daniélou presents a convincingly perspicacious analysis of Tatian's theology, as expressed in the *Oratio,* and argues that it "derives fundamentally from his teacher Justin and from the mainstream of Christian tradition, and the deviations are peripheral only."[5] Nevertheless, the *Oratio* is unusual not only for its often vicious tone but also for its sometimes peculiar emphases, one of which is a discussion of pharmacology that is unique in early Christian literature and has attracted at least the passing attention of various scholars who have sought to understand and describe the role of medicine in early Christianity.

Scholarly Interpretations of Tatian's Attitude toward Medicine

Although it should be clear to any reader of the Greek text of the *Oratio* that Tatian's concern with medicine is limited to pharmacology, nevertheless, irrespective of the language in which they were writing, modern scholars, myself included, have typically been semantically imprecise by using a generic term such as *medicine* without limiting it to medicinal drugs, or by specifying that Tatian condemned the use of drugs but then speaking of his rejection of "medicine." Other scholars have been more precise semantically but have not raised the question of why Tatian chose only to condemn pharmacology but not the other parts of medicine. Hence Owsei Temkin's recent analysis of Tatian's attitude toward secular medicine is quite salutary. He writes,

Tatian is concerned with theology, not with medicine. The words "medicine" and "physician" do not occur in the *Address against the Greeks* at all.[6] Tatian does not express what he thinks about medicine as a whole, for his criticism does not go beyond pharmacology; neither directly nor indirectly does it touch upon the other two branches of medicine: diet and surgery. . . . Dietetic medicine essentially is a reordering of the way of life; it does not ascribe healing power to any particular remedy. Nor does surgery, as long as it consists of cutting, cauterizing, bandaging, and manipulating the body without the aid of drugs.

Hence, Temkin goes on, "Tatian should not be quoted as a witness for early Christian hostility to medicine."[7] Temkin is absolutely right.[8] Any suggestion that Tatian is a bona fide example of a patristic source who rejects the Christians' use of all secular medicine on theological grounds is worse than an overstatement. It is patently wrong.

In an earlier essay I discussed Tatian's rejection of "medicine." My concern was to argue two points. First, Tatian's attitude toward "medicine" was conditioned by a dualism that was essentially Pauline but tempered by Middle Platonism (hence a dualism that was far from that of Marcion and even farther from Gnostic dualism, and well within the realm of orthodoxy). Second, it was Tatian's extreme, although entirely orthodox, demonology that, combined with his distinct dualism, accounts for his attitude toward "medicine."[9] Temkin's significantly longer discussion of Tatian provides a much more thorough analysis of Tatian's understanding of disease, his attitude toward various modes of healing, his perception of the role of demons in disease and healing, the broader theological context of these considerations, and the sorely needed caveat that Tatian's condemnation of pharmacology must not be exaggerated into, or presented so ambiguously as to seem to be, a wholesale rejection of the art of medicine.[10] Temkin then asks, "Did Hippocratic doctors also fall under his censure?"[11] His answer is essentially that Tatian implied no censure of physicians except insofar as they may have sought to effect cures through the employment of magic.[12]

Why Did Tatian Single Out Pharmacology for Condemnation?

Nevertheless, a specific question still needs to be asked that no scholar, including Temkin, has raised; and that is, why did Tatian condemn pharmacology? Of course, it can be said that Temkin and I both raised and answered that question, Temkin more thoroughly than I, but only at one level, and that is, since Tatian did in fact condemn pharmacology, how are we to understand this condemnation in light of Tatian's theology? In other words, how does one make accessible to the reader the theological basis, that is, the logical basis within Tatian's theological system, for his condemnation of pharmacology? But there is another question that needs to be raised and answered. Since one could expunge Tatian's condemnation of pharmacology from his *Oratio ad Graecos* without detracting from the treatise's coherence, and, correlatively, since nothing in the work would cause the reader to feel that Tatian would have been inconsistent if he had not condemned pharmacology along with, for example, astrology and magic, what is there about pharmacology that, in Tatian's mind, made pharmacology worthy of condemnation as demonic and, consequently, as wrong for Christians to employ? In other words, what attracted Tatian's attention to pharmacology in the first place?

All of the Christian apologists recognized the extraordinary power of demons, the fallen angels whom the pagans worshipped as their gods.[13] All of the apologists, especially Tatian, were positively convinced that demons were set on one goal: to keep fallen humanity in a state of ignorance and error, deluded and without salvation. To accomplish this end, the demons devised *antisophisteumata.*[14] Tatian's purpose was to unmask these antisophisteumata, one of which was the demons' use of matter, *hylē,* to entrap fallen man. To Tatian, hylē appears to be essentially the same as the various constructs used in the New Testament and patristic literature to designate the carnal and material world as it is contrasted with the spiritual, to distinguish the temporal from the eternal, the things that are on the earth from the things above. It is imperative that we recognize how great is the gulf between Tatian's understanding of matter and Marcion's and the Gnostics'. Matter to Tatian is not inherently evil. He emphasizes that God through the Logos is the Creator of matter. Hence matter itself cannot be evil.[15] His belief in the Incarnation and in a bodily resurrection would militate against classifying matter as evil.[16] But, in Hawthorne's words, "since . . . matter is so susceptible to perversion and to becoming an instrument of evil, though in itself it is not an evil, Tatian urges men to repudiate matter and thus nullify the power of demons."[17] The demons, who are themselves material, although (like air and fire) ethereal,[18] contrive numerous carnal deceptions, some of which are essentially and inherently sinful, as, for instance, a belief in fate as explicated and enforced by astrology.[19] Tatian does not deny the reality of fate or the power of astrology. But he rejoices in his assurance that "we are above fate, and instead of planetary[20] demons we have come to know one lord who does not err; we are not led by fate and have rejected its lawgivers."[21] Another demonic counterfeit is magic in all its forms.[22] Directly consorting with demons is the most blatant and obvious form of magic. But not all magic necessarily involves a recognition or acknowledgment of the direct involvement of demons by those who employ it. The use of the occult powers of various substances is a case in point. Many exploiters of such substances would recognize the direct involvement of demons, while others would see the occult power as accessible without demonic activity. For Tatian, such a distinction simply did not matter. Either way, it was demonic delusion and deceit.

The same holds true for the principles of sympathy and antipathy that Tatian associates with Bolos of Mendes, whom he confuses with Democritus. According to Tatian, "A disease is not destroyed[23] by antipathy, nor is a madman cured by wearing leather amulets. They[24] are visitations of demons, and the sick man and the man who claims to be in love, the man who hates and the man who wants revenge, all take these as their helpers. . . . the varieties of roots and sinews and bones are not efficacious in themselves, they are the elemental matter of the demons' wickedness."[25] One could easily be sidetracked here into a discussion of Tatian's definition and understanding of magic or into a perusal of the increasingly common examinations by medical historians of the fluidity of the lines between medicine and magic in classical antiquity.[26] Nevertheless, Tatian seemed to know pretty well—for his purposes, that is— what magic was and what it was not.

While sympathy and antipathy and the use of amulets were magic in Tatian's view, the use of drugs was not. And, of course, it is his denunciation of pharmacology that renders him unique in early church history. This brings us directly to the question of why Tatian chose to include medicinal drugs among those substances that demons used to deceive people and keep them from faith in God, hence rendering medicinal drugs unsuitable for use by Christians.

Tatian begins his discussion of pharmacology by saying, "Pharmacy in all its forms is due to the same artificial devising."[27] He had just been discussing magic, including principles of sympathy and antipathy. "The same artificial devising" *(hē autē epitechnēsis)* is synonymous with antisophisteumata, the demons' counterfeits.[28] We should note that Tatian attributes all forms of *pharmakeia* to the same artificial devising. Then, after saying, "If anyone is healed by matter because he trusts in it, all the more will he be healed if in himself he relies on the power of God," he returns to the subject of the first sentence and asserts, "Just as poisons [*ta dēlētēria*] are material concoctions, so remedies [*ta iōmena*] too belong to the same substance." It is not enough to "reject the baser matter" (by which he appears to mean *ta dēlētēria*) since

yet in practice some often set about healing by mixing one evil with another and will use evil means even to produce good. Just as a man who has supped with a bandit, even if he is not a bandit himself, shares his punishment because he shared his meal, so the man who is not bad himself but keeps low company and uses it for a supposedly good end will be punished by the Divine Judge, because of his association.[29]

So also, for Tatian, there is guilt by association with *pharmaka* that are *dēlētēria* even when one uses them as *iōmena*.

The Greek word group that includes *pharmakeia* and *pharmakon* (Latin *venenum*) enjoyed a wonderfully confusing range of meanings, for laymen especially, that included poison, magic, sorcery, and medicinal drugs. Popular confusion was probably not marked during the period under consideration. Nevertheless, it was always present, even if only latent. Furthermore, whereas the Old and New Testaments have nothing unequivocally negative to say about medicine, the *pharmakeia* word group in *all* its occurrences denotes sorcery or witchcraft in both the Septuagint[30] and the New Testament.[31] And even though Galen and others insisted on the unity of the three parts of medicine (pharmacology, dietetics, and surgery),[32] not all physicians and laymen agreed. There was no unanimity of opinion among the various medical sects regarding the proper use of drugs.[33] Some physicians rejected their use altogether.

It is impossible to determine how high a percentage of physicians refused to administer pharmaka during the late Hellenistic and early Roman Imperial eras. There certainly was a large enough number to arouse Scribonius Largus' concern. In the proem to his *Compositiones* he speaks of "certain humble, and indeed otherwise unknown, men [who] are clearly greatly skilled in terms of experience, although . . . far removed from the discipline of medicine and not associated with that profession. Often they can instantly free the sick from all pain and danger . . . by administering efficacious drugs."[34] A much greater problem was presented by two extreme groups of physicians. The first, who greatly aroused Scribonius' righteous indignation, tended to administer irresponsibly "so-called" drugs that had not been tested. The second group, worthy of equal condemnation, entirely refused to administer drugs:

I have been unable to discover why anyone should exclude the use of drugs from medicine unless it is that they would uncover their ignorance thereby. Yet if they have no experience of this type of remedy they must stand accused for having been grossly negligent in a most necessary part of the art. And if in fact they have mastered the use of drugs but nevertheless deny their use they are even more blameworthy.[35]

These physicians apparently were attempting to force other physicians to reject drug therapy also: "Therefore, let those men, who either do not wish or are not able to help the afflicted, also cease from preventing others from offering help to the sick. Such aid is frequently produced through the power of drugs."[36] Although some laymen were nearly obsessively fascinated with drug lore, especially that dealing with magical and poisonous drugs, others were very suspicious even of drugs that were administered by physicians; hence Scribonius Largus' perceived necessity to preface his pharmacological text, probably written for laymen, with a defense of both the ethical propriety of the administration of drugs and an assurance of their safety when taken properly.[37]

This ambiguity in medical circles and in the popular mentality about the use of pharmaka renders pharmacology categorically different from the other branches of medicine. In one sense, a Christian such as Tatian who condemned the use of medicinal drugs is similar to a physician who did so: neither, of course, was condemning medicine per se. But in one very significant sense the two are dramatically different: the reasons for their condemnations come from strikingly separate areas of concern. The physician who condemned the use of drugs did so because his theory of disease and healing or his concern for safety and responsible medical practice prompted his condemnation of pharmaka. Tatian's theology, specifically his belief in the subtle machinations of demons to entrap and deceive, made drugs strong candidates for inclusion in his litany of forbidden matters. There were two reasons for this.

The first is intimately related to Tatian's anthropology and epistemology. He continues his discussion of pharmacology with the rhetorical question, "Why is the man who puts his faith in the material system [*hylēs oikonomia*] unwilling to trust in God?"[38] This is a crucial concern that Tatian had already raised and answered in a variety of ways thus far in the *Oratio*. And the most basic answer for Tatian or any church father is central to historical Christianity. Although different sources express their answer in different ways, essentially it is that all humanity is separated into two distinct categories, the saved and the lost, the children of God and the children of Satan, the children of light and the children of darkness, the spiritually alive and the spiritually dead, spiritual men and natural men. With this quite incomplete list Tatian would have been in complete agreement. He would also have concurred with various church fathers who maintained that although man was created in the image and likeness of God he had lost this partaking of the divine nature by virtue of the Fall.

Tatian's doctrine of creation is based on the principle that God is spirit and that he is the "creator[39] of material spirits [*pneumata hylika*] and the shapes that are in matter," but he himself does not pervade matter. "For the spirit that pervades matter is inferior to the more divine spirit *(pneuma theioteron)*."[40] Man, before the Fall, possessed not only the *pneuma hylikon* but also the *pneuma theioteron*. "The celestial Word . . . made man an image of immortality, so that just as incorruptibility belongs to God, in the same way man might share God's lot and have immortality also."[41] But with the Fall all this changed. "We have knowledge of two different kinds of spirits, one of which is called soul, but the other is greater than the soul; it is the image and likeness of God. The first men were endowed with both, so that they might be part of the material world, and at the same time above it."[42] Fallen man no longer possesses the image and likeness of God. He possesses or, better, is pervaded by, the *pneuma hylikon*, as are all objects of creation, both animate and inanimate. But man also possesses a soul, which "is not in itself immortal but mortal."[43] The soul will be resurrected with the body to be judged and suffer eternal punishment with it. By contrast, the soul of the man who "has obtained knowledge of God" is immortal, for it has gained "union with the divine spirit."[44] Hence "we ought now to search for what we once had and have lost, and link the soul to the Holy Spirit and busy ourselves with the union ordained by God."[45]

Clearly there are for Tatian two categories of men: (1) those who have gained union with the divine spirit (literally the Spirit of God), who have regained the image and likeness of God, and who, since they are in the light, can perceive and ascertain the things of the Spirit; and (2) those who have only the material spirit and a mortal soul and who, since they are in the darkness, cannot perceive and ascertain anything higher than matter. One must keep these distinctions clear to understand the following passage:

Man is not, as the croakers[46] teach, a rational being capable of intelligence and understanding (for according to them even the irrational creatures will be proved capable of intelligence and understanding), but man alone is "the image and likeness of God." I mean by man not one who behaves like the animals, but who has advanced far beyond his humanity towards God himself. We have written about this in greater detail in our treatise "On animals."[47] [Otherwise] man is superior to the beasts only in his articulate speech; in other respects his way of life is the same as theirs, for he is not a likeness of God.[48]

This passage has been much discussed by patristic scholars whose concern is to determine wherein Tatian resembles and wherein he differs from pagan and other Christian sources in his understanding of the ontological distinctions between humans and animals. Often a convenient basis of comparison is provided by the debate between Origen and Celsus.[49] Celsus had posed the question of how, if one were to look down on the earth from heaven, men's actions would appear different from those of ants and bees. Origen argues that what distinguishes men from animals is that the former are rational and the latter irrational. While men are capable of reason, animals act on impulse, experience, or some natural power of apprehension, a natural constitutional tendency implanted by the Logos so that their species may survive. But in Celsus' view animals are rational. It is interesting to note how Robert M. Grant, a prominent historian of early Christianity, appreciates Tatian's position vis-à-vis those of Origen and Celsus. In 1952 he maintained that "Tatian insists on the resemblance of man to the animals, just as Celsus does. . . . Tatian agrees with Celsus rather than with Origen."[50] In 1988, without making any reference to his previous assessment, he asserted that Celsus "insisted that 'irrational animals' were rational, but Origen rejected the notion. . . . Here Origen agrees with Tatian."[51] Which of Grant's statements is correct? Both are half true. Unfortunately, both are also half false. It is, of course, fallacious to compare Tatian's position with the positions of Origen and Celsus. The argument of Origen and Celsus is entirely ontological and compares two entities, man and beast. Tatian's discussion involves both ontology and potentiality and contrasts three entities: man who possesses the image and likeness of God, man who possesses only a mortal or material soul, and beast.

The argument between Origen and Celsus centered on the phenomenon that animals are sometimes able to cure themselves when ill by having recourse to substances of which they would not otherwise avail themselves.[52] Returning now to Tatian's attack against pharmacology, we recall that he had last exclaimed, "Why is the man who puts his faith in the material system unwilling to trust in God?" He continues, "For what reason do you not resort to the lord of superior power, but choose rather to heal yourself like a dog with grass, or a deer with a snake, a hog with river crabs, or a lion with monkeys?"[53] The implication is that the demons, by their lies and deceptions, keep fallen man in the same lowly state as animals. And animals, of course, resort to matter for healing, whether through instinct or through a form of "rationality" that they have in common with men who are spiritually dead, irrational, and, in their fallen state, incapable of intelligence and understanding.[54] How clever and subtle are the demons to continue to keep fallen man in a state of dependence on matter, following the precedent of brute beasts!

Tatian now presents the second reason for his belief that demons contrived antisophisteumata to entrap and deceive men and so made drugs strong candidates for inclusion among forbidden matters. He asks, "Why, pray, do you make gods [*theopoieis*] out of this world's things?"[55] This is a gnawing frustration and a central, recurring theme in his attacks against Greek gullibility and vulnerability to demonic deceits. "I refuse to worship [God's] work of creation, brought into being for our sake," he exclaimed early in the *Oratio*. "It is for us that sun and moon have come into being; then how can I worship my servants? How can I proclaim sticks and stones as gods?"[56] Later he berates the Greeks for worshipping demons "though they were generated from matter."[57] And still later he vows, "I would neither be persuaded myself nor would I try to persuade my neighbour to worship the substance of the elements."[58] But, one may ask, were drugs particularly likely to be the objects of deification or of worship? The answer is really quite obvious.

For those who advocated and used them, *iōmena pharmaka* were indeed quite marvelous, awe-inspiring substances, potent, mysterious, dangerous if used improperly, and sometimes thrillingly effective if used properly. Scribonius Largus exudes enthusiasm for the wondrous power of drugs. Speaking of those who are "greatly skilled in terms of experience although . . . far removed from the discipline of medicine," he says, "Often they can instantly free the sick from all pain and danger, as if by divine intervention, by administering efficacious drugs."[59] Later, he remarks in regard to drug therapy, "we consider the ability . . . to restore . . . anyone whomsoever to good health to be a great thing and beyond the nature of man."[60] He had opened his treatise with the remark that the great Alexandrian physician, anatomist, and physiologist Herophilus "is reported to have said that drugs are like 'divine hands.'"[61] This appears to have been a somewhat popular idea. Plutarch attributes this phrase to Erasistratus (or perhaps to Herophilus),[62] and Marcellus to Herophilus.[63] Ludwig Edelstein comments, "This statement is not mere rhetoric. If nature is divine, the plants are divine too. Almost all physicians seem to agree with this. Some [physicians such as Antipatrus, Andromachus, and Archigenes] compose[d] special remedies which [they] called sacred."[64]

Immediately after asking, why "do you make gods out of this world's things?" Tatian continues his discussion of pharmacology with another question: "Why if you heal your neighbour are you called a benefactor [*euergetēs apokalēi*]?"[65] This is Whittaker's translation. Ryland[66] and Osborne[67] also take *apokalēi* as passive. Temkin, however, treats it as middle and translates, "Why do you call yourself a benefactor when healing your neighbor?"[68] Both translations, of course, are possible. Temkin justifies his by remarking, "Although outsiders rather than the healer are likely to apply this praise, this translation would shift the guilt away from the addressee."[69] Temkin's emphasis may well convey Tatian's intent.

Coming a close second to Tatian's anger against the demons themselves, their antisophisteumata, and the gullibility of the Greeks in that regard, is his contempt for the intellectual arrogance of the Greeks, especially of their philosophers. Sections 3 and 4 of the *Oratio* contain some of the most vitriolic and sarcastic ridicule of Greek philosophers in ancient literature. Tatian contrasts their pride, boasting, and self-display with their inconsistencies, foibles, and stupidities. Among several others there is Diogenes, who "by boasting of his tub prided himself on his self-sufficiency; he ate raw octopus, was seized with pain and died of an internal obstruction because of his intemperance."[70] And then, of course, Heraclitus:

I have no use for Heraclitus and his boast "I educated myself," because he was self-taught and arrogant. . . . His manner of death showed up his ignorance, for he was stricken with dropsy, and being a practitioner of medicine on the same lines as his philosophy he smeared himself all over with excrement; when it hardened it caused cramp all over his body, and after convulsions he died.[71]

Very likely Tatian would also have regarded Galen as worthy of condemnation for his intellectual pride. Galen writes,

Each of two things Herophilus said is true: for, if you say that drugs alone *per se* are nothing, you will make an appropriate statement, since they are nothing if they do not have a person who employs them correctly; and again, if you say drugs are just like the hands of the gods, this, too, will be a correct statement. For they effect great things if they have as their utilizer a person who is trained in the "rationalist" method and, along with this, is also intelligent by nature.[72]

For Galen the pharmaka are divine because the intellect of the human being who applies them also is divine. If Tatian were presented with Galen's statement, he would simply find confirmation of his belief that the demons are very subtle in their deceptions. Especially rankling for Tatian would be the self-assurance that the naturalist (like Galen) and those who administer or take medicinal drugs display by thinking that the drugs are within their control and subordinate to their lofty intellects. The demons have indeed been exceptionally clever in this subtle but spiritually deadly deception. It is easy to imagine how Tatian would react to Galen's poorly veiled desire to appear godlike to his patients,[73] and to material of the following ilk: In a letter, ostensibly written to Claudius or Nero, that is attributed (probably falsely)[74] to the physician and astrologer Thessalus of Tralles, introducing an astrological work on botanical pharmacology, the author recounts how, after he had failed to discover the occult virtues of various plants, he sought an interview with the god Asclepius. He claims that the god appeared to him and said, "Oh blessed Thessalus! Today you are honored by a god and soon, after men have heard of your success, they will revere you with the same reverence as a god. Question me about whatever you wish and I shall gladly answer anything about which you ask." Thessalus then asks for divine revelation concerning the mysteries of certain botanical concoctions.[75] Similarly, a magical papyrus contains a formula for adjuring a spirit who "will tell you about the illness of a man, whether he will also give [you both] wild herbs and the power to cure, and you will be [worshipped] as a god since you have a god as a friend!"[76] And with this we have returned to magic, but with pharmacology as a focal point of the magician's concern. It is not surprising, then, that pharmacology attracted Tatian's attention.

Conclusion

All of the Christian apologists were keenly alert to the fundamental differences between all pagan cosmologies, on the one hand, and the Christian cosmology, on the other. Religion was, in Greek philosophy, essentially an ennobled form of naturalism, and for all intents, nature was the supreme being, apart from which nothing was able to exist. Even the gods (or whatever there is that transcends man) are subordinate to nature and limited by it, and thus must work within it. And Tatian considers those gods to be demons who would use whatever power or influence was available to deceive and ensnare. These wondrous substances, medicinal drugs, whether their users saw them as part of deified nature or viewed them in the most rationalistic and naturalistic fashion, lured people away from faith in, trust in, and dependence on God.[77]

All of the church fathers who comment on medicine and physicians admonish their readers not to put their faith in medicine and not to rely on physicians alone. With this Tatian would ardently agree. But he goes further than they. There is one part of medicine (that is, pharmacology) that is especially dangerous. It is not dangerous for the reasons that the physicians who refused to administer drugs would give, but it is spiritually dangerous. We should note the highly spiritual language that Tatian uses when he pleads with his readers not to trust in pharmaka. "Why is the man who puts his faith in the material system not willing to put his faith in God?"[78] The dominant word is *pisteuō.* The realm is faith, trust, indeed dependence. And throughout the *Oratio,* Tatian warns against any and every antisophisteuma that can become the focus of one's faith and trust, thereby replacing or perverting one's dependence on God.

It is understandable why Tatian was convinced that pharmacology was especially dangerous for Christians, who were not likely to be lured into deterministic astrology and magic. If they were lured into astrology and magic, they would soon realize that they were doing wrong, as would those pagans who were willing to listen to Christian reasoning. But this was not so in the case of pharmacology. Here the involvement of demons was very subtle. Irrational animals treated themselves with "drugs" when ill. Those men who knew God were the only human beings who were above the level of brute beasts. So, Tatian reasons, do not be lured into imitating animals. Furthermore, the very ambiguity of the words for pharmacy—medicine, poison, sometimes even sorcery—should have alerted the perceptive Christian, especially since even some physicians refused to administer drugs. But more than that, the very marvelous nature of drugs—"the hands of the gods"—should have provoked suspicion. The demons, after all, were most dangerous when they were most subtle, especially when cloaked by philosophical naturalism or a Galenic style of rationalism. It is, I suggest, because Tatian believed that what should have been obvious to the Christian about pharmakeia was not sufficiently recognized, that he felt it necessary to warn against its dangers.

NOTES

1. E.g., by Irenaeus, *apud* Eusebius, *Historia ecclesiastica* 4.29. Irenaeus accuses Tatian of denying that Adam was saved, fantasizing "about invisible aeons," and repudiating "marriage as being depravity and fornication."

2. Several specialized studies, or at least portions of broader works, are devoted to Tatian. Robert M. Grant, "The Heresy of Tatian," *J. Theol. Stud.* 5 (1954): 62–68; and idem, *Greek Apologists of the Second Century* (Philadelphia: Westminster, 1988); Martin Else, *Tatian und seine Theologie,* Forschungen zur Kirchen- und

Dogmengeschichte, no. 9 (Göttingen: Vanderhoeck und Ruprecht, 1960); and R. W. Barnard, "The Heresy of Tatian—Once Again," *J. Ecclesiast. Hist.* 19 (1968): 1–10, provide a good starting point. Jean Daniélou, *Gospel Message and Hellenistic Culture*, trans. J. A. Baker (Philadelphia: Westminster, 1976), furnishes very profitable analyses of Tatian's place in various aspects of early Christian thought.

3. Several editions of the Greek text and translations into modern languages are available. I shall follow the edition and translation by Molly Whittaker: *Tatian: Oratio ad Graecos and Fragments* (Oxford: Clarendon, 1982). Several studies of the *Oratio* are worth perusing, especially those of Gerald F. Hawthorne, "Tatian and His *Discourse to the Greeks*," *Harvard Theol. Rev.* 57 (1964): 161–88; Alfred E. Osborne, "Tatian's Discourse to the Greeks: A Literary Analysis and Essay in Interpretation" (Ph.D. diss., University of Cincinnati, 1969); and the introduction and notes in Whittaker, *Tatian* (n. 3).

4. It should be noted that his denunciations of classical culture were merely an extreme version of those of other Christian apologists. His attacks not only against Homeric polytheism, the contradictions among various philosophers, and the grosser moral turpitudes of some pagans but also against classical culture generally were no more extreme than those of several classical sources (for which see Hawthorne, "Tatian" [n. 3] 180–81). As Osborne remarks, "Those who have criticized Tatian for his antagonism toward even what was best in the ancient world should remember that he was an accomplished craftsman in a previously developed art" ("Tatian's Discourse" [n. 3], 45), i.e., the Cynic *diatribē*.

5. Daniélou, *Gospel Message* (n. 2), 395.

6. While this is true of the section of the *Oratio* that is devoted specifically to pharmacology, it is not strictly correct. *Hē iatrikē* does occur in *Oratio* 3.1 in the description of Heraclitus' death.

7. Owsei Temkin, *Hippocrates in a World of Pagans and Christians* (Baltimore: Johns Hopkins University Press, 1991), 122.

8. But even Temkin can be misunderstood when, in a later chapter and in a different context, he says, "God was the supreme healer of the Old Testament; according to Tatian, man should rely on the power of God's word." Ibid., 144. This innocent statement could easily be taken to imply a rejection by Tatian of any form of healing other than direct reliance on God.

9. Darrel W. Amundsen, "Medicine and Faith in Early Christianity," *Bull. Hist. Med.* 56 (1982): 345–46; reprinted in slightly altered form as chap. 5, above.

10. Temkin, *Hippocrates* (n. 7), 119–23.

11. Ibid., 123.

12. Ibid., 123–25.

13. There is an extensive modern literature on demonology in early Christianity. A good starting point specifically treating demonology in the apologetic literature is Daniélou, *Gospel Message* (n. 2), chap. 18, "Demonology," 427–41. According to Daniélou, Tatian "unquestionably emphasised more than any other the demonic character of paganism" (430).

14. Whittaker, *Tatian* (n. 3), renders it as "hostile devices"; J. E. Ryland, "Tatian's Address to the Greeks," in *The Ante-Nicene Fathers*, vol. 2 (1884; reprint,

Grand Rapids: Eerdmans), as "trickeries"; and Osborne, "Tatian's Discourse" (n. 3), as "counterfeits," the latter of which I find preferable.

15. See especially Tatian, *Oratio* 4, 5, 11, 12, 17, 19.

16. Herbert Butterfield asserts that it "has always been realised in the main tradition of Christianity that if the Word was made flesh, matter can never be regarded as evil in itself." Herbert Butterfield, *Christianity and History* (New York: Scribner's, 1949), 121. D. S. Wallace-Hadrill adds, "If there is any true continuity between the earthly and the risen bodies, then matter, of which the former is composed, cannot be intrinsically evil." D. S. Wallace-Hadrill, *The Greek Patristic View of Nature* (New York: Barnes and Noble, 1968), 71. Tatian, insofar as he is known through the *Oratio,* is in full agreement with both of these statements of historical orthodoxy.

17. Hawthorne, "Tatian" (n. 3), 174.

18. Tatian, *Oratio* 12.3.

19. Ibid., 8–11.

20. Whittaker adds parenthetically, "i.e. erring" to convey the force of *planē-tōn* in the clause *anti planētōn daimonōn.* Tatian was probably playing with the common expression *planētes asteres.*

21. Tatian, *Oratio* 9.2.

22. Ibid., 16–17. Arthur Darby Nock remarks, "It is significant that Tatian, while ridiculing mythology, directs his serious attacks against astrology and magic." Arthur Darby Nock, *Early Gentile Christianity and Its Hellenistic Background* (New York: Harper and Row, 1964), 3 n. 2.

23. Whittaker translates *apollumenon* as "killed."

24. Whittaker's translation reads "there."

25. Tatian, *Oratio* 17.2–3.

26. On which see Ludwig Edelstein, "Greek Medicine in its Relation to Religion and Magic," in *Ancient Medicine: Selected Papers of Ludwig Edelstein,* ed. Owsei and C. Lilian Temkin (Baltimore: Johns Hopkins Press, 1967), 205–46; Temkin, *Hippocrates* (n. 7), 123–25, 234–35; and Vivian Nutton, "From Medical Certainty to Medical Amulets: Three Aspects of Ancient Therapeutics," *Clio Medica* 22 (1991): 19.

27. Tatian, *Oratio* 18.1.

28. See the text to nn. 14–15, supra.

29. Tatian, *Oratio* 18.1–2.

30. Exod. 7:11 (bis), 7:22, 8:7, 8:18, 9:11, 22:18; Deut. 18:10; 4 Kings 9:22; 2 Chron. 33:6; Ps. 57:5 (bis); Isa. 47:9, 47:12; Jer. 34:9; Dan. 2:2; Mic. 5:12; Nah. 3:4; Mal. 3:5.

31. Gal. 5:20; Rev. 9:21, 18:23, 21:8, 22:15.

32. There were several other *schemata* of the "parts of medicine." See the excellent discussion by Heinrich von Staden, *Herophilus: The Art of Medicine in Early Alexandria* (Cambridge: Cambridge University Press, 1989), 89–114.

33. Celsus, for example, charged Herophilus and his followers with excessive and irresponsible use of drug therapy. See ibid., 400, 419–20. Such accusations probably were not uncommon.

34. Scribonius Largus, proem to *Compositiones,* in J. S. Hamilton, "Scribonius Largus on the Medical Profession," *Bull. Hist. Med.* 60 (1986): 213.

35. Ibid.

36. Ibid., 214. It is interesting to note that centuries earlier Plato, *Republic* 459C, had distinguished between inferior physicians who used only dietetics and regimen and the "more manly" physicians who were able to apply drugs properly.

37. Temkin, in a context different from his discussion of Tatian, maintains that "the little pharmacological text by Scribonius Largus is best understood as written for laymen, with a preface on the ethics of medicine and the use of drugs intended to dispel Roman fear of poisoning and of physicians' experimenting on the patient." Temkin, *Hippocrates* (n. 7), 61; see also 40 n. 10. For the motif of the physician as poisoner, see Vivian Nutton, "Murders and Miracles: Lay Attitudes to Medicine in Classical Antiquity," in *Patients and Practitioners: Lay Perceptions of Medicine in Pre-Industrial Society*, ed. Roy Porter (Cambridge: Cambridge University Press, 1985), 23–53.

38. Tatian, *Oratio* 18.2.

39. Whittaker translates *kataskeuastēs* as "constructor."

40. Tatian, *Oratio* 4.2.

41. Ibid., 7.1.

42. Ibid., 12.1.

43. Ibid., 13.1.

44. Ibid., 13.1–3.

45. Ibid., 15.1.

46. I.e., the Stoics.

47. This work is not extant.

48. Tatian, *Oratio* 15.1–3.

49. Origen, *Contra Celsum* 4.85–87.

50. Robert M. Grant, *Miracle and Natural Law in Graeco-Roman and Early Christian Thought* (Amsterdam: North-Holland, 1952), 99.

51. Grant, *Greek Apologists* (n. 2), 131.

52. This subject excited the imagination of various philosophical schools and some classical authors, e.g., Aelian, *De natura animalium* 5.39 and 5.46; Plutarch, *Moralia* 991E-F; and Sextus Empiricus, *Pyrrhōneioi hypotypōseis* 1.57 and 1.70–72.

53. Tatian, *Oratio* 18.2. Tatian, incidentally, treated the Cynics with a bemused contempt: "You, sir, behaving like a dog—you have no knowledge of God and have sunk to imitating irrational creatures!" Tatian, *Oratio* 25.1.

54. Cf. Tatian, *Oratio* 15.1–2.

55. Ibid., 18.2.

56. Ibid., 4.2.

57. Ibid., 12.4.

58. Ibid., 21.3.

59. Hamilton, "Scribonius" (n. 34), 213.

60. Ibid., 215.

61. Ibid., 212. He goes on to say, "And indeed, I believe that this is a reasonable description, for it is possible to produce such a divine touch, and thus those drugs stand out which have been tested by use and experiment" (212–13).

62. Plutarch, *Moralia* 663B–C. The text reads "Erasistratus." Von Staden (*Herophilus* [n. 32], 417), following Max Wellmann and Karl Deichgräber, emends to "Herophilus."

63. Ibid.
64. Edelstein, "Greek Medicine" (n. 26), 231.
65. Tatian, *Oratio* 18.2
66. Ryland, "Tatian's Address" (n. 14), 73.
67. Osborne, *Tatian's Discourse* (n. 3), 200.
68. Temkin, *Hippocrates* (n. 7), 121.
69. Ibid., 121 n. 81. Whittaker's comment seems to me rather farfetched: "It is tempting to think, as Wilamowitz suggested, that personal knowledge of the great medical spa at Pergamum, birthplace of Galen, and a favourite resort of the hypochondriac Aelius Aristides, may have added animus to his polemic against the successful doctor who is called 'benefactor'" (*Tatian* [n. 3], xiii).
70. Tatian, *Oratio* 2.1.
71. Ibid., 3.1. We have no way of determining the extent, if any, of Tatian's awareness that, as von Staden says, "Hippocratic physicians too made fairly liberal use of the excrement of pigeons, poultry, goats, cows, donkeys, and mules, prescribing the external application of some and the internal consumption (in potions) of others." Von Staden, *Herophilus* (n. 32), 19.
72. Galen, *De compositione medicamentorum secundum locus* 6.8. The translation is von Staden's. Von Staden, *Herophilus* (n. 32), 418.
73. See Fridolf Kudlien, "Galen's Religious Belief," in *Galen: Problems and Prospects,* ed. Vivian Nutton (London: Wellcome Institute for the History of Medicine, 1981), 117–30 (nn. 78 and 89 for references).
74. Ibid., 126.
75. See A. J. Festugière, "L'expérience religieuse du médecin Thessalos," in *Hermétisme et mystique païenne* (Paris: Aubier-Montaigne, 1967), 162; Arthur Darby Nock, *Conversion: The Old and the New in Religion from Alexander the Great to Augustine of Hippo* (Oxford: Oxford University Press, 1933), 108–9; and Peter Brown, *The Making of Late Antiquity* (Cambridge: Harvard University Press, 1978), 63–64.
76. Quoted by Temkin, *Hippocrates* (n. 7), 123, from Hans Dieter Betz, ed., *The Greek Magical Papyri in Translation* (Chicago: University of Chicago Press, 1986), 7–8.
77. Tatian does not deny the efficacy of drugs. In a section well after his discussion of pharmacology, he writes, "Even if you are healed by drugs (I grant you this by way of excuse *[kata syngnōmēn]*), you should make your witness to God. For the world still drags us down, and it is weakness which makes me turn to matter." Tatian, *Oratio* 20.1. Tatian's nosology was primarily naturalistic rather than demonic. See Tatian, *Oratio* 16.3, 18.2–3. 19.3, 20.2.
78. Ibid., 18.2.

SEVEN

Caring and Curing in the Medieval Catholic Tradition

The date that marks the beginning of Roman Catholicism is a matter of some debate. Surely its roots go back to the earliest decades of Christianity, but the distinct identity of that enormously complex structure that was medieval Catholicism developed only gradually. In 380, in response to the teaching known as Arianism, which held that Christ was a created being neither co-equal nor co-eternal with God the Father, the Roman emperor Theodosius I decreed that all people of the empire must adhere to that religion "which the divine Peter the Apostle transmitted to the Romans . . . that is followed by the Pontiff Damasus and by Peter, bishop of Alexandria." That religion was the historical Christianity that had, during the preceding centuries, formulated among numerous other dogmas the doctrine of the Trinity as finally expressed in the Nicene Creed (325). Damasus is significant as the first bishop of Rome to articulate the conviction that the holder of that office was the direct successor to the apostle Peter, upon whom it was claimed that Christ had said that he would build his church (Matt. 16:18–19). This principle, which was the foundation of the papacy, was even more forcefully advanced by two subsequent bishops of Rome, Leo I (440–61) and Gelasius I (492–96), the latter of whom insisted that the bishop of Rome (later known as the pope) had the authority to judge secular rulers but was himself subject to no man.

The fundamental feature of the Catholic Church in the Middle Ages was its nearly complete identification with organized society in western

Europe, at least in theory if not always in practice. The church became possibly the most thoroughly integrated religious system in human history. It was not a voluntary association because, from the late fourth century, all members of organized society in the West, except for a small number of Jews who were tolerated and a few heretics who were excluded from society and intermittently persecuted, had to be part of it. Only obedient believers could enjoy full rights within it and, consequently, rights within the various secular states of western Europe, whose relationship with the church was often fraught with tensions and conflicting claims of authority and jurisdiction. As many scholars have observed, the church was "the ark of salvation in a sea of destruction." Being in this ark provided the only assurance of meaning and purpose in this life and confidence in respect to the next, which was the exclusive possession of the ark's occupants. All of life, indeed the entire cosmos and people's place within it, could be understood only with reference to the church, which had the obligation to direct and regulate the details of human life. The medieval Catholic Church had as its head a single spiritual and temporal power, the pope, who sometimes claimed ultimate and absolute power within western European society.

Pope Gregory I (590–604) gave to the medieval papacy its distinct character, claiming universal (catholic) jurisdiction over all Christendom and proclaiming a Christian commonwealth in which the pope and the clergy were to exercise authority and responsibility for ordering society. He was a significant figure also for being the first pope zealously to support monasticism and to stress the cult of saints and relics, ascetic virtues, and demonology, which were the most distinctive features of early medieval Catholicism. Additionally he was active in sponsoring missionary activity to the pagans, sending Augustine (who was later consecrated as archbishop of Canterbury) to convert the pagan English in 596.

The Middle Ages began as classical civilization was nearing collapse in western Europe and ended when the conversion of western Europe to Christianity was nearly complete. At the beginning of the fourth century, Christianity in the West was a religion of a small minority. By the end of that century, most of the aristocracy and the urban population had been converted. It took centuries more, however, before Christianity meaningfully penetrated the peasant population of western Europe, who, even when ostensibly converted, still continued to practice some form of ancestral paganism, however modified by Christian influence. The barbarian invasions of western Europe in the fifth century complicated the life of the church. The barbarians were almost all pagan. Many were converted to the Arian form of Christianity; others were gradually converted to Catholicism through missionary activity. Arians were finally brought into the Catholic fold by the end of the sixth century.

The centuries from about 500 to 1050 were, for the most part, chaotic and unsettled in western Europe, with the notable exception of the time of the so-called Carolingian Renaissance. Poverty, famine, plague, disorder, and commercial atrophy typified much of the early Middle Ages. Numerous monasteries provided a symbol of stability in the midst of instability, an image of eternal order in a world of change; when supplemented by local parishes, they represented the intrusion of the licit supernatural into the life of a society riddled by the reality of the evil supernatural. It was an age in which the ostensibly miraculous was common and expected, but never any less awe-inspiring on that account. The locus of the licit supernatural was the cult of saints and relics.

The high Middle Ages (1050–1300) were marked by enormous economic and religious changes. The period opened with a rapidly accelerating growth of economic development: the rise of urbanization, colonization on all frontiers, expanding commercial enterprise within western Europe, and trade with the East, stimulated in part by the Crusades. It was a time of significant population growth, an age in which numerous complex problems produced by rapid social change gave rise to the need for more sophisticated solutions than old secular and religious mechanisms were able to provide. Expert knowledge and competence were being demanded in every sphere of life. Education was still dominated by the clergy but was increasing dramatically, especially owing to the creation and growth of universities. Theological debate stimulated by renewed philosophical analysis captured the minds of intellectual giants, for example, Thomas Aquinas (1225–74). Canon law, which was virtually in a state of chaos at the beginning of this period, had developed into a vastly complex and intricate science before 1300.

Although the aspects of life controlled by direct appeal to the supernatural were decreasing in number, the authority of the church over the individual was broadening through its increasingly efficient mechanisms of moral coercion and social control. The catalyst of much of this development was the papacy. This period opened with popes who were zealous to put into practice the papal authority that had been usually present only in theory, and closed with a succession of lawyer-popes, who were the embodiment of a strong papal monarchy.

The late Middle Ages (1300–1545) began with a strong papal monarchy that may have seemed indestructible but was soon weakened significantly. Papal hegemony was decreased by the rise of strong national monarchies headed by kings who coveted absolute jurisdiction over their lands, which were inhabited by people whose sense of national and ethnic identity was increasing. In 1309 the papacy moved to Avignon, France, where it remained until 1377, appearing to many as simply a tool of the French monarch. The Avignonese Papacy led to the Great Schism, lasting from 1378 to 1417, a time that saw two, and then (from 1409) three, concurrent lines of popes. All claimed exclusive rights to the papal office and excommunicated each other. By the time this division ended, the prestige and authority of the papacy had been enormously weakened. Shortly thereafter, the effects of the Italian Renaissance were evidenced in the beginning of a line of "Renaissance popes." Some were pious and distinguished humanists; others were of very questionable spiritual qualifications and moral integrity.

In 1348–49 a plague called the Black Death ravaged Europe, killing at least a quarter of the population. The impact of this and subsequent epidemics of pestilential disease, combined with numerous social, economic, and political developments, contributed to a laicization of European society. The towns and cities became hotbeds of dissent, both political and religious. Varieties of subversive religious movements surfaced. Corruption in the medieval church, both real and alleged, became increasingly a matter of concern to a growing number of clerics and laymen. Attempts to remove certain abuses, periodically initiated by various popes and by some monastic movements, met usually with limited success. Other reform efforts within the church were unsuccessful because those seeking reform did not limit their efforts to dealing with the spiritual and moral laxity so prevalent within the church, but also sought to change some of the theology of the church that seemed to contradict Scripture. Such were John Wycliffe (ca. 1329–84), Jan Hus (1373–1415), and Martin Luther (1483–1546), the last of whom in great part perpetrated the Protestant Reformation, which brought to an end the medieval Catholic Church, a structure that had exercised nearly exclusive authority in religion in western Europe for a millennium. The reaction of the Catholic Church to the Protestant Reformation was the Counter Reformation, through which the church removed many abuses that had been weakening it internally and created a structure of practice and belief embodied in the decrees of the Council of Trent, which convened in 1545.

The Early Middle Ages (500–1050)

The Conversion of Western Europe and the Residues of Paganism

Early in the fourth century (313), official persecution of Christians by the imperial government ceased. By the end of the century (391), Christianity became the official religion of the empire, and all public forms of paganism were outlawed. That which had been the religion of a small minority in the western half of the empire now became the religion of all, at least in form. Church and state joined hands, the latter in an effort to suppress, and the former in an attempt to replace with Christian ideas and practices, whatever expressions of paganism remained.

The nature of Christian practices and even some beliefs undergirding those practices seem to have changed in late antiquity. It is a commonplace to attribute this change to the entry into the church, after the legalization of Christianity, of a vast number of pagans, who brought with them a rich diversity of pagan superstitions that were soon clothed in quasi-Christian garb. In this view a small theological elite, frustrated in their efforts to suppress the superstitious beliefs and practices of this horde of "converts," sought to accommodate, adapt, and gradually Christianize their religious expression. This interpretation, although correct to a limited extent, is inaccurate and simplistic. Before the Christianization of the empire, indeed even by the late third century, discernible changes had begun to occur in the Mediterranean ethos, affecting Christians and pagans alike. These changes affected people's perception, understanding, and definition of the supernatural and their relationship and access to it.[1] New relationships were evident both at a sociopolitical level, as the structure of late Roman society was undergoing enormous change, and at the religious level, as contact with the supernatural assumed new forms. New religious expressions emerged as people sought to relate to bewilderingly varied manifestations of the supernatural that were an integral part of even their most mundane affairs. The church clearly distinguished between the licit and illicit supernatural. And any contact with the supernatural was illicit if the church did not dispense it.

While the battle against the residue of paganism in the Mediterranean ethos of late antiquity was being waged by state and church, the western half of the empire was slowly falling to incursions of primarily Germanic barbarians, some of whom had already been converted to the Arian heresy and were, within two centuries, to be won over to Catholicism. The rest were pagans who were gradually converted by Catholic missionaries. In spite of enormous diversity among the coverted barbarian peoples of Europe during the early Middle Ages, two factors created a significant degree of homogeneity. First, all had their distinct ancestral religions, that, although greatly varied, possessed commonalities of thought and expression typical of folk paganism generally. This folk paganism, essentially pantheism, was so much a part of the very rhythm of their lives that it remained, for most of them, a vitally real, if officially suppressed and experientially submerged, current of their subconscious being and identity. Secondly, all had in common the same alternative to their folk paganism. That was Roman Catholicism, which consistently declared their folk paganism to be both real and evil, and could tolerate no alternative to itself. Accordingly, the church sought to channel their individual and communal impulses and wants into sources of actualization and fulfillment that were within the ordered structure of Catholic liturgy, sacraments, and the cult of saints and relics.

There were of course some, who usually became clerics, who embraced Christianity with such fervency and commitment that they utterly repudiated all association with their ancestral paganism, seeing all folk religious practice as magical and demonic. In a sense it is proper to speak of the clergy as an elite. But without significant qualifications, so to speak would be grossly misleading, for, when reading the literature written during the early Middle Ages, one is struck by "the common credulity and lack of critical sense which underlay the observances of literate and illiterate alike."[2] We may call the clergy a theological elite, an intellectual elite (especially because nearly the only literate people were clerics), and, to an extent, a social elite. But their eliteness was not manifest in their belief in a practice of religion that was, at a functional level, theological while that of the masses was superstitious, that was sophisticated while that of the masses was vulgar. Granted, the former had a theologically reasoned structure that could not be articulated in the latter; but at a functional level there was often very little significant difference except that the former was licit while the latter was not, and the licit declared the illicit to be evil and fought against it vigorously. While the early medieval church never denied the reality of the supernatural power that undergirded folk paganism, it did seek to meet the needs of pagan converts by substituting beliefs and practices that had already become part of the Christian experience in the West. It also permitted certain strictly pagan practices to continue as long as they were conducted in the vicinity of churches and not in traditional sites such as sacred groves.

The conversion of western Europe during the early Middle Ages hinged on combating one form of the supernatural with another. Gaining the religious loyalty of pagans depended upon missionaries convincing them that Christianity's power to aid them was greater than that of their pantheistic folk paganism. And the greatest display of Christianity's power was in the miracles worked by the cult of saints and relics. One of the most spectacular manifestations of this cult was the shrine of Saint Martin at Tours. Between 563 and 565, Nicetus, bishop of Trier, wrote to Clotsinda, Catholic queen of the Arian Lombards, urging her to help win her Arian husband, King Alboin, to the Catholic religion. Among other things, he suggested:

If the King chooses let him send his men to [Gaul], to the Lord Martin [at Tours], at his feast . . . where every day we see the blind receive their sight, the deaf their hearing, and the dumb their speech. What shall I say of lepers of of many others, who, no matter with what sickness they are afflicted, are healed there year after year? . . . What shall I say of the [shrines of the] Lord Bishops Germanus [of Auxerre], Hilary [of Poiters], or Lupus [of Troyes], where so many wonders occur every day, so great that I cannot express them in words: where the afflicted (those having demons) are suspended and whirled round in the air and confess the [power of the] Lords I have named? You have heard how your grandmother . . . led the Lord Clovis to the Catholic Law, and how, since he was a most astute man, he was unwilling to agree to it until he knew it was true. When he saw that the things I have spoken of were proved he humbly prostrated himself at the threshold of the Lord Martin [at Tours] and promised to be baptized without delay.[3]

Condemnation and Accommodation

The cult of saints and relics was the single most important force in the conversion of western Europe. The literature of the early Middle Ages is rife with examples of miracles wrought through the relics of the saints. In 601 Pope Gregory I wrote to Augustine of Canterbury, a missionary whom he had sent to England, congratulating him on his successes in converting through his miracles the Anglo-Saxons, whose souls "are drawn by outward miracles to inward grace."[4] Gregory recognized that when pagans were converted to Christianity, the process of transformation was often both precarious and lengthy. He wrote to Mellitus, who was en route to England, that "it is doubtless impossible to cut out everything at once from their stubborn minds: just as the man who is attempting to climb to the highest place, rises by steps and degrees and not by leaps." Accordingly, Gregory ordered that their idols should be destroyed but that their temples should be allowed to stand, purified with holy water, and furnished with altars and relics, so that

they should be changed from the worship of devils to the service of the true God. When this people see that their shrines are not destroyed they will be able to banish error from their hearts and be more ready to come to the places they are familiar with, but now recognizing and worshipping the true God. And because they are in the habit of slaughtering much cattle as sacrifices to devils, some solemnity ought to be given them in exchange for this. So on the day of the dedication or the festivals of the holy martyrs, whose relics are deposited there, let them make themselves huts from the branches of trees around the churches which have been converted out of shrines, and let them celebrate the solemnity with religious feasts. Do not let them sacrifice animals to the devil, but let them slaughter animals for their own food to the praise of God, and let them give thanks to the Giver of all things for his bountiful provision.[5]

Gregory's letter advocated both condemnation and accommodation. While accommodation involved a degree of condescension, condemnation did not, and throughout the early Middle Ages, condemnation of pagan practices was incessant.[6]

During the frequent outbreaks of plague that afflicted Europe in sixteen waves from 541 to 767, and especially during early episodes, people fled to pagan alternatives.[7] In the British Isles, Cuthbert (ca. 634–87) sought to convert the people "from a life of foolish habits to a love of heavenly joys. For many of them also at the time of the plague, forgetting the sacred mystery of the faith into which they had been initiated, took to the delusive cures of idolatry"[8] In France, 150 years later, Jonas of Orleans complained that people hastened to sorcerers when sick.[9]

Attempts to deal with relapses into paganism or participation in pagan practices varied. Early medieval law was concerned with any unauthorized religious or superstitious practice. Like Roman law,[10] the secular codes of the early Middle Ages adamantly forbade the use of malicious magic. But they differed from Roman law in prohibiting a wide variety of pagan practices such as "nocturnal sacrifices to devils," "infamous rites," going to a soothsayer for divination, incantation, performing sacrilege generally, worshipping at "a tree which the rustics call holy and at springs."[11] One of Charlemagne's laws specified some thirty superstitious practices as illicit;[12] another directed that "every bishop carefully visit his diocese each year and that he take pains . . . to prohibit pagan celebrations and diviners or soothsayers or auguries, amulets, incantations, and all kinds of pagan filth."[13] A half century earlier, Pope Gregory II had commended Bishop Boniface to the Christians of Germany. Boniface's mission was to deal with those who had been "led astray by the wiles of the devil and now serve idols under the guise of the Christian religion." Boniface was enjoined to enlighten them with his preaching.[14] Twenty years later (742) Boniface presided over a church council that decreed that "in accordance with the canons each bishop should take care . . . that the people of God should not do pagan things but should abandon and repudiate all the filthy practices of the gentiles, be it sacrifices to the dead or divination or immolation of sacrificial animals, things which ignorant people do in the pagan way next to churches in the name of the holy martyrs or confessors."[15]

Numerous church synods and councils had addressed the problem of continuing pagan practices. Walter Ullmann writes that the conciliar "decrees against superstition are so numerous that one is justified in the assumption that [the practices that they repeatedly prohibited] were general and widespread." Commenting on the motivation behind these conciliar actions, he asserts that the promulgators of such decrees "cared for what may be termed the public health of society, public health understood not in terms of physical well-being, but in terms of protecting and if necessary immunizing and inoculating the mind of the people against infectious diseases of a pandemic kind."[16]

Throughout the Middle Ages, the well-being of the corporate body of Christ was, above all else, the major concern of those who sought to protect the community from all incursions of contaminating influence, whether of paganism (including magic in its manifold varieties) or heresy. For salvation was only through the church; all else led to damnation. For the hierarchy of the church, and for those clerics about whom we have information, well-being found expression in personal piety, self-denial, ascetic practices, missionary zeal, and a deep pastoral concern for the well-being of the large numbers of people, mostly peasants, whose conception of well-being was significantly different from their own. Tension between these two groups arose from their markedly discordant conceptions of well-being. The well-being that was common probably to the majority of the laity during the early Middle Ages was essentially mundane. But this mundane sphere was intimately connected with the supernatural that permeated all aspects of their lives. Their well-being depended upon a sustained harmony with their whole environment, a harmony of well-being congruous with the very rhythm of their lives. When this harmony was marred by any cacophony, it could be restored only through rituals and magical manipulations that had proven efficacious in bringing their lives back into harmony with the properly integrated order for their world. Sometimes the church, through its liturgy and sacraments, and especially through the cult of saints and relics, was able to contribute to this process. But it was seldom able to satisfy the deepest cravings of the peasant population for sustained periods; life was too tumultuous and uncertain during these centuries. For them, well-being was the state of being in the right relationship with the totality of their environment. The well-being that Christianity offered was to be in a right relationship with God, which depended upon being in a right relationship with the church. Although the church provided mechanisms for sustaining and restoring equilibrium at a mundane level, the ultimate orientation and objective was always with a view to eternity, whereas the deepest yearnings of the peasants were predominantly temporal. Hence the tension illustrated by the efforts of the clergy, law, and councils to deal with the continued recurrence of illicit practices.

Sin and Penance, Sickness and Healing

Although this tension endured throughout the Middle Ages, at least in remote areas, it gradually diminished, particularly in the last century of the primitive age of medieval Catholicism. This process was aided by the organization of rural parishes (effective in few areas before the tenth century),[17] which made possible relatively close contact between the clergy and the majority of the people generally. The people needed to be protected from themselves, from Satan, from all evil influences, from sin itself. This was accomplished in part through pastoral teaching and exhortation. Even more intimate, however, was the personal encounter of clergy with laity in systematic efforts to identify and deal with specific sins. These efforts took the form of interrogation by the clergy, and confession, repentance, and penance by the laity. The most useful tool for this process was the penitential literature that was produced in abundance during the early Middle Ages. These handbooks of penance essentially were guides for clerics that enumerated and discussed a wide and imaginative variety of sins, for which specific acts of penance were prescribed. Probably more than any other, sexual sins aroused the attention of the authors of these handbooks. Adultery, fornication, sodomy, homosexuality, masturbation, and bestiality were treated with great thoroughness.[18]

Significantly less attention was paid to categories of sin other than sexual, but concern with superstitious practices was a strong contender for second place in these handbooks. Wilfrid Bonser writes of the penitentials that "the magical practices especially attacked may be divided into the following categories: (1) idolatry and worship of 'demons' in general; (2) the cult of the dead; (3) the worship of nature (trees, wells, stones, fire, etc.); (4) pagan calendar customs and festivals; (5) witchcraft and sorcery; (6) augury and divination; and (7) astrology."[19] Beginning with *The Penitential of Finnian* (ca. 525–50), the prescribing of penance for any kind of pagan practice became a constant feature.[20] With some regularity, pagan methods of healing or preserving health were mentioned. The placing of a child upon a roof or into (or on) an oven for the cure of a fever was frequently condemned.[21] The oven (or hearth) was the place where the guardian spirits of the house dwelt; spirits who might aid healing also resided on the roof.[22] One penitential condemns a woman's tasting her husband's blood as a remedy,[23] and another prescribes penance for drinking blood or urine, probably consumed for health-related reasons.[24] Two penitentials condemn the practice of burning grain at the place where a man has died, for preserving or restoring the health of the living.[25] One also assigns penance if on account of illness a person has bathed below a mill. The penance is much more severe if this act was accompanied by an incantation.[26] The same penitential also deals with the sin of uttering incantations while collecting medicinal herbs. Instead of incantations, one should recite the Creed or the Lord's Prayer while gathering the herbs.[27] Three centuries later, the same advice appears in *The Corrector and Physician* of Burchard of Worms.[28] In this work there are, among numerous interrogations regarding superstitious practices, the following, concerning sickness and healing:

Have you come to any place to pray other than a church or other religious place which your bishop or your priest showed you, that is, either to springs or to stones or to trees or to crossroads, and there in reverence for the place lighted a candle or a torch or carried there bread or any offering or eaten there or sought there any healing of body or mind? If you have done or consented to such things, you shall do penance for three years on the appointed fast days. Have you done what some do when they are visiting any sick person? When they approach the house where the sick person lies, if they find a stone lying nearby, they turn the stone over and look in the place where the stone was lying [to see] if there is anything living under it, and if they find there a worm or a fly or an ant or anything that moves, then they aver that the sick person will recover. But if they find there nothing that moves, they say he will die. If you have done or believed in this you shall do penance for twenty days on bread and water.[29]

Only two penitentials referred to permitted means of healing. The prologue to *The Penitential of Cummean* (ca. 650) quotes James 5:14–16, suggesting anointing with oil for healing.[30] The so-called *Roman Penitential of Halitgar* (ca. 830) included a prayer to be said over the sick: "O God, Who gave to Your servant Hezekiah an extension of life of fifteen years, so also may Your greatness raise up Your servant from the bed of sickness unto health. Through our Lord Jesus Christ."[31] Because the penitentials were concerned with sin, it is not remarkable that they had so little occasion to speak of licit means of healing. It would not be surprising, however, if they had much to say about sickness, especially given the assumed relationship of sin and sickness in medieval Christian thought. This, however, is not the case, for the penitentials mentioned sickness very little. One stipulated that any individual who became ill during penance should be permitted to receive the sacrament of communion.[32] There is no indication that the sickness was regarded as a punishment for sin, because the penitent was to resume penance if he or she recovered from his or her illness. Nothing here was even implied about causality.

The penitentials addressed the issue of causality only when insanity led to suicide.[33] *The Penitential of Theodore* (668–90) specified that "if a man is vexed by the devil . . . and slays himself, there may be some reason to pray for him if he was formerly religious."[34] Other reasons for insanity leading to suicide were then given: despair, fear, unknown reasons, or a sudden seizure.[35] *The Burgundian Penitential* (ca. 700–725) referred to wizards taking away the minds of men by the invocation of demons or by rendering them mad.[36] Here the emphasis was on the sin of practicing wizardry, whereas in *The Penitential of Theodore* the concern was with the sin of self-destruction, while insanity was only a mitigating factor. Because it is so common to assume that in the early Middle Ages demonic causality was accepted for most disease, and certainly for mental illness, such natural causes as despair, fear, sudden seizure, and "unknown reasons" may surprise us. Such explanations, however, occur with some frequency. For instance, when Richer of Rheims wrote his *Historia* between 991 and 998, he thus described the death of King Odo: "On account of his extreme nervousness he began to suffer from insomnia, the aggravation of which brought about the loss of reason . . . He died from what some call mania, others madness."[37] And in 1023, Fulbert of Chartres, when comparing the functions of priests and physicians, said that "it is a physician's duty to offer those who are suffering from depression, insanity, or any other illness what he has learned in the exercise of his art."[38] Jerome Kroll is undoubtedly right when he says of this period that "mental and spiritual illnesses were attributed as much to overwork, overeating, and overindulgence in sexual activity as to climatic conditions, magic spells, and demonic possession."[39] There is, however, considerable ambiguity in the literature. This ambiguity arises from two different sources. First, there was much imprecision in identifying the causes of mental illness. The second source of ambiguity is the failure of the modern reader to enter sufficiently into the early medieval structure of reality, in which ultimate and proximate causality may be spoken of in the same breath without any distinction being made, and an intermediate (usually demonic) causality mingled in with the former two. Any one of the three may be mentioned as the cause of a particular condition, and taken by the modern reader as the author's perceived sole cause, whereas the choice of that cause was simply determined by the author's desire to emphasize one, with no intention of making it appear exclusive. This applies not only to considerations of madness but also, indeed even more so, to sickness generally.

A degree of demonic causality was seen in many conditions, and some people may have attributed nearly every adverse condition to demons. But the sources adequately demonstrate that on the whole God was viewed as the ultimate dispenser of human suffering, including sickness. As a general rule, when early medieval sources mentioned direct demonic involvement, which they frequently did, the condition was clearly regarded as possession, whether accompanied by sickness or not. They delighted in relating stories of exorcisms, but they were equally eager to tell of healings through relics, healings from which exorcism is absent. Furthermore, the most holy of the saints could not conceivably have been possessed by demons, but yet were frequently ill; some indeed seemed to gain a high degree of sanctity through their sicknesses.

Another commonplace encountered in modern assessments of the early Middle Ages is the assertion that early medieval people saw sin as the cause of most sickness. Here there is room for much confusion because the relationship of sin with sickness can appear at three different levels. First, sin was certainly regarded by early medieval authors as the cause of sickness in the sense that without sin there would have been no material evil. This, although not expressed, was an underlying assumption of the sources. Second, one's own general sinfulness was often given as the cause of one's own sicknesses. Third, sickness, it was thought, might result from specific sin. This last statement is very seldom encountered except in denunciations of and warnings to entire communities, and then the emphasis was often on general moral laxity, which makes it nearly indistinguishable from the second category. We should also note that it is one thing to maintain that a person is sick as a punishment for a specific sin to which he or she is obstinately and tenaciously clinging, but it is quite another matter to attribute one's own sickness to one's general sinfulness and see the sickness as part of God's punitive and refining process.

There is, in the literature, a definite appreciation of God's hand in a Christian's suffering and of the salutary effects of sickness in the Christian's life. Pope Gregory I, in his pastoral handbook, wrote that "the sick are to be admonished to realise that they are sons of God by the very fact that the scourge of discipline chastises them." They were also exhorted to "preserve the virtue of patience."[40] We must bear in mind that the concept of discipline here was by no means limited to punishment. Indeed, the predominant emphasis in the term was on training or edification. For example, Bede, a contemporary of the events he described, said of the Abbess Aethelburh: "Now in order that her strength, like the apostle's, might be made perfect in weakness, she was suddenly afflicted with a most serious bodily disease and for nine years was sorely tried, under the good providence of our Redeemer, so that any traces of sin remaining among her virtues through ignorance or carelessness might be burnt away by the fires of prolonged suffering."[41] Aethelburh died of her disease. Bede also saw benefit derived from acute conditions. For example, he wrote that the merits of the saintly Germanus were increased by the suffering caused by an injury. Germanus was miraculously healed after a short period.[42] Bede's account of the suffering of Bishop Benedict and one of his colleagues is typical of the attitudes expressed in the literature:

And not long after, Benedict also began to be wearied by the assault of illness. That the virtue of patience might be added, to give conclusive proof of such great zeal for religion, Divine Mercy laid them both up in bed by temporal illness that, after sickness had been conquered by death, God might restore them with the endless rest of heavenly peace and light. Sigfrid, punished . . . by long internal suffering, drew toward his last day, and Benedict, during three years, gradually became so paralyzed that all his lower limbs were quite dead . . . to exercise him in the virtue of patience. Both men sought in their suffering ways to give thanks to their Creator, and always to be occupied with the praises of God and with teaching the brethren.[43]

Such attitudes, of course, were not typical of all people during the early Middle Ages. Some might admire the spiritual fortitude manifested in the sanctified suffering of a select, holy few whose actions were much more admired than emulated. Although the well-being of these few might be enhanced by suffering, the perceived well-being of the semi-Christianized pagans of the early Middle Ages was destroyed or at least disrupted by sickness. Their eager, indeed frantic, quest for the healing that was itself a restoration of well-being indicates that their sense of wellness was tied to temporal and material considerations.

In their efforts to deal with the spiritual needs of the majority, the clerical minority sought to maintain a delicate balance between meeting the people's temporal and material wants, on the one hand, and meeting their eternal and spiritual needs, on the other. There was a long and evolving tradition of physical healing in Christianity. There was an equally long tradition in Christianity to provide for spiritual healing; indeed, the very essence of Christianity had that as its goal. This tradition also assumed new forms, or at least was manifested in new emphases, in late antiquity and even more so in the early Middle Ages, when the expectation of Christ's return, which had always been present to some degree in Christianity, assumed an air of impending destruction and doom precipitated by God's wrath. While the mechanisms for physical healing were exploited in missionary activities and in pastoral efforts to keep the flock from reverting to pagan healing methods, the message of impending doom was proclaimed in an attempt to wean the flock from the temporal to the eternal, and from the material to the spiritual, to realign their well-being from a present horizontal to a future vertical orientation. Plague proved to be most useful in this effort. We have noted earlier that Europe was afflicted by sixteen waves of plague from 541 to 767, during the early occurrences of which Christians often relapsed into pagan practices. But plague was a two-edged sword, and in the long run the effect was less to stimulate people to concern for the well-being of their bodies than to direct their concern to escaping the eternal consequences of the wrath of God. Plague "mainly had the effect of making them more amenable to certain Christian beliefs and practices. Seen as one element in a whole set of calamities and signs, the plague settled in people's minds a concrete expectation of the Last Judgement. . . . [It] explained calamities as retribution for collective sin, instilled notions of a wrathful God . . . and gave rise to an apocalyptic and millenarian mentality."[44] Pope Gregory I was obsessed by the plague. Gregory assumed the papacy during a time of plague (590) and "preached a sermon . . . declaring the plague to be a punishment from God and calling upon the people to do penance and repent of their sins. He ordered them to pray and sing psalms for three days, and at the end of that time arranged for a massive city-wide litany. . . . No less than eighty people dropped dead of the plague during the procession."[45]

About 150 years later, Bede, in his *Ecclesiastical History*, marveled that the Anglo-Saxons were not turned from their wicked ways by a devastating visitation of the plague,[46] and in his *Life of St. Cuthbert* he referred to the plague as "a blow sent by God the Creator."[47] Bede was interested not only in the theological nature of plague but also in its natural explanation. In his *De natura rerum* he asserted that plague was generated by corrupted air, and then hastened to add parenthetically that this was in accord with men's deserts.[48] Although Gregory, Bede, and churchmen generally saw the plague as punishment imposed by God, it does not follow that they also viewed those stricken by the plague as especially great sinners. When the pestilence hit Britain, Bede recorded the death of the "blessed Boisil," who had predicted three years earlier that he himself would die of the plague. Cuthbert also came down with the plague at the same time but did not die of it.[49]

Personal sanctity was no guarantee of avoiding plague. Being afflicted with it was no sign of personal sin. Plague and all other sicknesses were designed for the purpose of adjusting people's minds to eternal and spiritual verities. And repentance, regardless of the level of one's own personal sanctity, was always appropriate. But such views were not always consonant with the heart of the masses and even of some clerics. Around 829, part of southern France was hit by a very painful epidemic. Terror-stricken people bringing offerings flocked to the shrine of Fermin, hoping to be cured. No one was cured. Agobard, bishop of Lyons, "was particularly critical of the willingness of the clergy who accepted these offerings to keep them to their profit. He suggested that plagues visited on men by God required not simply payment but repentance."[50] Bishop Agobard's criticism of the lack of repentance on the part of those who hoped to be healed at the shrine of Fermin was consistent with the theology of the time. It was, however, discordant with the emphasis and orientation of the thriving cult of saints and relics during the early Middle Ages.

Miraculous Healing

As Christianity expanded northward during the early Middle Ages, the cult of saints and relics was imported into the realm of the barbarians, and for many who were converted, the bones of holy men and their relics became the very core of Christianity, taking the place of theological subtleties that they could not hope to understand. For a millennium the beliefs and miraculous practices associated with the cult of saints and relics dominated western Christianity. Each shrine and its immediate vicinity were viewed as being inhabited by a powerful presence, and it was believed that the saints were especially responsive to prayers made near their relics. For the physically ill or maimed or the demon-possessed, these shrines became a focal point for hope, comfort, healing, and a social and spiritual reintegration throughout the Middle Ages. But especially during the early Middle Ages, when the cult of saints and relics was a substitute for some of the pagan practices that had provided security by maintaining or restoring social cohesiveness, the importance of the cult is best understood in view of its identity with the welfare of the community rather than the welfare of the individual. The festival of a saint, celebrated at his shrine, as Peter Brown says, "made plain God's acceptance of the community as a whole: his mercy embraced all its disparate members, and could reintegrate all who had stood outside in the previous year. . . . The terror of illness, of blindness, of possession . . . resided in the fear that, at that high moment of solidarity, the sinner would be seen to have been placed by his affliction outside the community. . . . Hence [these were] miracles of reintegration into the community."[51] The cult of saints and relics provided stability and safety for a society in which individuals were of little importance, because individuals' meaning, security, indeed their well-being itself, derived from their oneness with their community.[52]

Although not the sole means of healing in the church's repertoire, the cult of saints and relics overshadowed all other sources of licit miraculous healing. Prayer was a mechanism for hope, but it lacked both the glamor and the efficacy of the cult of saints and relics. Even prayer itself was so frequently made to or through saints and their relics that it seems to be nearly subsumed under the cult. Another healing medium was the practice of anointing with oil for healing, as directed in James 5:14–16. The practice prescribed there appears to have received little attention in the post-apostolic church. Perhaps the earliest direct application was in a letter by Pope Innocent I in the early fifth century.[53] This letter addressed the question of whether consecrated oil could be taken home and used privately for healing (as was the practice, apparently) or could only be administered by a priest. Innocent allowed this nonclerical practice to continue, which it did for much of the early Middle Ages.[54] It is difficult to tell how popular this procedure was with the common people. When Caesarius of Arles, in the early sixth century, complained about people reverting to pagan practices when sick, he said: "How much more right and salutary it would be if they made haste to the church . . . and piously anointed themselves and their family with holy oil; and in accordance with the words of the Apostle James received not only health of the body but also pardon of their sins."[55] The connection between physical healing and the forgiveness of sin, the latter being under the exclusive province of the clergy, caused the demise of anointing with oil for the healing of the sick in medieval Catholicism. Through a rather circuitous route, the anointing of the sick for physical healing became associated in practice with penitential anointing, which could be administered only by a priest. Because penitential anointing carried with it several stipulations as to conduct (including a permanent renouncing of marital relations and of the eating of meat), it was quite understandably put off until the last moment. It became known in the tenth or eleventh century as extreme unction and for the most part lost any of its effective connection with physical healing, usurping the significance of the *viaticum*, the administration of communion to those in danger of death.

Secular Healing

We see in Caesarius' statement a desire for the cure of the body to be combined with the cure of the soul. This is by no means peculiar to him or to his time. It has been and remains at least a latent source of tension in Christianity. Spiritual models for physical healing controlled by the church were least productive of tension. Pagan or magical models obviously went beyond simple tension because they were declared illicit. The greatest tension was produced by natural or medical healing models. They were sometimes essentially neither strictly medical nor magical:

quasi-medical healing models, as it were. A good example is provided by the *De Medicamentis* of Marcellus of Bordeaux (fifth century) which was designed to show people how to treat their own ills by learning to employ the occult virtues of plants, gems, and other natural properties. This curious mixture of classical pharmacology, local herb lore, and Greco-Roman and Celtic spells offered, in the words of Peter Brown, "a model of direct and unmediated dependence of the individual on his environment."[56] And it was an environment regarded as alive with hidden but exploitable powers.[57] Basically this kind of healing effort could be something as innocent as simple folk-medicine, but when it employed any means that were, or appeared to be, magical or pagan, it assumed a dangerous ambiguity. Against such sometimes ambiguous practices the early medieval church waged considerable combat. It was particularly the use of spells or incantations in connection with herbs, gems, and the like, that frustrated the church. We have already seen mention of this in the penitential literature that recommended the substitution of the Creed and the Lord's Prayer for pagan utterances.[58]

The tension between the church and such folk medicine arose from the potential for even temporary dependence upon a source that either was not compatible with Christianity or could be employed without reference to it. Most obviously, the use of incantations and spells in conjunction with folk remedies had to be replaced with Christian formulae. But even if folk medicine were employed without the use of any illicit procedures, the attitude of the one using the remedies was important, because a dependence upon the power of herbs and gems without reference to their Creator was regarded as improper for a Christian. The latter of these two objections to folk medicine could also be applied to the secular medicine practiced by physicians.

It is not uncommon to see in modern discussions of the Middle Ages assertions or implications that the medieval church was hostile to science, especially to medicine, and disparaged its practice as a threat to the spiritual health of the physically ill. Such a picture is false. It may, however, appear on the surface to be at least partially true. For example, miraculous healing abound in much of the literature. The spectacular nature of these healings is highlighted when the failures of physicians are mentioned in particular cases. Several times in the two accounts of the life of Cuthbert, individuals were miraculously healed whom doctors could not help "with their compounds and drugs" or "with all their care."[59] One of the most enthusiastic recorders of miracles was Gregory of Tours (sixth century). He especially seemed to delight in describing the abysmal failures of physicians whose patients subsequently found healing at the shrine of Saint Martin. But Gregory definitely used Greco-Roman medical handbooks and pharmacological guides himself.[60] Likewise, Pope Gregory I, who more than any other individual shaped the ethos of early medieval Catholicism, with its emphasis on miraculous healings, the cult of saints and relics, and demonology, had a fascination with medicine. Because of his almost constant illnesses, he kept an Alexandrian physician in permanent attendance. When a friend of his living in Ravenna was sick, Gregory solicited the opinions of all the physicians he knew and passed them on to his ill friend. Tradition also has it that he cured a Lombard king's stomach ailment by prescribing a milk diet.[61]

Medicine was a standard part of the medievel curriculum, and it is not uncommon to encounter educated clerics requesting medical handbooks[62] and both seeking and giving medical advice. Bishop Fulbert of Chartres (early eleventh century) outdid Pope Gregory I by sending not only medical advice but also a variety of medicines to a sick friend.[63] On another occasion he wrote to a fellow bishop: "Believe me, father, I have not prepared any ointments since I was raised to the bishopric. But the little that is left of what a doctor gave to me I am sending as a gift . . . with the prayer that Christ, the author of good health, may make it help you."[64]

The closing comment in this letter is important: The cure comes from God. This theme was a constant undercurrent, and occasionally voices were raised to remind people that when they are ill their hope should be placed not in drugs and remedies but in God, who gave these substances their efficacy. Physicians likewise were urged to place their faith in God and to extend charity to the destitute ill. This latter advice appeared in some treatises on medical etiquette from the early Middle Ages. One of these, from the eighth century, urged the physican to serve rich and poor alike, and to look for eternal rather than material rewards.[65] The identity of the authors and the intended audience of these treatises is unknown. These writings are part of a fairly large body of medical manuscripts that reflect a sustained tradition of Greco-Roman medicine. References to physicians are frequently encountered in all genres of literature. These physicians were of two basic categories: strictly secular practitioners and cleric-physicians, often monks. Occasionally, physicians schooled in Constantinople or Alexandria appear. Now and then we also encounter Jewish or Islamic physicians, who were trained in the much more medically sophisticated environment of the East. But the vast majority undoubtedly were Catholics born and trained in western Europe, who were little more than craftsmen who had acquired their medical skills by apprenticeship. Even those who were trained at Salerno in Italy, of whom we hear a little by the tenth century, were essentially craftsmen. Our knowledge is very inadequate of the wide variety of secular physicians who tended the ills of the probably relatively small minority of the population who could pay for their services. The vast majority of people who sought nonmiraculous healing had to rely upon traditional folk remedies or seek help from such clerics as possessed medical knowledge or skill.

The duty to visit and care for the sick is clearly given in the gospel and is repeatedly encountered in the literature of early Christianity.[66] Care of the poor and infirm was enjoined by various councils throughout these centuries.[67] It was the bishop's responsibility to administer the funds for the care of the poor and sick. Bishops were directed to provide accommodations for the destitute. These buildings were originally called *xenodochia*, a term that eventually gave way to *hospitia* or *hospitalia*. These were usually attached to a cathedral or other church.[68] It is a mistake to envision these facilities for the most part as hospitals in anything approaching the modern sense.[69] Some, particularly in the sixth and seventh centuries, were designed for the extension of medical care by a staff of trained physicians, but these were probably an exception.[70] The vast majority of xenodochia simply provided refuge in the form of shelter, food, and a few amenities.

The xenodochia that survived the chaos of the disintegration of the Carolingian Empire usually became the property of monasteries. In the early Middle Ages, monasteries were also places of refuge for the poor and the sick. The *Rule* of Benedict (sixth century), which governed the vast network of Benedictine monasteries that spreaad throughout western Europe during these centuries, addressed health needs. One passage specified that the cellarer give care to fellow monks who were ill.[71] In another passage he was admonished to "take the greatest care of the sick, of children, of guests, and of the poor, knowing without doubt that he will have to render account for all these on the Day of Judgement."[72] The availability of those qualified to give medical care certainly varied from monastery to monastery. Both accounts of the life of Cuthbert tell of a young paralytic monk who was sent by his abbot to Cuthbert's monastery, not to be healed by Cuthbert's relics but because there were "very skilled" physicians there. All their medical skills availed nothing, however, and the youth finally cried out for aid from the "heavenly Physician" and was cured through the relics (in this case the shoes) of the deceased Cuthbert.[73] This incident tells us that there were physicians who were viewed as "very skilled" at the monastery at Lindisfarne in the seventh century. Their work on this youth was undoubtedly performed in the infirmary, which was reserved for clerics. It tells us nothing about the availability of health care provided by monks for the needy laity. We do know that in the sixth century the sick came to the monastery at Iona for medical attention.[74] It is unlikely that the destitute sick were refused help when they presented themselves at a monastery, and the monasteries to which the sick would most likely have come were those known for their competent physicians. Such care as was extended was ideally motivated by Christian charity and not by a desire for financial gain.

The High and Late Middle Ages (1050–1545)

The Practice of Medicine by Clerics

The Cistercian abbot Bernard of Clairvaux (1090–1153) wrote to an abbot of another monastery in response to the latter's demand that a monk who had fled to Clairvaux be returned to his former monastery. This monk's complaint was that his abbot "used him not as a monk but as a doctor" and forced him "to serve not God but the world; that in order to curry favour with the princes of this world he was made to attend tyrants, robbers, and excommunicated persons." His work apparently had resulted in much financial gain for his monastery. The monk had fled for the health of his soul. His abbot accused him of having left, "drawn away by his cupidity and curiosity to run around here and there selling his art." Bernard refused to force him to return.[75] It should be noted that shortly after Bernard's death the Cistercians adopted a rule that none of the order's physicians could practice outside their monasteries or treat laymen.[76] That there were indeed monks who practiced medicine for their monasteries' or their own profit is clear from a canon promulgated by the Second Lateran Council of 1139 having the rubric, "Monks and canons regular are not to study jurisprudence and medicine for the sake of temporal gain." This canon condemned the impulse of avarice that caused some monks to pursue such studies: "The care of souls being neglected . . . they promise health in return for detestable money and thus make themselves physicians of human bodies."[77] Although the canon also mentioned that when acting as physicians monks would see shameful things that were not appropriate for them, the major concern was that the study and practice of medicine and secular law were not appropriate for those whose lives were to be devoted exclusively to a religious life, if their motivation were financial gain. Two matters should be noted. First, this canon applied only to monks and canons regular and not to most clerics. Second, this canon was never incorporated into any official collection of canon law.

In 1163, at the Council of Tours, Pope Alexander III enacted a canon considerably weaker than the one just mentioned, which simply forbade monks and other regular clerics to leave their religious institutions for the study of medicine or secular law.[78] This canon, which said nothing about the practice of medicine by clerics, was included in the first officially promulgated major collection of canon law, the *Decretales* of Gregory IX (1234).[79] Another piece of papal legislation, a rescript of Honorius III issued in 1219 and also included in the *Decretales*,[80] extended the prohibition of the study of medicine and secular law essentially to all clerics whose livelihood was provided by the performance of spiritual duties. A vast number of clerics, however, still would not have been affected by this legislation. Even its prohibitions were significantly lessened by subsequent legislation.[81] At the end of the Middle Ages there was still no prohibition of the practice of medicine by clerics in canon law. Surgery, however, was a different matter, because it involved the shedding of blood and much greater risk of harm to a patient, thus heightening the danger that a clerical practitioner might be held responsible for a patient's death. In 1215, at the Fourth Lateran Council, the practice of surgery was forbidden to clerics in major (holy) orders (subdeacons, deacons, and priests) but still permitted to those in minor orders (porters, acolytes, exorcists, and lectors).[82]

While medieval canon law never prohibited the practice of medicine by clerics, there was obvious uneasiness on the part of the church about their motivation for engaging in such pursuits and the effects such endeavors would have on their spiritual obligations. The issue eventually grew nearly moot as more and more secular physicians were trained in the universities, one of many examples of the increasing involvement of the educated laity in areas previously dominated by the clergy. Medical and surgical practice by clerics, however, continued to an extent throughout the Middle Ages, but the major motivation appears to have been charity. For instance, a medical treatise was written in the thirteenth century by a member of a religious order to instruct his fellow clerics in medicine so that they could treat the poor gratis. They could receive fees from the rich.[83] Such treatises were fairly common. Numerous medical handbooks were also written by clerics in order to help the poor help themselves. For example, Peter Hispanus, who became pope in 1276 as John XXI, was the probable author of the *Treasury for the Poor*, which listed simple but salubrious herbs that the poor could gather for themselves.

It was especially in response to the widespread suffering and disease in the growing towns and cities of the late eleventh and twelfth centuries that Augustinian canons (who were like monks in that they lived under a rule but unlike them in that they did not remove themselves from society) and various lay brotherhoods established houses of charity that included institutions or facilities for the succor of the destitute ill.[84] A variety of what may be called hospitals were founded by kings, bishops, feudal lords, wealthy merchants, guilds, and municipalities as endowed charitable institutions that were then staffed by members of various orders, some of which, like the Knights Hospitallers of Saint John of Jerusalem, were, as their nomenclature indicates, given to the tasks of charity. Numerous nursing orders arose whose members devoted their lives to caring for the destitute ill in these institutions. By the beginning of the thirteenth century, many hospitals had one or more trained physicians. The hospitals themselves were owned by church orders. During the thirteenth and fourteenth centuries, especially in Italy and Germany, the control of many of these institutions passed into the hands of municipal governments, as part of the general laicization of European society.[85]

The Church and Medical Ethics

The rapidly changing character of society in the high Middle Ages stimulated churchmen to subject the vagaries of the contemporary scene to both abstract and practical moral analyses. The theologians who engaged in such efforts during the twelfth century were the founding fathers of moral theology. The Parisian theologian Peter the Chanter is a good example.[86] His major work[87] consists of three parts, the first dealing with sacraments, the second with penance and excommunication, and the third with ways of resolving cases of conscience. Peter wrote this work in part to aid priests in the increasingly difficult task of determining what constituted sin in a society enormously more complex and confusing than that which had prevailed during the preceding centuries, when the penitential handbooks had proved quite adequate. The genre of aids to confessors, of which Peter's work is an early example, was significantly stimulated by a canon promulgated in 1215 by the Fourth Lateran Council, which a leading historian of the last century called "perhaps the most important legislative act in the history of the Church."[88] This canon,[89] which was soon incorporated into the *Decretales,*[90] required, under pain of excommunication, annual confession to one's own priest. This thoroughly publicized decree reached every level of medieval society.[91] The literature that arose in response to this need consisted of lengthy, finely reasoned tomes and short, practical confessional manuals (or *summae*) to be used by confessors in their systematic interrogations of penitents. One summa, the *Astesana* (ca. 1317), instructs the confessor to "scrutinize the conscience of the sinner in confession as a physician scrutinizes wounds and a judge a case."[92] Confessional examination was to penetrate into every area of life: birth, marriage, sex, the rearing of children, and vocational obligations.

The writers of these summae appear to have been concerned with sexual morality more than with any other area. The thoroughness and interrogatory ingenuity of the probing of confessors into the sexual activities of penitents are really quite remarkable. Sexual sins were thus graded in order of gravity: unchaste kiss; unchaste touch; fornication; simple adultery; double adultery; rape or abduction of a virgin, of another's wife, or of a nun; incest; masturbation; unnatural relations within marriage; homosexuality; and bestiality. The last five of these were regarded as sins against nature. Thomas Tentler, an authority on the confessional literature of the late Middle Ages, writes: "Taken as a whole, the practical literature on sin and confession gave considerable attention to sins against nature. Medieval churchmen were devoted to the idea of the moral goodness of procreation and mistrustful of doing anything for pleasure. They accordingly conceived a horror of unnatural practices, which they sometimes defined with a startling comprehensiveness."[93]

Other sins against nature, such as contraception and abortion, were regarded both as sexual sins and, under some circumstances, as homicide. Both were fraught with interpretive problems during the period under consideration and have been discussed extensively by modern scholars.[94] Contraception and abortion, although treated separately, were oftentimes confused owing to the primitive understanding of fertilization and fetal development. The statements of Jerome and Augustine, made several centuries earlier than the period under consideration, that abortion was not counted as homicide unless the fetus was "formed," were incorporated into the early medieval penitentials and taken by Gratian, in the twelfth century, as meaning "vivified" or "ensouled,"[95] along the lines of Aristotelian embryonic theory. In the *Decretales,* two canons deal with abortion. One follows Gratian;[96] the other applies the penalty for homicide to contraception and to the induced abortion of a fetus at any stage of development.[97] Theologians, canonists, and the authors of summae were split between these two positions. The more liberal of the two did not regard induced abortion as a mortal sin if performed within the first forty days in the case of a male fetus, eighty (or, according to some, ninety) days in the case of a female; it permitted abortion during these periods under a variety of extenuating circumstances. The stricter position generally forbade abortion at all times and under all circumstances. The conflict of interpretations between these two camps was not resolved until long after the period under consideration. Both, however, clearly condemned contraception and abortion as reprehensible if performed simply to vitiate normal procreative functions.

The writers of the summae often had to interpret and apply fine points of canon law. While the summae were not always totally consistent with one another, they were usually as consistent with canon law and theological opinion as these were with themselves. Some scholars say that the effect of canon law and confessional interrogation on private morality was probably negligible. There is, however, good reason to believe that the hortatory impact of the pulpit and the coercive force of the confessional proved to be significant factors in shaping the moral attitudes, if not always the behavior, of a large portion of the population. Tentler writes that "it would have been impractical and self-defeating" for the authors of the summae "to appeal to ideas and expectations that were novel, irrelevant, or unintelligible." He sees in this literature "the practicality of men who understood the inherent power of the system placed at the disposal of every rank of ecclesiastical authority."[98] He considers the confessional system of the late Middle Ages to have been a "most effective means of social control" because of its "clear and explicit expectations, clear and direct accountability." He says of the summae that "they are, if any books ever were, devoted to the clarification, definition, and publication of expectations, as well as to the assertion of the legitimacy of the authority of priest over penitents and the hierarchy

Amundsen p. 196-214, 222-239, 289-304

Black p. 243-244, 249-256, 257-262,
197-205

Rider Article
Caesarius p. 1-3, 21, 22, 30-36, 303-307,
366-368, 453-455, 531-534, 456, 479,
487-492
Chs: 14, 21-27, 98, 36, 1-2, 47-49, 3-16, 22-24
    book 1   1   4   5   7   7

Diane Watt Articl

John Aberth, The Black Death p. 19-32, 40-45

Medicine in Christianity

~~Wolfgang Chagalla~~

Black #66

Arnald of Villanova : quote

over the church."[99] It was perhaps due to the educational efficacy of the confessional, supplemented by the pulpit, that such conditions of religious law and order prevailed in the western church that the Greek Orthodox monk Barlaam in the early fourteenth century was moved to remark: "The whole people is ruled by laws, even the smallest matters are subject to regulation and orderly administration." He was struck not only by the all-pervasive character of canon law but also by the reverence that people seemed to have for it "as the ordinances of Christ himself."[100]

Sometimes this reverence was for religious principles, whether or not they had been specifically embodied in canon law and inculcated through the church's mechanisms or moral instruction. A good example of this involves the attitudes of physicians toward an obligation made in 1215 by the Fourth Lateran Council that required physicians, before undertaking treatment, to ensure that their patients make a confession to a priest.[101] This canon, which was included in the *Decretales*,[102] reads:

Since bodily infirmity is sometimes caused by sin, the Lord saying to the sick man whom he had healed: "Go and sin no more, lest some worse thing happen to thee" (John 5:14), we declare in the present decree and strictly command that when physicians of the body are called to the bedside of the sick, before all else they admonish them to call for the physician of souls, so that after spiritual health has been restored to them, the application of bodily medicine may be of greater benefit, for the cause being removed the effect will pass away. We publish this decree for the reason that some, when they are sick and are advised by the physician in the course of the sickness to attend to the salvation of their soul, give up all hope and yield more easily to the danger of death. If any physician shall transgress this decree after it has been published by the bishops, let him be cut off from the church till he has made suitable satisfaction for his transgression. And since the soul is far more precious than the body, we forbid under penalty of anathema that a physician advise a patient to have recourse to sinful means for the recovery of bodily health.[103]

Even before this obligation was imposed, we find the author of an anonymous twelfth-century treatise dealing with medical etiquette suggesting the following to his fellow physicians: "When you reach [a patient's] house and before you see him, ask if he has seen his confessor. If he has not done so, have him either do it or promise to do it. For if he hears mention of this after you have examined him and have considered the signs of the disease, he will begin to despair of recovery, because he will think that you despair of it too."[104] The author, of course, was part of a society that believed in the absolute necessity of confession before death for the health of the soul. Although he may not have considered it his spiritual duty to look after his patients' spiritual welfare, he certainly considered it potentially dangerous to patients to advise them to confess only when in dire straits. He makes no mention, however, of the relationship of sickness and sin.

In the late thirteenth or early fourteenth century, a treatise was written, later attributed to the physician Arnald of Villanova, that contains the following advice: "When you come to a house, inquire before you go to the sick whether he has confessed, and if he has not, he should immediately or promise you that he will confess immediately, and this must not be neglected because many illnesses originate on account of sin and are cured by the Supreme Physician after having been purified from squalor by the tears of contrition, according to what is said in the Gospel: 'Go, and sin no more, lest something worse happens to you.' "[105]

This so strikingly resembles the canon of Lateran IV that it demonstrates the direct influence of canon law on a strictly secular piece of medical literature, as does the following passage in an anonymous plague tractate composed in 1411: "If it is certain from the symptoms that it is actually pestilence that has afflicted the patient, the physician first must advise the patient to set himself right with God by making a will and by making a confession of his sins, as is set forth according to the Decretals: since a corporal illness comes not only from a fault of the body but also from a spiritual failing as the Lord declares in the gospel and the priests also tell us."[106] The author of this passage includes a provision not in medieval canon law, that the physician advise the patient to make a will. About a century earlier, similar advice was given by the physician Henri de Mondeville: "Do not let the patient be concerned about any business except spiritual matters only, such as confession and his will and arranging similar affairs in accordance with the rules of the Catholic faith."[107] The injunction concerning the making of a will was not in canon law, but was in the confessional literature.

The summae, as already mentioned, probed into all aspects of life, including one's vocation. Several professions, including medicine, were regarded as worthy of scrutiny because of their potential for sin.[108] Two matters raised by the canon of Lateran IV were considered by the authors of the summae. The first was the physician's obligation to advise a patient to call a priest to hear his confession. The second was to refrain from advising sinful means to bring about a cure. The summae specify as sin a physician's advising fornication, masturbation, incantations, consumption of intoxicating beverages, breaking the church's fasts, and eating meat on forbidden days. More problematic, however, was the question of calling a confessor, as is evident from the involved discussions in the summae. Two reasons are given in the canon for the requirement: First, because confession had a curative effect, it would make physicians' attendance either superfluous or more efficacious. Second, the practice of calling a confessor as a matter of course before undertaking treatment would dispel the notion that physicians only call for a confessor when they have given up hope for the recovery of a patient. The variety of problems that would arise in practice are very obvious. The authors of the summae raised and discussed several questions: Does this apply to each and every case undertaken? Is it the physician's responsibility to ensure compliance? Must the physician withdraw from the case if the patient refuses to call a confessor? The authorities seldom agreed on the answers to these and related questions.

They were much more in accord on a variety of other matters. They agreed, for example, that a physician sins by practicing without being competent according to the accepted standards of the art; by failing to keep abreast of medical developments or to consult colleagues when in doubt about a case; by harming patients owing to ignorance or negligence; or by experimenting on patients. Rash treatment was condemned, as was the giving of medicines about which the physician is in doubt. They felt that patients would be much better off, under such circumstances, to be left in God's hands. In the case of patients for whom there was little hope of recovery, if the physician was unsure about the state of the patients' temporal affairs, he was obliged to inform them of impending death and advise them to make a will. A physician sinned if he withheld effective treatment so that he could increase his fee by prolonging the illness. The physician was obligated not to desert his patients even if there was virtually no hope of recovery, and to extend care even if the patient refused to pay, if without such care the patient would die. The authors of summae dealt with the question of treating the poor by following Thomas Aquinas' principle that because "nobody can possibly help out all those in need," charity ought first to be given to those with whom one is united in any way. "There still remains the question whether somebody is in such dire straits that it is not immediately obvious how else he is to be helped. And in such a case, one is bound to come to his assistance." Accordingly, a physician was not obligated always to treat the destitute, "otherwise he would have to give up all other work and devote himself exclusively" to them.[109] Most summae maintained that the physician must treat the poor gratis only if it were evident that otherwise they would die. The sometimes crass expectations of some members of society for free medical care were a source of much frustration for many secular physicians in the high and late Middle Ages.[110]

There was considerable popular sentiment against physicians during this period. While physicians' greed topped the list of complaints,[111] their lack of concern for spiritual affairs came in a close second. The ill will that was felt appears to have been generated in great part by concern for the potential spiritual damage a physician could cause if he put the health of the patient's body ahead of the health of his soul. Undergirding this concern was the suspicion that, as the Latin adage goes, *Tres medici, duo athei* (Out of three physicians, two will be atheists). In the thirteenth century, the preacher Jacque de Vitry told his auditors that the advice of the physicians was deleterious to their souls: "God says keep vigils; the doctors say go to sleep. God says fast; the doctors say eat. God says mortify your flesh; the doctors say be comfortable."[112] Such sentiments occurred with regularity in the homiletical literature and represented an extreme antipathy to secular medicine. More consonant with late medieval theology and canon law was a thirteenth-century sermon of Humbert de Romans to the brethren and sisters of the hospitals, in which he briefly directed his attention to physicians, urging them never to perform an operation

that is doubtful without grave consultation and deliberation. So let them deal faithfully with their patients as to cause them as little expense as possible; let them take a moderate fee that their consciences be not hurt. Above all let them beware of doing aught in their art against God in themselves or in others, lest whilst they heal bodies they kill souls, others' or their own. Finally, let them have not as much confidence in their medicines as in their prayers, and let them have most in God.[113]

Humbert's advice, although given before many of the summae had been written, bears some clear resemblance to their categories. Much of the criticism of the medical profession in late medieval literature seems to have been closely modeled on the concerns expressed in the confessional literature.[114]

Given the interests of the church in the spiritual well-being of its people, as illustrated by the canon of Lateran IV dealing with the spiritual obligations of physicians, it is not surprising that church authorities sought to impose and enforce a policy of restricting medical practice on Christian patients to Christian physicians, especially because the conduct of non-Christian physicians could not be checked by the confessional. Particularly during the thirteenth century we find church councils strictly forbidding Christians to obtain medical or surgical services from Jewish or Islamic physicians, under pain of excommunication.[115] Nevertheless, many people, including religious leaders, continued to employ the services of non-Christian physicians in spite of such prohibitions.

In the confessional literature there was a much greater emphasis on the responsibility of a physician not to advise sinful means for restoring health than on the responsibility of the patient to refuse to follow such advice. However, several summae discussed the obligations of patients.[116] A composite includes the following matters: Patients do not sin if they disobey their physicians, because physicians have no real authority over them but can only advise and exhort. It is, however, good to trust one's physician to the extent to which he is an expert in the art. If patients knowingly or by gross (thus inexcusable) ignorance consume something deadly, they sin. They do not sin mortally, however, if they intentionally consume a substance that they believe is not deadly if by so doing they are attempting to aggravate their illness.

Medicine and Late Medieval Catholicism: Tensions and Compatibilities

The small amount of attention in the confessional literature to the sins of patients should not lead one to believe that theologians were unconcerned about the moral responsibilities of the sick. A good example of late medieval attitudes toward the conduct of patients is found in the sermons preached in 1498 and 1499 by Johann Geiler von Kaiserberg, a German priest and professor of theology. In one sermon, entitled "Sick Fools," Geiler discussed seven follies of the ill.[117] The first four involved their relations with the medical art and its practitioners. Ill fools scorned medicine; deceived or disobeyed their physician; followed the physician's advice belatedly or distorted it so that it did not help. These four follies were simply foolish. The confessional literature did not classify them as sins. The remaining three involved sin, although the first of these was potentially neutral, being pivotal in this list. The ill sought medicine and advice from "old women and from others who have never learned medicine." They searched "for medicine and health from witches and exorcisoresses of the devil." The most serious folly was "to neglect one's duty to God—to make use of medicine and not desire the help of God."

The last of these seven follies of the sick was a frequently repeated concern of medieval authors. It showed an attitude of independence, of sufficiency to maintain or restore one's health without reference to one's Creator. The church could exhort, threaten, and plead against that attitude but could not effectively regulate or control the attitudes of the sick or of physicians toward the medical art, which was regarded both as a gift of the Creator and as a potential lure away from submission to him.

Geiler complained that people sought the help of "old women and . . . others who have never learned medicine," and searched "for medicine and health from witches and exorcisoresses of the devil." During the twelfth and thirteenth centuries, the practice of medicine had changed from a right to a privilege, with the introduction of medical licensure and the development of medical and surgical guilds that sought and obtained monopolies in medical and surgical care in exchange for guarantees of high ethical standards and requisite training for all practitioners, which was the basis for the assurance of competence. When guilds petitioned for monopolies, they always emphasized that this was for the public good. Those who granted such monopolies concurred. In some communities (e.g., Montpellier) the church granted and enforced the monopoly. In others, even though it had not granted the guild's charter, it helped enforce the guild's rights. In Paris, for example, both the medical and surgical corporations maintained a constant struggle against unlicensed practitioners. They often appealed to the church. The accused would be tried by a church court, which would either excommunicate the defendant or threaten excommunication for a second offense. Very often the alleged charlatans were women.[118]

The majority of unlicensed practitioners probably employed techniques and substances typical of folk medicine without any magical formulae and charms. But because so many of these unlicensed practitioners were women, they readily evoked suspicion of engaging in witchcraft or other illicit practices. In dealing with the subject of illicit healing in the high and late Middle Ages, we enter a maze of confusion.[119] Beginning with the revival of learning in the twelfth century, scholars were increasingly interested in those realms of inquiry that we probably would label superstition. Their definitions of the demonic, magic, miracle, natural properties, and occult virtues seem to blend in with the pertinacious endurance of various strata of folk and pagan practices. In a hazy middle ground between magic and miracle was the realm of "natural medicine" or the exploitation of occult virtues, to which Geiler's fifth and sixth points both have reference. "Natural medicine" was not simply the folk medicine that unlicensed people practiced without proper medical training, but possessed the additional ingredient of techniques for releasing the occult virtues contained within the natural objects. This could be done illicitly through incantations or licitly through formulae prescribed by the church.

Penitential handbooks continued condemning pagan practices through the twelfth century.[120] But beginning in that century we find magic denounced less as paganism than as heresy. From the quagmire of definitional confusions that prevailed arose a renewed interest in astrology. Astrology had usually been either condemned by the church fathers as demonic or dismissed as banal, and these attitudes prevailed during the early Middle Ages. In the twelfth century, however, Hugh of Saint Victor distinguished between "natural astrology" and "superstitious astrology." William McDonald explains: "The former, also called scientific astrology, concerned itself with the constitution of physical bodies like illness and health, which varied according to the mutual alignments of the astral bodies. In contrast, superstitious astrology, also designated judicial and divinatory astrology, was concerned with chance happenings or future contingent events and with matters of free will."[121] This distinction, which did not originate with Hugh, was the basis for much of the discussion that continued well beyond the period under consideration. Various questions arose. Were the stars agents of action or simply its harbingers? If the licit branch of astrology was concerned with such physical matters as illness, could prognostication be made without dabbling in the illicit branch, especially if one did not presume upon the spiritual realm, which included reason and free will? Different answers were given by different people, and debate raged. The physician who did not use astrology was regarded by many as either incompetent or negligent. In the late thirteenth century, Roger Bacon, in his *On the Errors of Physicians*, says that "a physician who knows not how to take into account the positions and aspects of the planets can effect nothing in the healing arts except by chance and good fortune."[122] Although there were some voices raised against the validity of "natural astrology," it had become so much a part of medicine by the close of the Middle Ages that in 1509 the English Franciscan monk Alexander Barclay could criticize medical quacks for their failure to heed astrological signs.[123]

The supposed prognostic benefits of astrology came to the fore, espe-

cially in attempts to explain and cope with the Black Death of 1348–49
and the subsequent waves of pestilential disease that periodically ravaged Europe well beyond the end of the Middle Ages. McDonald thus
paraphrases the conclusion of a treatise written in the fifteenth century
by Conrad Bosner: "Everything is subservient to the divine will. God
[ordains] the celestial bodies to carry out their influence and does not
hinder the natural forces on earth as a consequence of man's offenses
against heaven. Following from this, the apparent decisive influence of
the stars is but a further manifestation of divine control, in that God
tolerates and uses that influence as an agent of his will to punish man for
sin and error."[124] Just as in the early Middle Ages, plague and all epidemic diseases were regarded as visitations of God's wrath. God was
commonly depicted showering arrows of vengeance on sinful humanity.[125] We have seen that in the early Middle Ages the plague had proved
to be a very effective illustration of God's wrath and of the importance of
eternal priorities and thus was instrumental in turning the peasants'
attention from their temporal concerns. Popular reactions to the plague
in the late Middle Ages demonstrated that the desires of the theologians
of earlier centuries had in great part been fulfilled.

The church's reaction to the Black Death of 1348–49, the most horrible pestilence ever to afflict Europe, is well illustrated by the actions
taken by Pope Clement VI as soon as the plague hit Avignon, then
the seat of the papacy. In addition to taking various measures to hinder
contagion, he hired physicians to care for the afflicted, gave special indulgences to encourage the clergy to minister to those stricken, and
instituted a special mass to implore an end to the plague.[126] Medical care
was viewed as an immediate form of assistance to be given in an attempt
to counter this affliction, of which God was viewed as the ultimate cause.
This was by no means regarded as inconsistent with the equally important effort to approach God through a special mass. This compatibility,
however, was marred when, on numerous occasions during the next
several centuries, physicians' concerns with contagion were overruled by
the church's popularly welcomed organization of massive processionals
to implore God's mercy.[127] There were, of course, some clerics and some
laymen who argued against the use of physicians during time of plague,
either on the spiritual grounds that such efforts were inconsistent or on
the pragmatic grounds that physicians' efforts at prophylaxis and treatment were obviouly of little or no value. Although physicians were able
to accomplish little or nothing for their patients who were afflicted with

the plague, their efforts to deal with this scourge were often supererog-atory.[128] "The prestige of doctors was not weakened by heavy plague mortality," writes Sylvia Thrupp, "for they could take credit for cases of recovery and by personal concern and courage they eased the atmo-sphere of fear. Popular devotion to a favorite doctor was expressed in terms of love and of the honor due a father by a son."[129]

In addition to providing medical care and instituting a special mass, Clement gave indulgences to clerics ministering to the stricken. These indulgences were regarded as absolving the sins of those to whom they were granted so that their sins would not require expiation in purgatory. Apparently death by plague came to be regarded by some as potentially expiatory in itself. John of Saxony, who wrote a treatise on plague during the first half of the fifteenth century, complained that some people disregarded the prophylactic advice of physicians during times of plague. He gave several reasons for this attitude, one of which was a prevailing fatalism, for some held that "the time of one's death has been estab-lished for every individual." Another reason was "the desire and hope for death. For I recall that in a certain great pestilence in Montpellier, when many men wished to die, on that acount the pope gave to the dy-ing absolution from punishment and guilt and thus they hoped to be carried to heaven immediately, and therefore they did not want physi-cians to prolong their lives."[130]

It was commonly held by all levels of society that one must suffer for one's sins, either in this life or in purgatory, although usually in both. This led to various reactions to the plague, one of which was the flagel-lant movement. Flagellation had existed in Christianity for centuries. It had been prescribed as a means of public penance in late antiquity and the early Middle Ages. It was also a part of monastic discipline. Addi-tionally, it was a form of voluntary penance that, during the eleventh century, became widespread among monks and laymen. In the thir-teenth century, owing in great part to the emphasis of the mendicant orders on identification with Christ's sufferings, the order of Penitents arose. Members of this order identified themselves so closely with Christ's sufferings that they believed they could contribute to the expiation of the sins of mankind by self-flagellation. In central Italy in 1260 a popular outbreak of flagellation was stimulated in part by a famine (1258) fol-lowed by an epidemic (1259). John Henderson remarks, "One can un-derstand how flagellation came to be seen as the obvious method of expiation when translated into the context of a mass movement characterized by a widespread belief that God was intent on punishing mankind. It provided immediate and violent release from guilt and in the very process of beating their bodies participants could feel that they were washing away their sins. Moreover, in this exercise they saw themselves as sharing the sufferings of Christ."[131]

Various officially authorized flagellant confraternities arose over the next century. While the Black Death was devastating Europe, the flagellant movement took on a popular fervor. Motivated by the hope of appeasing God, groups of people formed who believed that by flagellating themselves for a period of thirty-three and one-half days they could bring about the end of the plague and then be themselves cleansed entirely of sin. This popular movement spread rapidly, beginning in June 1349, apparently in Germany, which was soon overrun by flagellant bands. Violence and disorder accompanied some of these groups, and when they reached Avignon in October 1349, Clement condemned their activities and ordered them to desist.[132] Although their disorder and the attendant violence contributed to Clement's decision to condemn them, his action should not be taken as a denial of their basic theology. Rather, his negative reaction was primarily precipitated by their having adopted a specific habit. He "saw the wearing of a habit as a sign of the flagellants' rejection of the authority of the church, believing they saw their exercise as an end in itself which led them to their salvation unaided by the priesthood."[133]

Sin was commonly regarded as the immediate cause of plague, or at least the catalyst behind God's sending the plague. This was collective sin. Individual sin was seldom seen as the cause of sickness, whether mental illness or physical ailments.[134] One notable exception was leprosy, which was associated with a variety of sins, but especially with lust and pride.[135] By a strange irony to which medieval Catholic theology was conducive, lepers were also regarded as chosen by God for the privilege of suffering in this life in lieu of purgatory.[136] Most people who suffered from sickness in the late Middle Ages were, of course, not afflicted with either leprosy or plague. Some people when ill may have been burdened with a sense of guilt. If medieval theology in some ways fostered such an attitude, it did not, however, encourage it as a morbidly obsessive response to illness.

The canon of the Fourth Lateran Council, which required physicians to have their patients make confession to a priest, began with the clause "Since bodily infirmity is sometimes caused by sin. . . ." Confession was thought to restore spiritual health. If the physical problem was exacerbated by a spiritual problem, medicine for the body would be more effective after confession. If the physical affliction was caused by spiritual sickness, physical healing would directly result from confession. Richard Palmer remarks, "In catholic theology confession was of fundamental importance in the treatment of disease. It was probably the church's nearest approximation in the medieval and early modern periods to a formal ritual of healing."[137] This observation, although essentially correct, is easily misleading. Confession was of "fundamental importance" to the formulators of canon law and to many theologians during the late Middle Ages. On the very eve of the Reformation, Dietrich Coelde, the author of a famous and highly influential manual of spiritual instruction, stressed that the ill should first seek such cures as confession and the mass because sickness "generally comes from sins."[138] It does not follow that confession was stressed, however, in even a significant minority of those varied procedures available for physical healing that were loosely under the auspices of the church. Mention was made earlier of a ninth-century French bishop's frustration at the lack of repentance evidenced by those who had flocked to the shrine of Fermin for healing. His reaction was atypical of that time. As Patrick Geary says of this period, "The miraculous rather than the penitential aspects of devotion to relics seem to have formed . . . the basis for popular devotion to local and religious pilgrimage sites."[139] But a significant change occurred in the eleventh and twelfth centuries as a motivation other than healing arose for visiting shrines. It was typically believed that expiatory pilgrimage to various shrines greatly contributed to the forgiveness of a pilgrim's sins. The age of the penitential pilgrimage had begun, a striking feature of the closing centuries of medieval Catholicism. The rapid social changes and population growth that marked the eleventh and twelfth centuries had led to a stark sense of alienation that is so evident in the literature of that time.[140] The deep sense of sin and the fear of purgatorial fires, coupled with a feeling of alienation, fostered penitential pilgrimages. The vast majority of pilgrims undoubtedly were not seeking physical healing during the late Middle Ages. But when the sick came as pilgrims to shrines for healing, there appears to have been as little concern on the part of the clerics at the shrines to deal with the ill persons' spiritual state as there had been during the early Middle Ages. We know of at least one shrine that required those who came for healing to have proof that they had confessed to their parish priest before leaving home,[141] but this was probably an exception to the practice that prevailed at most shrines, because the shrine in question was of Mary, a rather late extension of the cult of saints and relics. The majority of the healing shrines of the late Middle Ages were repositories of the bones or relics of saints.

Ronald Finucane, a leading authority on the English shrines of the late Middle Ages, has found that 90 percent of the miracles that were recorded at English and Continental shrines from the twelfth through the fifteenth centuries involved healings and alleviations of physical ills. Many of those seeking healing had first tried other available means. The clerics at these shrines responded to the failures of physicians with the same enthusiasm and motivation as had Gregory of Tours earlier. Finucane concludes that "it is clear that in practice most sick people called on both the power of saints and of trained physicians. This was as true at the very top of the social ladder as at the bottom; as true for laymen as for clerics."[142]

Trafficking in relics was an enormously lucrative business. So numerous were the healing shrines of this period that control was difficult. The church made gallant efforts to authenticate miracles and to limit canonization of individuals whose remains were potential relics.[143] At the same time, a concerted effort was made to direct popular devotion away from often quite minor, nondescript, or simply unapproved saints to Christ and Mary. This was eminently practical: They did not require canonization, and their shrines needed no relics, only a crucifix or a statue of Mary.[144] This seems to have resulted in some redirecting of attention from the shrines of saints to these new focal points of devotion and miracles. Also, the relic value of the elements in the sacrament of communion was exploited by the "exposition" of the Host in a container in which it could be viewed and venerated during the mass.[145] Stories of healing miracles that occurred during the mass were very common in the late Middle Ages.

Although some voices in late antiquity questioned the theological validity of the cult of saints and relics, opposition to the cult was extremely rare in the Middle Ages. Individual relics were often discredited, and abuses abounded. A good example of a critic of the abuses of the cult of saints and relics is Guibert of Nogent, who wrote *The Relics of the Saints* around 1120. He was a critic of the abuses, not of the theology underlying the cult itself. "Guibert did not object in principle to their veneration, but he was profoundly uneasy about some of the features of the developing cult," observes Colin Morris. "In the eyes of God, he believes, it is genuine faith which counts, and a prayer made through a false saint will still be of avail if the petitioner honestly believes in his sanctity."[146] Many Catholics, ranging from Guibert in the twelfth century to Erasmus in the sixteenth, expressed concern about particular relics, shrines, or supposed saints, and indignation about widespread abuses, while yearning for a reform of medieval Catholicism within the grounds of accepted orthodoxy. Others, however, voiced a more general skepticism about the whole range of supposedly miraculous occurrences. Such were, for example, John Wycliffe (ca. 1329–84) and the Lollards in England, and Jan Hus (1373–1415) and his followers on the Continent. Their desire for radical reform struck so deeply at the core of late medieval Catholic theology and practice that they appeared heretical in their denunciations of what they regarded as gross abuses, including allegedly miraculous performances under the auspices of corrupt clerics. In short, the cult of saints and relics and the cults of Christ and Mary were undergirded by the same theology that approved and stimulated the sale of indulgences, an abuse that incensed both Luther and Erasmus.

The removal of the healing shrines from countries that became Protestant left a void filled in part by the rise of a wide variety of practices that were labeled as magic and witchcraft, and were associated with "cunning men and wise women."[147] Interestingly, Lionel Rothkrug has suggested that in the Reformation in Germany, "areas rich in pilgrimage places remained Catholic, and those showing a paucity of sites embraced the Protestant faith."[148] This phenomenon had its roots in the differing religious emphases and cultural variations within Germany that contributed to the popularity of the rather sensationalistic shrines as an expression of lay piety in some areas and the rather quiet piety of, for example, the Brethren of the Common Life, in others. This is but one example of the enormous diversity that existed within Catholicism during the late Middle Ages. After commenting on Finucane's study, Richard Palmer remarks that "far less is known about the shrines of continental Europe [than about those of England]. In Italy the bodies of the saints were venerated. . . . But shrines . . . do not seem to have been places of healing in any way comparable to those of medieval England. In Italy if a sick person travelled at all he was probably *en route* to one of the flourishing medicinal spas."[149] The reader should be aware that the present study stresses the commonalities and homogeneity of medieval Catholicism. Finucane, who was himself quite aware of the enormous diversity within late medieval Catholicism, rightly emphasizes that "the Church" is really a convenient expression almost devoid of meaning. At its extremes it embraced the Church of the Lateran in Rome and the Church as known, say, to the medieval villagers of Oxenton in rural Gloucestershire. There was not only an Italian and an English medieval Church, as a modern historian has emphasized,[150] there was a French Church and a Spanish, an Icelandic and a German, each with its own history, traditions, liturgical uses and saints. Within these Churches were hundreds of divisions subdivided again into thousands of smaller units, ending at last with a semi-literate cleric in some rude chapel in the midst of inhospitable forests or fields, surrounded by peasants who muttered charms over their ploughs and whispered magic words at crossroads. It was a very long way from pope or prelate to peasant-priest, a long way in distance, education, and attitude.[151]

NOTES

1. See the numerous works of Peter Brown, especially *The Making of Late Antiquity* (Cambridge: Harvard University Press, 1978); and idem, *The Cult of the Saints: Its Rise and Function in Latin Christianity* (Chicago: University of Chicago Press, 1981).

2. Derek Baker, "*Vir Dei:* Secular Sanctity in the Early Tenth Century," in *Popular Belief and Practice,* ed. G. J. Cuming and Derek Baker, Studies in Church History, no. 8 (Cambridge: Cambridge University Press, 1972), 43.

3. Nicetus, translation in J. N. Hillgarth, ed., *The Conversion of Western Europe, 350–750* (Englewood Cliffs, N.J.: Prentice-Hall, 1969), 78–79.

4. Bede, *Ecclesiastical History* 1.31, trans. B. Colgrave and R. Mynors (Oxford: Clarendon, 1969). Subsequent quotations of Bede's *Ecclesiastical History* are from this translation.

5. Ibid., 1.30. For a fascinating discussion of the survival of paganism in Anglo-Saxon England, see Wilfrid Bonser, *The Medical Background of Anglo-Saxon England: A Study in History, Psychology, and Folklore* (London: Wellcome Historical Medical Library, 1963), 117–57.

6. See, for example, the sermons of Maximus of Turin and Martin of Braga in Hillgarth, ed., *Conversion of Western Europe* (n. 3), 54–63.

7. For a discussion of the nature and effects of plague in the early Middle Ages, see J.-N. Biraben and Jacques LeGoff, "The Plague in the Early Middle Ages," in *Biology of Man in History: Selections from the Annales: Economies, Sociétés, Civilisations,* ed. R. Forster and O. Ranum, trans. E. Forster and P. M. Ranum (Baltimore: Johns Hopkins University Press, 1975), 48–80.

8. Bede, *Life of St. Cuthbert* 9, in *Two Lives of Saint Cuthbert,* ed. and trans. B. Colgrave (1939; reprint, New York: Greenwood, 1969), 185.

9. Jonas of Orleans, *Institutio laicalis* 3.14.

10. See Clyde Pharr, "The Interdiction of Magic in Roman Law," *Trans. Am. Philol. Assoc.* 63 (1932): 269–95.

11. Thus the laws of the Visigoths and Lombards. See Hillgarth, ed., *Conversion of Western Europe* (n. 3), 103–4.

12. Walter Ullmann, "Public Welfare and Social Legislation in the Early Medieval Councils," in *Councils and Assemblies,* ed. G. J. Cuming and Derek Baker, Studies in Church History, no. 7 (Cambridge: Cambridge University Press, 1971), 35.

13. *The First Capitulary of Charlemagne* 7, translation in John T. McNeill and Helena M. Gamer, *Medieval Handbooks of Penance* (New York: Columbia University Press, 1938), 389.

14. A translation of this letter of Pope Gregory II is in Hillgarth, ed., *Conversion of Western Europe* (n. 3), 133.

15. Quoted in Patrick J. Geary, "The Ninth-Century Relic Trade: A Response to Popular Piety?" in *Religion and the People, 800–1700,* ed. James Obelkevich (Chapel Hill: University of North Carolina Press, 1979), 11.

16. Ullmann, "Public Welfare" (n. 12), 35–36.

17. Janet L. Nelson, "Society, Theodicy and the Origins of Heresy: Towards a Reassessment of the Medieval Evidence," in *Schism, Heresy, and Religious Protest,* ed. Derek Baker, Studies in Church History, no. 9 (Cambridge: Cambridge University Press, 1972), 75–76.

18. See McNeill and Gamer, *Handbooks of Penance* (n. 13), passim.

19. Bonser, *Medical Background* (n. 5), 128–29.

20. See, e.g., McNeill and Gamer, *Handbooks of Penance* (n. 13), 78, 90, 120, 198, 206–7, 228–29, 246, 255, 288–89, 292, 302, 311, 318, 330–35.

21. *The Penitential of Theodore* (ca. 668–90), 1.15.2; *The Penitential Ascribed to Bede* (possibly early eighth century), 10.2; the so-called *Confessional of Egbert* (ca. 950–1000); penitential canons from Regino's *Ecclesiastical Discipline* (ca. 906), sec. 304.

22. Bonser, *Medical Background* (n. 5), 248.

23. *The Penitential of Theodore* 1.14.16.

24. *The Irish Canons* (ca. 675), 12. See McNeill and Gamer, *Handbooks of Penance* (n. 13), 120 n. 22 (and references there to secondary literature).

25. *The Penitential of Theodore* 1.15.3; *The Penitential of Silos* (ca. 800) 11.

26. *The Penitential of Silos* 11.

27. Ibid., 7.

28. Burchard of Worms, *The Corrector and Physician* 65; cf. *The Penitential of Theodore* 2.10.5.

29. Burchard of Worms, *The Corrector and Physician* 66, 102; adapted from the translation in McNeill and Gamer, *Handbooks of Penance* (n. 13), 331, 335.

30. McNeill and Gamer, *Handbooks of Penance* (n. 13), 100.

31. *Roman Penitential of Halitgar,* adapted from the translation in ibid., 302.

32. *Roman Penitential of Halitgar* 81, 82. See the discussion, with other references, in John T. McNeill, *A History of the Cure of Souls* (New York: Harper and Row, 1951), 129.

33. With the possible exception of a totally enigmatic statement in the *Old Irish Penitential* (ca. 800) 1.20, in McNeill and Gamer, *Handbooks of Penance* (n. 13), 159.

34. *The Penitential of Theodore* 2.10.1; cf. 2.10.2, 2.10.4; translation in McNeill and Gamer, *Handbooks of Penance* (n. 13), 207. A similar passage occurs in *The Judgement of Clement* (ca. 700–750), 15, in ibid., 272.

35. *The Penitential of Theodore* 2.10.2, 2.10.3.

36. *The Burgundian Penitential* 36. A similar passage occurs in the *Roman Penitential of Halitgar* 39.

37. Loren C. MacKinney, "Tenth-Century Medicine as Seen in the *Historia* of Richer of Rheims," *Bull. Inst. Hist. Med.* 2 (1934): 361–62.

38. Fulbert of Chartres, *Letters* 71, in *The Letters and Poems of Fulbert of Chartres,* ed. and trans. Frederick Behrends (Oxford: Clarendon, 1976), 121.

39. Jerome Kroll, "A Reappraisal of Psychiatry in the Middle Ages," *Arch. Gen. Psychiatry* 29 (1973): 281.

40. Gregory the Great, *Pastoral Care* 3.12, trans. Henry Davis (New York: Newman, 1950), 122, 125.

41. Bede, *Ecclesiastical History* 4.9.

42. Ibid., 1.19.

43. From Bede, *Vita beatorum abbatum,* translation in Hillgarth, ed., *Conversion of Western Europe* (n. 3), 121.

44. Biraben and LeGoff, "Plague" (n. 7), 61.

45. Jeffrey Richards, *Consul of God: The Life and Times of Gregory the Great* (London: Routledge and Kegan Paul, 1980), 41–42.

46. Bede, *Ecclesiastical History* 1.14.

47. Bede, *Life of St. Cuthbert* 9, in *Two Lives* (n. 8), 185.

48. Bede, *De natura rerum* 37.

49. Bede, *Life of St. Cuthbert* 8.

50. Geary, "Relic Trade" (n. 15), 12.

51. Brown, *Cult of the Saints* (n. 1), 100.

52. For a discussion of healing by means of relics in Anglo-Saxon England, see Bonser, *Medical Background* (n. 5), 178–210.

53. See Bernhard Poschmann, *Penance and the Anointing of the Sick,* trans. F. Courtney (New York: Herder and Herder, 1964), 239–40.

54. See H. B. Porter, "The Origin of the Medieval Rite for Anointing the Sick or Dying," *J. Theol. Stud.,* n.s., 7 (1956): 211–25.

55. Caesarius of Arles, *Sermon* 279.5, quoted by Poschmann, *Penance* (n. 53), 241–42.

56. Brown, *Cult of the Saints* (n. 1), 117.

57. See Benedicta Ward, *Miracles and the Medieval Mind: Theory, Record, and Event, 1000–1215* (Philadelphia: University of Pennsylvania Press, 1982), 11.

58. See the statements of Aelfric (ca. 955–1020), quoted by Bonser, *Medical Background* (n. 5), 118–19, 138.

59. *Anonymous Life of St. Cuthbert* 1.4, 4.4; Bede, *Life of St. Cuthbert* 4, 23, 32; both in *Two Lives* (n. 8), 67–69, 117, 165–67, 231–35, 257–59.

60. See Pierre Riché, *Education and Culture in the Barbarian West: Sixth through Eighth Centuries,* trans. J. J. Contreni (Columbia: University of South Carolina Press, 1976), 204–6.

61. See Richards, *Consul of God* (n. 45), 47; and Riché, *Education and Culture* (n. 60), 142–43.

62. For a discussion, see Darrel W. Amundsen, "Medicine and Surgery as Art or Craft: The Role of Schematic Literature in the Separation of Medicine and

Surgery in the Late Middle Ages," *Trans. Stud. Coll. Phys. Philadelphia,* n.s., 1 (1979): 49–52; and Riché, *Education and Culture* (n. 60), 386.

63. Fulbert of Chartres, *Letters* 47, 48. For a more reticent attitude, see *The Letters of Gerbert with His Papal Privileges as Sylvester II,* trans. H. P. Lattin (New York: Columbia University Press, 1961), 188.

64. Fulbert of Chartres, *Letters* 24, pp. 45–47 in the edition cited in n. 38.

65. Loren C. MacKinney, "Medical Ethics and Etiquette in the Early Middle Ages: The Persistence of Hippocratic Ideals," *Bull. Hist. Med.* 26 (1952): 1–31.

66. Matt. 25:35–46; see Adolf Harnack, *The Expansion of Christianity in the First Three Centuries,* trans. J. Moffatt (1904–5; reprint, Freeport, N.Y.: Books for Libraries, 1972), 199.

67. See Ullmann, "Public Welfare" (n. 12), 8.

68. See ibid., 9–10.

69. This caution is convincingly expressed by Timothy S. Miller, "The Knights of St. John and the Hospitals of the West," *Speculum* 53 (1978): 709–33, especially 709–12.

70. See ibid., 710–11.

71. Benedict, *Rule* 36.

72. Benedict, *Rule* 31, trans. and ed. Justin McCann (London: Burnes and Oates, 1952), 83. Cf. the very elaborate and atypical instructions by Cassiodorus, *Introduction to Divine and Human Readings* 1.31.

73. *Anonymous Life of St. Cuthbert* 4.17; Bede, *Life of St. Cuthbert* 45; both in *Two Lives* (n. 8), 137–39, 299–31.

74. See *Vita Sancti Columbae auctore Adamnano,* ed. W. Reeves (Dublin: Bannatyne Club, 1857), 55 ff.

75. Bernard of Clairvaux, *Letters* 70 and 71, in *The Letters of St. Bernard of Clairvaux,* trans. Bruno Scott James (London: Burnes and Oates, 1953), 95–99.

76. Miller, "Knights of St. John" (n. 69), 714.

77. Lateran II 9, translation in R. J. Schroeder, *Disciplinary Decrees of the General Councils* (St. Louis: Herder, 1957), 201–2.

78. A translation, as well as a discussion of all pertinent legislation, may be found in Darrel W. Amundsen, "Medieval Canon Law on Medical and Surgical Practice by the Clergy," *Bull. Hist. Med.* 52 (1978): 22–44; reprinted in slightly altered form as chap. 8, below.

79. Gregory IX, *Decretales* 3.5.3.

80. Ibid., 3.50.10.

81. See Amundsen, "Canon Law" (n. 78), 36–38.

82. Lateran IV 18 = *Decretales* 3.50.9. See Amundsen, "Canon Law" (n. 78), 40–43.

83. C. H. Talbot, *Medicine in Medieval England* (London: Oldbourne, 1967), 96.

84. Miller, "Knights of St. John" (n. 69), 714–17.

85. On hospitals and hospital orders in the high and late Middle Ages, see the secondary literature cited by Miller, in ibid.; and by Brian Tierney, *Medieval Poor Law: A Sketch of Canonical Theory and Its Application in England* (Berkeley: University of California Press, 1959), notes accompanying pp. 85–87.

86. See John W. Baldwin, *Masters, Princes, and Merchants: The Social Views of Peter the Chanter and His Circle* (Princeton: Princeton University Press, 1970).

87. Peter the Chanter, *Summa de sacramentis et animae consiliis.*

88. Henry Charles Lea, *A History of Auricular Confession and Indulgences in the Latin Church*, 2 vols. (Philadelphia: Lea Brothers, 1896), 1:230.

89. Lateran IV 21. For a translation, see Oscar Watkins, *A History of Penance*, 2 vols. (London: Longmans, Green, 1920), 2:748–49.

90. Gregory IX, *Decretales* 5.38.12.

91. Thomas N. Tentler, "Response and Retractatio," in *The Pursuit of Holiness in Later Medieval and Renaissance Religion*, ed. Charles Trinkaus (Leiden: Brill, 1974), 134.

92. *Astesana*, as quoted by Thomas N. Tentler, "The *Summa* for Confessors as an Instrument of Social Control," in Trinkaus, *Pursuit of Holiness* (n. 91), 115.

93. Thomas N. Tentler, *Sin and Confession on the Eve of the Reformation* (Princeton: Princeton University Press, 1977), 207.

94. See especially John T. Noonan, Jr., *Contraception: A History of Its Treatment by the Catholic Theologians and Canonists* (Cambridge: Harvard University Press, 1966); idem, "An Almost Absolute Value in History," in *The Morality of Abortion: Legal and Historical Perspectives*, ed. John T. Noonan, Jr. (Cambridge: Harvard University Press, 1970), 1–59; and John Connery, *Abortion: The Development of the Roman Catholic Perspective* (Chicago: Loyola University Press, 1977).

95. Gratian, *Decretum* C. 32 q. 2 c. 7.

96. Gregory IX, *Decretales* 5.12.20.

97. Ibid., 5.12.5.

98. Tentler, *Sin and Confession* (n. 93), xv.

99. Tentler, "Response and Retractatio" (n. 91), 137.

100. Barlaam, quoted by Bernard J. Verkamp, *The Indifferent Mean: Adiaphorism in the English Reformation to 1554* (Athens: Ohio University Press, and Detroit: Wayne State University Press, 1977), 6, 9.

101. Lateran IV 22 (*Cum infirmitas* [or *Quum infirmitas*]).

102. Gregory IX, *Decretales* 5.38.13 (*Cum infirmitas* [or *Quum infirmitas*]).

103. Translation in Schroeder, *Disciplinary Decrees* (n. 77), 236.

104. Latin text in S. DeRenzi, *Collectio Salernitana*, 5 vols. (Naples: Filiatre-Sebezio, 1852–59), 2:74; translation is mine.

105. Translation in Henry E. Sigerist, "Bedside Manners in the Middle Ages: The Treatise *De Cautelis Medicorum* Attributed to Arnald of Villanova," *Quart. Bull. Northwestern Univ. Med. School* 20 (1946): 141.

106. Anonymous plague tractate, translation in Darrel W. Amundsen, "Medical Deontology and Pestilential Disease in the Late Middle Ages," *J. Hist. Med. Allied Sci.* 32 (1977): 416; reproduced with minor changes as chap. 10, below.

107. Latin text in Paul Diepgen, *Die Theologie und der ärztliche Stand* (Berlin, 1922), 51 n. 287; my translation.

108. For a discussion, see Darrel W. Amundsen, "Casuistry and Professional Obligations: The Regulation of Physicians by the Court of Conscience in the Late Middle Ages," *Trans. Stud. Coll. Phys. Philadelphia*, n.s., 3 (1981): 22–39, 93–112; reproduced with minor changes as chap. 9, below.

109. Thomas Aquinas, *Summa theologiae* 2–2.71.1, various translators (Westminster: Blackfriar, 1964–80), 38:145.

110. See Darrel W. Amundsen and Gary B. Ferngren, "Philanthropy in Medicine: Some Historical Perspectives," in *Beneficence and Health Care*, ed. Earl E. Shelp (Dordrecht: Reidel, 1982), 22–23.

111. See the discussion in G. R. Owst, *Literature and Pulpit in Medieval England: A Neglected Chapter in the History of English Letters and of the English People*, 2d ed. (Oxford: Blackwell, 1961), 349–51.

112. Jacque de Vitry, quoted by Jonathan Sumption, *Pilgrimage: An Image of Medieval Religion* (Totowa, N.J.: Rowman and Littlefield, 1975), 80.

113. Humbert de Romans, Sermon 40, quoted by Bede Jarrett, *Social Theories of the Middle Ages, 1200–1500* (1926; reprint, Westminster, Md.: Newman Book Shop, 1942), 223.

114. E.g., in the early fifteenth century John Mirfield, and late in the same century the various authors of different versions of *The Ship of Fools*.

115. See P. Delaunay, *La médecine et l'Eglise: Contribution à l'histoire de l'exercise médical par les clercs* (Paris: Editions Hippocrate, 1948), 11–12; and Darrel W. Amundsen, "Medical Legislation of the Assizes of Jerusalem," in *Proceedings of the XXIIIrd International Congress of the History of Medicine* (London: Wellcome Institute, 1974), 521 n. 16.

116. The following works have a section devoted to the subject: Bartholomaeus de Sancto Concordio, *Summa casuum* (ca. 1338; Venice, 1473), copy at University of Pennsylvania, generally cited as *Pisanella;* Antoninus of Florence, *Summa theologica* (1477; reprint of 1740 edition, Graz, Austria, 1959), also known as *Summa moralis;* Baptista Trovamala de Salis, *Summa de casibus conscientiae* (ca. 1480; Venice, 1495), copy at College of Physicians of Philadelphia, generally cited as *Baptistina;* Angelus Carletus de Clavasio, *Summa angelica de casibus conscientiae* (ca. 1486; Lyons, 1494), copy at Free Library of Philadelphia generally cited as *Angelica.*

117. See Thomas G. Benedek, "The Image of Medicine in 1500: Theological Reactions to *The Ship of Fools*," *Bull. Hist. Med.* 38 (1964): 332–33.

118. See Pearl Kibre, "The Faculty of Medicine at Paris, Charlatanism, and Unlicensed Medical Practices in the Later Middle Ages," *Bull. Hist. Med.* 27 (1953): 1–20.

119. See the discussion in Ward, *Miracles* (n. 57), chap. 1, especially 10–13.

120. E.g., *The Penitential of Bartholomew Iscanus*, in McNeill and Gamer, *Handbooks of Penance* (n. 13), 350.

121. William C. McDonald, "Death in the Stars: Heinrich von Mügeln on the Black Plague," *Mediaevalia* 5 (1979): 97.

122. Roger Bacon, *On the Errors of Physicians* 144–45, as quoted by John M. Riddle, "Theory and Practice in Medieval Medicine," *Viator* 5 (1974): 169–70 n. 51.

123. Benedek, "Image of Medicine" (n. 117), 336–37.

124. McDonald, "Death in the Stars" (n. 121), 101–2.

125. Richard Palmer, "The Church, Leprosy, and Plague in Medieval and Early Modern Europe," in *The Church and Healing*, ed. W. J. Sheils, Studies in Church History, no. 19 (Oxford: Blackwell, 1982), 83.

126. C. Mollat, *The Popes at Avignon, 1305–1378* (London: T. Nelson, 1963), 40.

127. See Palmer, "The Church, Leprosy, and Plague" (n. 125), 94–99; and Carlo M. Cipolla, *Faith, Reason, and the Plague in Seventeenth-Century Tuscany* (Ithaca, N.Y.: Cornell University Press, 1979); and idem, *Public Health and the Medical Profession in the Renaissance* (Cambridge: Cambridge University Press, 1976).

128. Amundsen, "Medical Deontology" (n. 106), 403–21.

129. Sylvia L. Thrupp, "Plague Effects in Medieval Europe," *Comp. Stud. Society Hist.* 8 (1966): 480–81. For the effects of the Black Death on the medical profession and on medical knowledge, see Robert S. Gottfried, *The Black Death: Natural and Human Disaster in Medieval Europe* (New York: Free Press, 1983), 104–28.

130. John of Saxony, treatise on plague, Latin text in Karl Sudhoff, "Pestschriften aus den ersten 150 Jahren nach der Epidemie des 'schwarzen Todes' 1348," *Sudhoffs Archiv* 16 (1924–25): 26; my translation.

131. John Henderson, "The Flagellant Movement and Flagellant Confraternities in Central Italy, 1260–1400," in *Religious Motivation: Biographical and Sociological Problems for the Church Historian*, ed. Derek Baker, Studies in Church History 15 (Oxford: Blackwell, 1978), 151. See also Norman Cohn, *The Pursuit of the Millennium* (London: Oxford University Press, 1970), for a discussion of the flagellant movement and related phenomena.

132. Mollat, *Popes at Avignon* (n. 126), 41.

133. Henderson, "Flagellant Movement" (n. 131), 160.

134. See Kroll, "Reappraisal of Psychiatry" (n. 39), 276–83; George Rosen, *Madness in Society* (Chicago: University of Chicago Press, 1968), chap. 7; and Ronald C. Finucane, *Miracles and Pilgrims: Popular Beliefs in Medieval England* (Totowa, N.J.: Rowman and Littlefield, 1977), 72.

135. Palmer, "The Church, Leprosy, and Plague" (n. 125), 82–83.

136. Saul Nathaniel Brody, *The Disease of the Soul: Leprosy in Medieval Literature* (Ithaca, N.Y.: Cornell University Press, 1974), 103.

137. Palmer, "The Church, Leprosy, and Plague" (n. 125), 85.

138. Quoted by Steven E. Ozment, *The Reformation in the Cities: The Appeal of Protestantism to Sixteenth-Century Germany and Switzerland* (New Haven: Yale University Press, 1975), 29.

139. Geary, "Relic Trade" (n. 15), 19.

140. Colin Morris, *The Discovery of the Individual, 1050–1200* (New York: Harper and Row, 1972), 122.

141. Sumption, *Pilgrimage* (n. 112), 144. See also Emma Mason, "Rocamadour in Quercy above All Other Churches: The Healing of Henry II," in Sheils, ed., *Church and Healing* (n. 125), 52.

142. Finucane, *Miracles and Pilgrims* (n. 134), 67.

143. See ibid., 52–53; and Eugene A. Dooley, *Church Law on Sacred Relics*, Canon Law Studies, no. 70 (Washington, D.C.: Catholic University, 1931).

144. Finucane, *Miracles and Pilgrims* (n. 134), 196–97.

145. Ibid., 198. See also Lionel Rothkrug, "Popular Religion and Holy Shrines: Their Influence on the Origins of the German Reformation and Their Role in German Cultural Development," in Obelkevich, ed., *Religion and the People* (n. 15), 28–29 and 36.

146. Colin Morris, "A Critique of Popular Religion: Guibert of Nogent on *The Relics of the Saints*," in Cuming and Baker, eds., *Popular Belief and Practice* (n. 2), 56, 58.

147. See Finucane, *Miracles and Pilgrims* (n. 134), 214–15. This is an important aspect of Keith Thomas' thesis in *Religion and the Decline of Magic* (New York: Scribner's, 1971).

148. Rothkrug, "Popular Religion and Holy Shrines" (n. 145), 56.

149. Palmer, "The Church, Leprosy, and Plague" (n. 125), 87.

150. Finucane is speaking of R. Brentano, *Two Churches: England and Italy in the Thirteenth Century* (Princeton, N.J.: Princeton University Press, 1968).

151. Finucane, *Miracles and Pilgrims* (n. 134), 10–11.

EIGHT

Medieval Canon Law on Medical and Surgical Practice by the Clergy

Were the medieval clergy ever forbidden to practice medicine or surgery? If an answer to this question is sought in secondary sources, the inquirer will soon find himself sinking into a quagmire of often conflicting and confusing statements usually alluding to but almost never citing, much less quoting, primary documents. The searcher may turn to a survey of medieval history and find the assertion that "at the beginning of the twelfth century, the medicine of the soul was declared incompatible with that of the body. The Church forbad monks to become professional doctors, a ban renewed in 1219 and extended at the same time to . . . cover the secular clergy."[1] Or he may look into a recent survey of the history of medicine and read, "By the late centuries of the Middle Ages, medicine . . . passed entirely into the hands of the laity: Pope Honorius III had in fact forbidden clergy to practise."[2] He may wish for more detailed information and turn to other medical history texts and find statements such as these:

Notably under Pope Innocent II edicts were given forth (Council of Clermont 1130, of Rheims 1131, Lateran Council 1139) against medical practice by ecclesiastics.[3]

The practice, and in fact the study and teaching, of medicine, were forbidden to the higher clergy by the Council of Rheims 1131, the Lateran 1139, Montpellier 1162, Tours 1163, Paris 1212, and the second Lateran 1215. Finally the lower monks were also restricted, and especially by the Council of Le Mans 1247 all burning and cutting (surgery) were forbidden them, on the principle "The Church shuns bloodshed."[4]

At the Councils of Rheims (1131), Montpellier (1162), Tours (1163), Paris (1212, at those of the Lateran (1139 and 1215) and also by the decretals of the Popes Alexander III (1180) and Honorius III (1219) medical practice and especially surgery were forbidden to priests.[5]

We find the Church instituting that long series of edicts, which, in the first instance, were aimed not so much at medicine as at its malpractice by monks. These were the decrees of the councils of Clermont (1130), Rheims (1131), the second Lateran (1139), Montpellier (1162), Tours (1163), Paris (1212), the Fourth Lateran (1215) and Le Mans (1247). The general effect was, unfortunately, not only to stop the monks from practising, but to extend the special odium of these decrees to the whole medical profession.[6]

If the searcher stops at this point, he will have a fairly consistent list of church councils, the mention of papal decrees, and the impression that the church had forbidden the practice of both medicine and surgery to monks and/or to priests, or perhaps, both to "the higher clergy" and to monks.

The inquirer may then turn to more specialized works on medical history and see a statement such as this:

Ecclesiastic law is exemplified by the action of the Fourth Lateran Council which, in 993, prohibited the regular clergy from performing any surgical operation involving the shedding of blood, thus leaving such operation to seculars and clerks. However, the priest-physicians were not prohibited from practicing medicine until 1131, at which time the Seventh Lateran Council forbade the monks and regular canons from pursuing the study of medicine. Later still, in 1163, the Council of Tours positively interdicted all surgical operations by the clergy.[7]

The dates and the names of some councils are now different, and new types of clerics are introduced unto the scene. If the searcher after truth has not yet become discouraged, he may look further into the secondary literature in the hope of some clarification, and read that "those in Orders were discouraged or forbidden by the Church from the practice of surgery, involving as it did the shedding of blood. In the practice of medicine the cleric had to compete with the experienced lay physician."[8] A new twist is now added: Clerics "in Orders" were forbidden to practice surgery, but clerics in general were allowed to pursue medicine.

The investigator may then wish to look further into the matter of the prohibition of the practice of surgery. He will find that "one of the main objections developed in the Middle Ages against anatomical studies was the maxim that 'the Church abhors the shedding of blood.' On this ground, in 1248, the Council of Le Mans forbade surgery to monks. Many other councils did the same. . . . So deeply was this idea rooted in the mind of the universal Church that for over a thousand years surgery was considered dishonourable."[9] Seeking to confirm that monks had been forbidden to practice surgery as of 1248, he may turn to a noted history of the relations of medicine and surgery and see that "the Rheims (A.D. 1125) and Lateran (A.D. 1139) Councils restricted the surgery of the clerical or, in other words, of the educated class, and no doubt feudal ideas did no less to abase its services; it was at Tours however that the sinister and perfidious 'ecclesia abhorret a sanguine' was first pronounced."[10]

If the conflict over the council responsible for the prohibition of surgery, as well as the question of whether only monks or all clerics were affected, stimulates the searcher to dig further into the problem, he will find that Tours of 1163 is more frequently mentioned than any other council in this regard and that the prohibition appears to have applied to all clerics. Additionally, it may have been this opprobrious action of the church that caused the great split between medicine and surgery in the late Middle Ages:

Another practical obstacle to the advance of medicine at this time was the prohibition formulated at the Council of Tours against the shedding of blood by ecclesiastics. Since the doctor until well into the Renaissance was generally also a priest, he was henceforward prohibited from the practice of surgery. This resulted in him having to send his servant, a lay-brother, who would generally be the barber who kept his tonsure shaved, to attend to those of his clients who wished to be bled or have a tooth drawn. As a result of this he completely abandoned his status as a craftsman and merged himself into the authoritarian scholastic hierarchy.[11]

If in doubt that this was how the barber-surgeons originated, the investigator might seek confirmation: "Surgery . . . was considered an unseemly practice for Monks. In 1163 the canon of Tours by its edict, Ecclesia abhorret a sanguine, had ordained that Monks should wholly abstain from manual operations of surgery; as a consequence this deserted profession fell into the hands of barbers and surgeons."[12]

Tours of 1163 remains the source; again it only affects monks. That it caused the separation of medicine and surgery remains clear, at least until the investigator reads further:

Innocent III . . . at the Lateran Council of 1215 . . . forbade all clerics in higher orders, that is, subdeacons, deacons and priests, to carry out surgical operations which involved cutting or burning. It was to be left to laymen. This decree has been constantly brought forward to show that from this point onwards surgery was thrown into the hands of the illiterate and that it led to the separation of medicine and surgery. . . . The separation of surgery from medicine was not an effect of ecclesiastical legislation: it was due not to the prohibition of medical practice to clerics.[13]

Yet a different council and date and different types of clerics were affected; and the church is no longer held responsible for separating medicine and surgery. In the hope that the author last cited said more on the subject elsewhere, the diligent inquirer will find him maintaining that "after the decree of the Lateran Council of 1215, when clerics in major Orders were forbidden to practice surgery and cautery, it became clear that physicians and surgeons could not be housed (at least in ecclesiastically dominated universities) under one and the same academical roof."[14] So, perhaps the church was partially responsible after all.

If the investigator stops here, pondering on the degree of the church's guilt in relegating surgery to barbers, or at least expelling it from the universities, will he at any rate have found an answer to the original question: were the medieval clergy ever forbidden to practice medicine or surgery? He certainly will have a variety of answers from which to choose. If he wishes to step back through the looking glass into the whirlwind of confusion of more secondary sources, the variations on the theme will continue to grow.[15] Nearly all that he reads on the subject will contain at least a small kernel of truth. Some will be essentially accurate in certain details. But he will probably look in vain for a study that will assure him that there had indeed been much inaccuracy and confusion on the question in secondary literature and that will then discuss systematically the relevant action of various church councils and, more importantly, the regulations in medieval canon law governing the involvement of the clergy in medicine and surgery.

It is my purpose in this paper to present and discuss the primary documents in order to demonstrate that the prohibitions were not nearly as restrictive as they usually appear in the secondary literature and that such broad statements as "clerics were forbidden to practice medicine or surgery in the late Middle Ages" are generally inaccurate and consequently misleading.

The Nature of the Primary Sources

The primary documents employed will be the canons of various church councils, both regional and general, and the official collections of canon law. In regard to church councils, it is important to be aware that the enactments of regional councils applied only to these councils' immediate area of jurisdiction and that those of general councils applied to all Christendom. If one looks only to the provisions of church councils in order to determine the law of the medieval church, the result will be distorted. In addition to the canons of church councils there are also papal rescripts or decretals, both of a universal and of a limited application, and the writing of the church fathers. From the fifth century on, many attempts were made to form collections of regulations from these materials. Thus, although the collections contained canons of church councils both general and local, they also included selections from letters of popes and other bishops and from patristic literature. These, the first canonical collections, were unofficial in nature, though they provided regulations for those dioceses in which they were used. Vast and disorganized, this array of conflicting sources provided no systematic treatment of the law of the church. The most spectacular effort at bringing order out of this chaos was the *Decretum* of Gratian, completed about 1140. Its original title, *Concordia discordantium canonum* (A harmony of disharmonious canons), graphically portrays Gratian's purpose. The method he employed was to state a specific problem, introduce authorities on both sides of the question, and then propose a solution that would bring the apparently conflicting positions into harmony or show the greater acceptability of one position. Although a monument of scholastic method, and of enduring significance, this dialectical treatise on the law of the church was entirely of an unofficial nature in the sense that it was never promulgated as an "authentic" source of canon law. The *Decretum* was not, however, only of academic value; it was used by canonical courts in reaching decisions and presumably guided bishops and other ecclesiastical officials in their administration. After Gratian completed his *Decretum*, many new laws were promulgated by general church councils, and many decretals having a universal application were issued by popes. These were collected by a variety of efforts, most being unofficial, that is, not having been promulgated as authentic collections. The first official collection was the *Compilatio tertia*,[16] composed of decretals issued during the first twelve years of Innocent III's pontificate, and promulgated in 1210. The second official collection was the *Compilatio quinta*, promulgated in 1226 by Honorius III and composed of decretals issued between 1216 and 1226. The most important collection having the force of law is the *Decretales* of Gregory IX, promulgated in 1234. This, the first official collection of a universal character not limited to decretals issued during restricted periods of time, rendered all previous collections, whether of an official or unofficial nature, obsolete,[17] and is part of what became known as the *Corpus iuris canonici*.[18]

In discussing the regulations bearing first on the practice of medicine and then on the practice of surgery by clerics, we shall look at the relevant canons of regional and general church councils dated before the promulgation of the *Decretales* of Gregory IX. We shall then turn to the *Decretales*, followed by a brief discussion of later decretal and conciliar developments.

Before pursuing the primary documents, some terminological distinctions should be made regarding the different classifications of clergy. On what may be called a horizontal plane, one must distinguish between regular and secular clergy. Some clerics lived under a rule and were called regular clergy, or religious. Monks and canons regular are in this category. The majority of clerics, however, were secular clergy who did not live under a rule but functioned within secular society. On a vertical plane, there were seven different orders: four minor orders (porters, acolytes, exorcists, and lectors) and three major orders (subdeacons, deacons, and priests). The major orders are sometimes referred to as holy orders, or sacred orders.

Canon Law on Medical Practice by Clerics

Canon 5 of the Council of Clermont of 1130,[19] canon 6 of the Council of Rheims of 1131,[20] and canon 9 of the Second Lateran Council of 1139,[21] are all identical, with minor textual variations. (The first two councils were regional, and the third was a general council under Innocent II.) Their common rubric reads: "Monks and canons regular are not to study jurisprudence and medicine for the sake of temporal gain."

An evil and detestable custom, we understand, has grown up in the form that monks and canons regular, after having received the habit and made profession, despite the rule of the holy masters Benedict and Augustine, study jurisprudence and medicine for the sake of temporal gain. Instead of devoting themselves to psalmody and hymns, they are led by the impulses of avarice to make themselves defenders of causes and, confiding in the support of a splendid voice, confuse by the variety of their statements what is just and unjust, right and wrong. The imperial constitutions, however, testify that it is absurd and disgraceful for clerics to seek to become experts in forensic disputations. We decree, therefore, in virtue of our Apostolic authority, that offenders of this kind be severely punished. Moreover, the care of souls being neglected and the purposes of their order being set aside, they promise health in return for detestable money and thus make themselves physicians of human bodies. Since an impure eye is the messenger of an impure heart, those things about which good people blush to speak, religion ought not to treat. Therefore, that the monastic order as well as the order of canons may be pleasing to God and be conserved inviolate in their holy purposes, we forbid in virtue of our Apostolic authority that this be done in the future. Bishops, abbots, and priors consenting to such outrageous practice and not correcting it, shall be deprived of their honors and cut off from the Church.[22]

Although there is a degree of uneasiness that these religious who practice medicine would encounter things that they ought not to see, the central matter of concern in this canon is the avaricious motivation behind entering into the study and, by extension, the practice of medicine and secular law. This was a time of great social and economic change, a period marked by the rise of commercial and professional activities of a wide variety. The church was engaged in an internal ideological struggle regarding the spiritual aspects of commercial activity, and the attitudes of canonists and the stipulations of church councils evidence an attempt at adaptation designed to cope with socioeconomic change. This is reflected in the fact that, while in the *Decretum* of Gratian all commercial profit seems to have been condemned, even his earliest commentators did not sustain his views on merchants' activities.[23] It is particularly during the twelfth century that there was a "shift in values within the traditional scheme of the cardinal vices."[24] The primacy of pride as the supreme vice was being displaced by the sin of avarice in theological and popular conceptions. This had its effect on the secular activities of the clergy. "In practice, clerics had engaged in secular pursuits from the time of the early Church onwards, and gradually, in theory, the canonists came to apply one criterion, i.e., of motive, whether such work was undertaken from a genuine need *(necessitas)* or selfish gain *(turpe lucrum)*."[25]

It is essential to note that the prohibitions contained in the canon common to the councils of Clermont, Rheims and Lateran II extended only to monks and canons regular, those who were professed religious, who had withdrawn from secular affairs. The study and practice of medicine and secular law were here not considered appropriate for those who should be devoted exclusively to a religious life, if the motivation behind medical or legal activity was financial gain. The specific prohibition against the study and practice of medicine did not apply to a sizable segment of the clergy and is hardly a wholesale condemnation of the practice of medicine by clerics. Even though it is also a canon of a general church council, its provisions were of little lasting significance. It simply was never included in any official collection of canon law. We shall find no further mention of any prohibition of the *practice* of medicine by any clerics in the canons of general church councils or in decretals.

The charge is made with some frequency that it was necessary for the church to repeat nearly incessantly its prohibition of the practice of medicine by clerics.[26] If all the church councils that issued canons regarding clerical involvement in medicine or surgery were simply listed chronologically, it would then appear that these were frustrated repetitions of previous legislation that had been ignored by obstreperous and recalcitrant clerics. This is a theme to which we shall return later in this chapter. For now, let us consider whether the charge holds true in the case of the first three relevant church councils. In 1130 a regional council (Clermont) issued the canon discussed above. Its provisions would have applied only to the specific region represented by the council. The same canon was, in the following year, adopted by another regional council (Rheims [1131]), still having only regional force. Both Clermont and Rheims were regional but also papal councils, two of four regional councils over which Innocent II presided.[27] Eight years later the canon was adopted by a general council (Lateran II [1139]), also under Innocent II, thus applying its provisions to all Christendom, at least until such time as it was superceded by other general church legislation. In fact, one-fourth of the canons adopted by Lateran II simply repeat verbatim canons enacted by regional but papal councils presided over by Innocent II between 1130 and 1135. This is hardly a case of frantic repetition of ineffective legislation.

In 1162, at the Council of Montpellier, a regional and papal council presided over by Alexander III, a canon appears to have been enacted pertaining to the study of medicine and secular law by monks, canons regular, or other religious. The records of this council are not extant, but in a later council in Montpellier (1195) reference was made to the earlier council: "He [sc. Alexander III] also prohibited under every severity of ecclesiastical discipline any monk or canon regular or other religious to depart in order to study secular laws or physic. Moreover, in consequence of the decree promulgated under Lord Alexander in the council at Montpellier and of Tours in accord with this article, let them be punished canonically by the diocesan bishops."[28]

The canon enacted by Alexander III at Montpellier in 1162 is linked with and may be identical to that of Tours. In 1163, at the regional and papal Council of Tours, Alexander III enacted a canon that had an immediate and enduring impact:

The ancient enemy's hatred does not strive with much effort to ruin the weak members of the Church, but he sends his hand against her more desirable members and attempts to trip up the elect, for the Scripture says, "The elect are his food." Therefore he thinks that he has caused the fall of many when he has drawn away a more precious member of the Church by his cunning. And, of course, it is then that, by his usual habit, he entices away from their cloisters certain regulars for the study of law and for pondering medical concoctions[29] under the pretext of aiding the bodies of their ill brothers and performing ecclesiastical affairs more proficiently. On this account, so that, by the pursuit of knowledge, spiritual men be not entangled again in the affairs of this world and be not lacking in things of the soul, believing themselves thereby to provide for others in external matters, we decree with the consent of the present council, that no one at all is permitted to depart for the purpose of studying[30] medicine or secular law after having taken the vow and profession of religion in any religious place. If he does depart and does not return to his cloister within the space of two months, let him be avoided by all as if excommunicate, and in no case, if he dares to present a defense, should he be heard. When he has returned, however, let him always be the last of the brothers in the choir, in the chapter, at table, and in the rest, and let him lose hope of every advancement, unless, perhaps, by the pity of the Apostolic See.[31]

This canon, although not of a general council, quickly was included in a variety of twelfth-century decretal collections. It is, for example, found in these major collections: *Appendix consilii Lateranensis*,[32] *Collectio canonum Lipsiensis*,[33] *Collectio canonum Bambergensis*,[34] *Collectio canonum Casselana*,[35] and *Compilatio prima*,[36] and also in several unedited English collections.[37] It is also the first document printed in the cartularies of the University of Paris.[38] Most importantly, it was included in the first officially promulgated major decretal collection, the *Decretales* of Gregory IX (1234).[39]

The section of the *Decretales* in which this canon of the Council of Tours is placed is entitled "Clerics and Monks Are Not to Involve Themselves in Secular Affairs." The major emphasis of this section is that some acts are forbidden to all Christians, some are permitted to all; others, although permitted to laymen, are prohibited to all clerics; and others still are forbidden only to certain groups of clerics. The canon under consideration falls into the last category. The study of medicine and secular law is here prohibited for the same groups as were included in the canon from Lateran II. Canons regular and monks were religious rather than secular clergy. They lived together under a rule and were bound by a vow of stability, an obligation of residence. It is the leaving of their cloisters for secular purposes rather than purely religious ones that was condemned, not the study of medicine or secular law. That these two disciplines are again mentioned together is interesting: the canon lawyers themselves were required to receive extensive training in secular law before advancing to canon law. The study of secular law obviously was not being condemned *eo ipso*. Nor was the study of medicine. Significantly, the canon did not forbid all members of the clergy to study medicine or secular law. The majority of clerics would not have been affected. Nor did it prohibit the *practice* of these arts even by monks and canons regular.

In 1213[40] the regional Council of Paris adopted the following canon:

Since certain regulars (to use the words of the Lateran Council), under the pretext of caring for the bodies of their sick brothers and conducting ecclesiastical affairs more proficiently, do not fear to leave their cloisters for the purpose of studying secular law and pondering medical concoctions in order to attend to jurisprudence and medicine, and are *eo ipso* deficient in things of the soul, although they believe themselves to be providing for others in exterior matters: following in the footsteps of that council, we order that, unless they return to their cloisters within the space of two months, even if they had the permission of their abbott (since he was not allowed to give such permission), let them be excommunicate and avoided by all, and in no case, if they wish to present a defense, are they to be heard.[41]

Note that, although the council cited is the Lateran, the canon that is paraphrased is that of Tours. This may be simply a *lapsus linguae*, but it is equally possible that the reference is to Lateran III of 1179. (It obviously is not to Lateran II.) Reference was made above[42] to the inclusion of Tours canon 8 in *Appendix consilii Lateranensis*, a collection of canons that is found associated with the canons of Lateran III. Canon 8 of the Council of Tours on that account may have been mistaken for a canon of Lateran III, which would have given it additional weight, as Lateran III was a general council while Tours was a regional, although papal, council.[43]

In 1219 Honorius III issued a lengthy rescript, usually called the *Super specula* (or *Super speculam*), which was designed to promote the study of theology.[44] The steps taken in this rescript were (1) to provide that teachers of theology (as long as they were teaching) and theological students (for a period up to five years) could receive the income of their prebends or benefices; (2) to repeat and extend the provisions of canon 8 of the Council of Tours; and (3) to forbid the teaching and study of civil (i.e., Roman) law at the University of Paris. The sections of the *Super specula* dealing with the above three matters were extracted and included in the *Compilatio quinta*,[45] the second official decretal collection, which was promulgated in 1226 by Honorius III. They were also included in the *Decretales* of Gregory IX (1234).[46] It is the second of the three actions taken by Honorius III in the *Super specula* that pertains directly to our subject. The text, as it appears in the *Decretales* of Gregory IX, reads:

Our predecessor, Alexander [III] once enacted in the Council of Tours in regard to religious persons leaving their cloisters to attend lectures on laws or physic,[47] that unless they return to their cloisters within the space of two months, they are to be avoided by all as if excommunicate, and in no case, if they wish to present a defense, are they to be heard. When they have returned, however, they are to be the last of the brothers in choir, at table, in the chapters and in the rest, and they are to lose hope of every advancement, unless, perhaps, by the pity of the Apostolic See. Indeed, because some of these, on account of the varied opinions of certain men, adopt any kind of excuse, we, wishing that they henceforth incur the sentence of excommunication *ipso facto*, as a warning strictly command that both by their diocesan [bishops] and by their chapters, and also by the other bishops in whose dioceses they study to this effect, such men be publicly announced as excommunicate [and] liable to the above stated penalties. Inasmuch as we desire the study of theology to be increased, so that, just as when the space for one's tent has been broadened one also lengthens its cords, the Catholic faith might be girded about by an impregnable wall of warriors, with which she will have the power to fend off those scaling up from outside: we wish and order that this [prohibition] be extended to archdeacons, deacons, rural deans, priors, cantors and other clerics having benefices, and also to priests, unless they desist from these things within the prescribed period, and that [this order] be firmly enforced, with the right of appeal having been rescinded.[48]

It is important to consider the tone and the intent of the entire rescript of which the section just quoted above is only a part. Honorius III's purpose in issuing the *Super specula* was to encourage theological study, not to condemn any activity. It could easily be argued that this rescript furnishes solid evidence of his open hostility to the study of civil law. Not only did Honorius extend the prohibition of its study (as well as of the study of medicine) to new groups of clerics but he also forbade its being taught or studied in the city of Paris. Hastings Rashdall comments that the teaching and study of civil law in Paris was forbidden "not (as is sometimes represented) in a narrow spirit of hostility to legal or to secular studies in general, but because it threatened to extinguish the study of theology in the one great theological school of Europe."[49] Indeed, the papacy was highly supportive of the faculty of civil law at the greatest center for legal studies, Bologna. On the University of the Roman Curia, Rashdall writes:

It is particularly worthy of notice that the civil law received especial encourage-ment in a school which was the absolute creature of the holy see, priests habitu-ally receiving dispensations to enable them to study it in spite of the prohibition of Honorius III—a sufficient refutation of the idea that the supreme pontiffs were systematically hostile to that study. Even Honorius III was no enemy to the civil law as such, though anxious to promote the study of theology and canon law by the priesthood and the religious orders. But the study of civil law soon became essential to the study of canon law; and the Popes themselves were usually lawyers rather than theologians.[50]

Nor is there any evidence that the papacy opposed the teaching and study of medicine at the universities under ecclesiastical control.[51]

With the issuance of the *Super specula,* the prohibition of the study of medicine extended to clerics whose major functions were spiritual and to those who possessed ecclesiastical benefices to which they owed their primary responsibilities. Extensive as the groups now forbidden to study medicine and secular law may appear at first glance, the prohibition still did not apply to a vast number of clerics: no mention is made of those in minor orders or of the major order of subdeacons. Nor is there any prohibition of the practice of medicine, even for those who are forbid-den to leave their ecclesiatical duties for the purpose of studying it.

In 1298 Boniface VIII promulgated the *Liber sextus,* designed to sup-plement the *Decretales* of Gregory IX.[52] The *Liber sextus* contains a decree that reduces somewhat the restrictions imposed by the *Super specula:*

Following in the footsteps of Pope Clement IV,[53] our predecessor of pious mem-ory, we declare that the statute of our predecessor, Pope Honorius III, of blessed memory (which forbade the study of laws and physic to deacons, archdeacons, rural deans, priors, cantors, and other clerics having benefices) does not extend, by the pronouncement of this present constitution in the interest of parochial churches, to those who are known to possess churches of this kind, unless the same churches are prebends having chapels under them in which are instituted permanent clergy who are not permitted to be removed from these except for reasonable cause.[54]

Another decree in the *Liber sextus* forbids religious to depart for the purpose of any study, then provides means whereby they may obtain permission to do so, and finally extends punishment to professors and teachers who knowingly take on as students religious who have laid aside their habit without permission:

In order that a dangerous pretext for wandering be removed from religious, we more strictly order that henceforth no one, who has silently or orally taken vows of a religious life, audaciously abandon the habit of his religious life in schools or elsewhere, or depart to any schools of learning whatsoever, unless permission is first given to him to depart for study by his prelate with the consent of his religious house or the majority of its members. If anyone, however, is a rash violator of these, let him incur the sentence of excommunication *ipso facto*. Also professors or teachers who knowingly presume to teach religious, who have laid aside their habit, attending lectures on laws or physic, or to retain them in their schools, shall have been implicated in a similar sentence *eo ipso*.[55]

These two statutes in the *Liber sextus* appear to be the last pronouncements of medieval canon law addressed to the study of medicine and secular law by clerics. Thus, in the officially promulgated collections of universal canon law of the Middle Ages there are four relevant statues. The first, issued originally in 1163, forbade monks and canons regular to leave their religious houses for the purpose of studying medicine or secular law and imposed stiff penalties on those who departed for that purpose and were absent for more than two months. The second, originally issued in 1219, extended the same prohibitions and penalties to clerics having specific spiritual functions and those possessing benefices. The third, promulgated in the *Liber sextus* of 1298, removed the prohibition from clerics having parochial churches; and the fourth, also in the *Liber sextus*, addressed only to religious, permits their departure for study if permission is first obtained from their prelates with the consent of the majority of members of their religious house.

These prohibitions of the study of medicine that affected certain groups of clerics would not have prevented them from practicing the art. It could be objected that if they were not permitted to leave their places of residence in order to study medicine, a prohibition of their practicing it would hardly be necessary. There is nothing in the actual legislation to suggest that clerics affected by the prohibition of being absent for extended study were not allowed to study medicine within the confines of their religious houses. There is a manuscript written by a religious in the late thirteenth century designed to instruct other religious in medicine so that they could treat the poor gratuitously, since the poor "are abandoned by the ordinary physicians and surgeons."[56] Clerics unaffected by the prohibition of formal study of medicine, that is, those in minor orders and subdeacons, unless they were monks or canons regular, could have obtained formal training in medicine without violating canonical injunctions. Those affected by the prohibition could seek and sometimes probably obtain permission to study.[57]

Being a practicing physician was not an impediment to clerical advancement. A famous example is Peter of Spain who was dean of the church of Lisbon, then physician to Pope Gregory X, next archbishop of Braga, and then cardinal of Tusculum; and who, in 1276 was elected pope under the name of John XXI. But the practice of medicine did present certain unique problems for the clergy, on which a rescript was written by Clement III. Between 1187 and 1191, Clement had received an inquiry from a *canonicus* concerned with this matter. Clement's reply reads:

You have brought to our attention that, since you are skilled in the art of physic, you have diligently treated many by the medical tradition of this art, although frequently it had happened to the contrary and those, to whom you thought you were applying a remedy, after taking the medicine, incurred the danger of death. But, because you desire to be advanced to sacred orders, you wished to consult us on this. We reply to you briefly that, if your conscience troubles you on account of those things said above, in our opinion you should not advance to major orders.

This papal rescript, known by its incipit, *Ad aures*, was included in the *Compilatio secunda*[58] and later in the *Decretales* of Gregory IX.[59] It clearly indicates that the major concern was whether the cleric as a physician had done anything that would prevent his fulfilling his spiritual functions with a clear conscience. If a cleric was responsible, even in a most peripheral way, for anyone's death, he incurred a canonical irregularity. If he was in major orders, this irregularity prevented him from fulfilling his most important ecclesiastical functions. If he was in minor orders, it was an impediment to his advancement to major orders.

Canon Law on Surgical Practice by Clerics

The risk of incurring responsibility for the death of a patient in surgical practice was much greater than in medicine. In the latter the treatment was viewed as primarily passive, as maltreatment was less readily suspected and much more difficult to prove. The practice of surgery, however, is active, and the death of a patient is much more easily credited to the practitioner. There is an interesting rescript, bearing the incipit *Tua nos,* written by Innocent III in 1212, included in *Compilatio quarta*[60] and later in the *Decretales* of Gregory IX,[61] that illustrates the problem as seen from an ecclesiastical vantage point:

Your brotherhood said that we should be consulted. You asked *to be advised by the Apostolic See* what must be decided concerning a certain monk who, believing that he could cure a certain woman of a tumor of the throat, acting as a surgeon, opened the tumor with a knife. When the tumor had healed somewhat, he ordered the woman not to expose herself to the wind at all lest the wind, stealing into the incision in her throat, bring about her death. But the woman, defying his order, rashly exposed herself to the wind while gathering crops, and thus much blood flowed out through the incision in her throat, and the woman died. *She, nevertheless, confessed that she was responsible because she had exposed herself to the wind.* The question is whether this monk, since he is also a priest, may lawfully exercise his priestly office. We therefore reply to your brotherhood that, although the monk himself was very much at fault for usurping an alien function which very little suited him, nevertheless, if he did it from piety and not from cupidity, and was expert in the exercise of surgery and was zealous to employ every diligence which he ought to have done, he must not be condemned for that which happened through the fault of the woman against his advice. Then, with no penance being required, he may be permitted to celebrate divine service. Otherwise, the fulfilling of the sacerdotal office must be strictly forbidden him.[62]

Although Innocent III was uneasy about the monk in question exercising the art of surgery and described him as having usurped an alien function that little suited him, nevertheless, it was the fact that this monk was also a priest that precipitated papal response. It is clear that if this monk-priest had been responsible in any way for the death of the woman in this case, he would have been prevented from fulfilling his spiritual functions as a priest (not as a monk). It is this concern that motivated action by a general church council just three years later. In 1215, the Fourth Lateran Council, under Innocent III, promulgated what is one of the most significant pieces of ecclesiastical legislation from the Middle Ages, a canon especially noted for its immediate effect on medieval secular law:

No cleric may pronounce a sentence of death, or execute such a sentence, or be present at its execution. If anyone in consequence of this prohibition should presume to inflict damage on churches or injury on ecclesiastical persons, let him be restrained by ecclesiastical censure. Nor may any cleric write or dictate letters destined for the execution of such a sentence. Wherefore, in the chanceries of the princes let this matter be committed to laymen and not to clerics.

Neither may a cleric act as judge in the case of the Rottarii,[63] archers, or other men of this kind devoted to the shedding of blood. No subdeacon, deacon, or priest shall practice that part[64] of surgery involving burning and cutting. Neither shall anyone in judicial tests or ordeals by hot or cold water or hot iron bestow any blessing; the earlier prohibitions in regard to dueling remain in force.[65]

This canon was included in *Compilatio quarta*[66] and later in the *Decretales* of Gregory IX.[67]

It is reasonable to ask why, in all these prohibitions except that against surgery, all clerics are included, while in the case of surgery just subdeacons, deacons and priests are mentioned. We should indeed hesitate to believe that the church held all the activities mentioned in this canon at the same level. If that were the case, there would have been no reason not to have included all clerics in the prohibition of the practice of surgery. But the church obviously did not view the practice of surgery in the same light as executions, trial by ordeal, and similar activities, in which no cleric was to participate. Surgery was forbidden only to those clerics who were in major orders, who would have been most severely affected by incurring a canonical irregularity. It is frequently claimed that the church forbade the practice of surgery to all clerics on the ground that *Ecclesia abhorret a sanguine*, that is, "The church abhors the shedding of blood." This maxim is sometimes attributed to canon 18 of Laterna IV, although usually to the Council of Tours, which took no action on the question of the practice of surgery by clerics. Talbot's comments on the maxim bear quoting:

It is a literary ghost. It owes its existence to Quesnay, the uncritical historian of the Faculty of Surgeons at Paris, who in 1774, citing a passage from Pasquier's *Recherches de la France* ("et comme l'église n'abhorre rien tant que le sang") translated it into Latin and put it into italics. No earlier source for this sentence can be found. Quesnay himself quoted a register from the archives of the Surgeons of Paris, in which it was stated that "at the time of Boniface VIII (1294–1303) and Clement V (1305–14) a decree was put forth at Avignon and confirmed by the council of Philip le Bel that surgery was separated from medicine." No such decree can be found in the register of Boniface VIII, whilst among the ten thousand documents contained in the register of Clement V only one refers to medicine, and that concerns itself with studies at Montpellier.[68]

Leaving the infamous maxim aside, it remains that many scholars cite canon 18 of the Fourth Lateran Council as the source of the church's prohibition of the practice of surgery to all clerics. It is easy to see how such a misinterpretation is so frequently repeated. Even in a history of the general church councils this summary of the canon in question is found: "Clerics are not to have any part in trials that involve the punishment of death. They are forbidden all military employment. They are not to act as surgeons. They are not to bless ordeals."[69] Such an error may not seem significant until one considers the fact that, since the prohibition applied only to those clerics in major orders, the majority of clerics were not affected.

Mention was made above of the charge that the church found it necessary to keep repeating its prohibitions of the involvement of clerics in medicine and surgery. Indeed, if the references to the prohibition regarding surgery were simply listed, as they often are, this would appear to hold true. The provision in canon 18 of the Fourth Lateran Council is in fact repeated at least four times in the next eighty-five years: In the Statutes of Le Mans (1247) appears "A subdeacon or a deacon or a priest shall not practise any part of surgery involving burning or cutting."[70] The Diocesan Synod of Nîmes (1284) includes, "Also no cleric established in sacred orders[71] shall practise any art of surgery including burning or cutting."[72] In the Diocesan Synod of Würzburg (1298) there is found a somewhat different version: "No cleric, deacon, subdeacon, or priest,[73] shall practise the surgical art or be present when it is practised."[74] The Diocesan Synod of Bayeux (1300) includes, "Nor shall a subdeacon, a deacon, a priest practise any part of surgery including burning or cutting."[75]

When these statements are isolated from the context in which they appear, and are neatly lined up in a row with the similar prohibition from canon 18 of Lateran IV at the head of the procession, weight surely seems to be lent to the argument that it was indeed necessary for the church incessantly to repeat this regulation, which must have been so flagrantly ignored. But it is dangerously misleading to snatch these prohibitions from their surroundings for such purposes. All four of these examples given above are found in the context of lengthy regulations governing the conduct and responsibilities of clerics. These regulations (usually given under the rubric *De vita et honestate clericorum*, [On the life and character of clerics]) range from general exhortations on moral probity to specific injunctions on types of activities expected of or denied to all clerics or to individual groups of clerics. The prohibition of the practice of surgery to subdeacons, deacons, and priests occurs in these four cases as simply a part of one sentence within broad, local summaries of general church legislation covering the spectrum of clerical morals and conduct. The prohibition of surgery was not singled out for special attention in these extensive guides; nor should it be by historians. If the repetition of this prohibition was prompted by its being flagrantly disregarded by those to whom it applied, then we must also assume that the repetitions of the entire range of regulations governing the conduct of clerics in which the prohibition of surgery appears were prompted by the same considerations.

Conclusions

It has been my purpose in this paper to present and discuss the regulations found in medieval canon law governing clerical involvement in medicine and surgery. It is evident that these regulations cannot be legitimately used to support the broad statements made to the effect that *clerics* were forbidden to practice medicine and surgery. But knowledge of the law does not equal knowledge of its interpretation and application. It is on these two aspects that considerable work remains to be done. First, in regard to interpretation: Around the different parts of the *Corpus iuris canonici* a vast literature of treatises and glosses grew up. It would be extremely rewarding to examine as much of this literature as possible in order to achieve a balanced appraisal of how the relevant regulations were interpreted by contemporary canonists. Citing the opinions of a small number of canonists here, however, might be misleading and should be held in abeyance until they can be juxtaposed to the opinions of similar sources. Second, on the matter of application: There is a vast quantity of primary documents of a regional nature (e.g., regional councils, diocesan synods, ecclesiastical correspondence) that should be investigated with a view toward determining the effect of the relevant regulations in canon law on local practice. It is here that the most concrete information can be sought on regional enforcement, extension and, perhaps, modification of the legislation surveyed in this paper.[76]

NOTES

All translations in this chapter are mine unless otherwise indicated.

1. Robert S. Lopez, *The Birth of Europe* (New York: Evans-Lippincott, 1967), 373.
2. Roberto Margotta, *The Story of Medicine* (New York: Golden, 1968), 146.
3. Max Neuburger, *History of Medicine*, trans. E. Playfair (London: Oxford University Press, 1925), vol. 2, pt. 1, 40.

4. J. H. Baas, *Outlines of the History of Medicine and the Medical Profession,* trans. H. E. Handerson (New York: J. H. Vail, 1889), 253.

5. Theodor Puschmann, *A History of Medical Education,* trans. E. H. Hare (1891; reprint, New York: Hafner, 1966), 280.

6. Fielding H. Garrison, *An Introduction to the History of Medicine,* 4th ed. (Philadelphia: W. B. Saunders, 1929), 168.

7. Benjamin Spector, "The Growth of Medicine and the Letter of the Law," *Bull. Hist. Med.* 26 (1952): 512 f.

8. Charles Singer, "Thirteenth-Century Miniatures Illustrating Medical Practice," *Proc. Roy. Soc. Med.* 9 (1915–16): 35.

9. Andrew Dickson White, *A History of the Warfare of Science with Theology in Christendom* (1896; reprint, New York: Dover, 1960), 2:31 f.

10. T. C. Allbutt, *The Historical Relations of Medicine and Surgery to the End of the Sixteenth Century* (London: Macmillan, 1905), 21.

11. W.S.C. Copeman, *Doctors and Disease in Tudor Times* (London: Dawson's of Pall Mall, 1960), 6. Copeman makes essentially the same assertion in "The Evolution of Anatomy and Surgery under the Tudors," *Ann. Roy. Coll. Surg. England* 32, no. 1 (1963): 11.

12. John F. Eustace, "The Dublin Guild of Barber Surgeons," *Industrial Med. Surg.* 32 (1963): 449.

13. C. H. Talbot, *Medicine in Medieval England* (London: Oldbourne, 1967), 51 ff.

14. C. H. Talbot, "Medical Education in the Middle Ages," in *The History of Medical Education,* ed. C. D. O'Malley (Berkeley: University of California Press, 1970), 80.

15. The more the researcher turns to secondary literature, the more he will become confused on the question. The contradictions *between* the secondary sources quoted above or cited here are extreme; individually, many of these are correct in certain details, but their authors apparently were not aware of the larger context of the development and relations of the various primary documents. See, e.g., E. Withington, "Roger Bacon and Medicine," in *Roger Bacon Essays,* ed. A. G. Little (Oxford: Clarendon, 1914), 339; Stephen D'Irsay, "On the Original Connection between Medicine and the University," *Johns Hopkins Hosp. Bull.* 46 (1930): 120 f.; Henry E. Sigerist, "The Physician's Profession through the Ages," originally published in 1933 and reprinted in *Henry E. Sigerist on the History of Medicine,* ed. F. Marti-Ibañez (New York: M D Publications, 1960), 9; David Riesman, *The Story of Medicine in the Middle Ages* (New York: Hoeber, 1936), 197 f.; Edward F. Hartung, "Medical Education in the Twelfth Century," *Med. Life* 41 (1934): 21; G. G. Coulton, *Medieval Panorama: The English Scene from Conquest to Reformation* (New York: Macmillan, 1938), 445; Gertrude M. Engbring, "Saint Hildegard, Twelfth Century Physician," *Bull. Hist. Med.* 8 (1940): 778; Edward F. McLaughlin, "The Guilds and Medicine," *Ann. Med. Hist.* 3 (1941): 389 f.; Mary Niven Alston, "The Attitude of the Church towards Dissection before 1500," *Bull. Hist. Med.* 16 (1944): 231; Pearl Kibre, "The Faculty of Medicine at Paris, Charlatanism, and Unlicensed Medical Practices in the Later Middle Ages," ibid., 27 (1953): 4; Monique Berry, "Les professions civiles dans le Décret de

Gratien" (diss., Facultée de Droit de Paris, 1956), 96 ff.; H. M. Karn, "The History of Medical Training and Licensure," *New Zealand Med. J.* 56 (1957): 328; Morris Fishbein, "The Barber Surgeons and the Liberation of Surgery," *J. Intern. Coll. Surg.* 27 (1957): 772; B. L. Gordon, "Lay Medicine during the Early Middle Ages," *J. Michigan State Med. Soc.* 57 (1958): 1006; E. A. Hammond, "Physicians in Medieval English Religious Houses," *Bull Hist. Med.* 33 (1958): 119 f.; idem, "Incomes of Medieval English Doctors," *J. Hist. Med. Allied Sci.* 15 (1960): 167; and idem, "The Westminster Abbey Infirmarers' Rolls as a Source of Medical History," *Bull. Hist. Med.* 39 (1965): 262; Vern L. Bullough, "Status and Medieval Medicine," *J. Health Human Behav.* 2 (1961): 206 n. 17; idem, *The Development of Medicine as a Profession: The Contribution of the Medieval University to Modern Medicine* (New York: Hafner, 1966), 109; Jacques Le Goff, "Métiers licites et métiers illicites dans l'Occident médiéval," *Ecole des hautes études, annals, études historiques* 5 (1963): 42 f. and 48; David Knowles, *The Monastic Order in England,* 2d ed. (Cambridge: Cambridge University Press, 1963), 518; George Clark, *A History of the Royal College of Physicians* (Oxford: Clarendon, 1964), 1:17, 22; Alessandro Simili, "Considerazioni storico-critiche sulla medicina monastica," *Minerva Medica* 65 (1974): 3106. Examples such as these could be increased substantially. Special mention should be made of Paul Diepgen, *Die Theologie und der ärztliche Stand* (Berlin-Grunwald: W. Rothschild, 1922). Diepgen's discussion of the problem (16–19), although excellent for what it covers, is cursory in its selection of primary documents.

16. This is one of the *Quinque compilationes antiquae,* the five most famous decretal collections composed between ca. 1187 and 1226. The actual sequence of composition was *prima, tertia, secunda, quarta,* and *quinta.* These were edited by E. Friedberg (1882; reprint, Graz: Akademische Druck- und Verlagsanstalt, 1956).

17. Excepting the *Decretum* of Gratian, which the official collections did not supplant but rather supplemented.

18. The title *Corpus iuris canonici* was first used in 1580 by Gregory XIII and refers to the *Decretum* of Gratian (ca. 1140), the *Decretales* of Gregory IX (1234), the *Liber sextus* of Boniface VIII (1298), the *Clementinae* (1317; named after Clement V), the *Extravagantes* of John XXII (1325), and the *Extravagantes communes* (1500 and 1503). These were edited by E. Friedberg under the title *Corpus iuris canonici,* 2 vols. (1879; reprint, Graz: Akademische Druck- und Verlagsanstalt, 1959).

19. *Sacrorum conciliorum nova et amplissima collectio,* ed. J. D. Mansi et al., new ed. (Florence and Venice, 1759–98), vol. 21, col. 438f. (Hereafter cited as "Mansi.")

20. Mansi, vol. 21, col. 459.

21. *Conciliorum oecumenicorum decreta,* ed. J. Alberigo et al., 3d ed. (Bologna: Istituto per le Scienze Religiose, 1973), 198 f. (Hereafter cited as "Alberigo.")

22. I have used the translation made by R. J. Schroeder, *Disciplinary Decrees of the General Councils* (St. Louis: Herder, 1957), 201 f. The Latin text in Alberigo reads:

Prava autem consuetudo, prout accepimus, et detestabilis inolevit, quoniam monachi et regulares canonici post susceptum habitum et professionem factam, spreta beatorum magistrorum Benedicti et Augustini regula, leges temporales et medicinam gratia lucri temporalis addiscunt. Avaritiae namque flammis accensi, se patronos causarum faciunt; et cum psalmodiae et hymnis vacare debeant, gloriosae vocis confisi munimine, allegationum suarum varietate iustum et iniustum, fas nefasque confundunt. Attestantur vero imperiales constitutiones, absurdum immo et opprobrium esse clericis, si peritos se velint disceptationum esse forensium. Huiusmodi temeratores graviter feriendos, apostolica auctoritate decernimus. Ipsi quoque, neglecta animarum cura, ordinis sui propositum nullatenus attendentes, pro detestanda pecunia sanitatem pollicentes, humanorum curatores se faciunt corporum. Cumque impudicus oculus impudici cordis sit nuntius, illa de quibus loqui erubescit honestas, non debet religio pertractare. Ut ergo ordo monasticus et canonicus Deo placens in sancto proposito inviolabiliter conservetur, ne hoc ulterius praesumatur, apostolica auctoritate interdicimus. Episcopi autem, abbates et priores tantae enormitati consentientes et non corrigentes, propriis honoribus spolientur et ab ecclesiae liminibus arceantur.

23. The subject is complex. A discussion of the economic doctrines of the canonists can be found in J. Gilchrist, *The Church and Economic Activity in the Middle Ages* (London: Macmillan, 1969), 53 ff.

24. L. K. Little, "Pride Goes before Avarice: Social Change and the Vices in Latin Christendom," *Amer. Hist. Rev.* 76 (1971): 16.

25. Gilchrist, *Church and Economic Activity* (n. 23), 55.

26. See, e.g., Puschmann, *History of Medical Education* (n. 5), 280 f.; Neuburger, *History of Medicine* (n. 3), 40; Hammond, "Physicians in Religious Houses" (n. 15), 120; Talbot, *Medicine in Medieval England* (n. 13), 51.

27. The other two were Piacenza (1132) and Pisa (1135).

28. Mansi, vol. 21, col. 1160, and vol. 22, col. 670. "Prohibuit praeterea sub omni severitate ecclesiasticae disciplinae, ne quis monachus, vel canonicus regularis, aut alius religiosus, ad saeculares leges vel physicam legendas accedat. Alioquin iuxta decretum sub domino Alexandro in concilio apud Montempessulanum et Turonis super hoc articulo promulgatum, a dioecesanis episcopis canonice puniantur."

29. This is a strange periphrasis that could also be translated "for weighing medical confections." See the comments of William D. Sharpe, *Isidore of Seville: The Medical Writings*, Transactions of the American Philosophical Society, n.s., 54 (2) (Philadelphia, 1964), 17, n. 64.

30. *Legendas* here means "studying," not "teaching," as some scholars misread it. Le Goff, "Métiers licites" (n. 15), for example, makes this general statement on the supposed action of the medieval church against the practice of medicine by clerics: "Il est clair qu'interdire une profession à un clerc dans une société religieuse et 'cléricale,' comme celle de l'Occident médiéval, n'est pas une recommandation pour cette profession, mais lui vaut au contraire un discrédit qui rejaillit sur les laïcs qui l'exercent" (42). Later (48), when discussing the provisions of the Council of Tours, he states that the prohibition against "clergy" in respect to medicine and law not only reduced clerics' profit potential but also reduced their prestige. His inconsistency can perhaps be explained by his mistranslation of the phrase "ad physicam legesve mundanas legendas" as "pour enseigner la médecine ou le droit civil." *Legendas* in the context of this canon surely does not mean teaching but, rather, learning. The canon states that

under the pretext of caring for the bodies of their ill brothers and handling ecclesiastical affairs more proficiently, certain regulars are lured out of their cloisters "ad legendas leges, et confectiones physicales ponderandas." For this to
imply teaching rather than learning would be an utter non sequitur.

31. Canon 8. Mansi, vol. 21, col. 1179.

Non magnopere antiqui hostis invidia infirma membra ecclesiae praecipitare laborat: sed
manum mittit ad desiderabilia eius: et electos quoque nititur supplantare, dicente scrip-
tura: Escae eius electae. Multorum si quidem causam operari se reputat, ubi pretiosius
aliquod membrum ecclesiae fuerit aliqua calliditate detractum. Inde nimirum est, quod se
in angelum lucis more solito transfigurans, sub obtentu languentium fratrum consulendi
corporibus, et ecclesiastica negotia fidelius pertractandi, regulares quosdam ad legendas
leges, et confectiones physicales ponderandas, de claustris suis educit. Unde ne sub occasione scientiae spirituales viri mundanis rursum actionibus involvantur, et in interioribus
eo ipso deficiant, et quo se aliis putant in exterioribus providere: de praesentis concilii
assensu, huic malo obviantes, statuimus, ut nullus omnino post votum religionis, post
factam in aliquo religioso loco professionem, ad physicam, legesve mundanas legendas
permittatur exire. Si vero exierit, et ad claustrum suum infra duorum mensium spatium
non redierit: sicut excommunicatus ab omnibus evitetur, et in nulla causa, si patrocinium
praestare praesumpserit, aut tentaverit, audiatur. Reversus autem ad claustrum, in choro,
capitulo, mensa, et ceteris, ultimus fratrum semper existat: et nisi, ex misericordia forsan
sedis apostolicae, totius spem promotionis amittat.

32. *Appendix consilii Lateranensis* 27.2, in Mansi, vol. 22, col. 373. The text
there is identical except for the addition of a final sentence: "Episcopi vero, abbates, priores, tantae enormitati consentientes, et non corrigentes, spolientur
propriis honoribus, et ab ecclesiae liminibus arceantur." (Bishops, abbots, and
priors consenting to such outrageous practice and not correcting it, shall be
deprived of their honors and cut off from the church.) This is, of course, with
minor variations, the concluding sentence of Clarmont 5, Rheims 6, and Lateran
II 9.

33. *Collectio canonum Lipsiensis* 14.2, edited with the *Quinque* (n. 16).

34. *Collectio canonum Bambergensis* 14.2, in *Die Canonessammlungen zwischen Gratian und Bernhard von Pavia*, ed. E. Friedberg (Leipzig: Tauchnitz, 1897).

35. *Collectio canonum Casselana* 24.2, in *Die Canonessammlungen* (n. 34).

36. See n. 16, above.

37. *Belverensis*, "Durham Collection," and "Fountains Collection." On these
see Charles Duggan, *Twelfth-Century Decretal Collections and Their Importance in
English History* (London: University of London Press, 1963), 72, 79 ff.

38. *Chartularium Universitatis Parisiensis sub auspiciis consilii generalis facultatum
Parisiensium*, ed. H. Denifle and A. Chatelain, vol. 1 (1899; reprint, Brussels: Culture et Civilisation, 1964).

39. Gregory IX, *Decretales* 3.50.3 (see n. 18). The text is essentially the same as
that given above (n. 31), with some omissions and verbal alterations:

Non magnopere antiqui hostis invidia . . . inde nimirum est, quod in angelum lucis se
more solito transfigurans, sub obtentu languentinum fratrum consulendi corporibus et
ecclesiastica negotia fidelius pertractandi, regulares quosdam ad legendas leges et confectiones physicales ponderandas de claustris suis educit. Unde, ne . . . occasione scientiae

spirituales viri mundanis rursus actionibus involvantur, . . . statuimus, ut nulli omnino post votum religionis, et post factam in aliquo loco religioso professionem ad physicam legesve mundanas legendas permittantur exire. Si vero exierint, et ad claustrum suum infra duorum mensium spatium non redierint, sicut excommunicati ab omnibus evitentur, et in nulla causa, si patrocinium praestare voluerint, audiantur. Reversi autem in choro, capitulo, mensa et ceteris ultimi fratrum . . . exsistant, et, nisi forte ex misericordia sedis apostolicae, totius spem promotionis amittant.

40. Mansi gives 1212.

41. Canon 20, in Mansi, vol. 22, col. 831.

Cum quidam regularium, ut verbis concilii Lateranensis utamur, sub obtentu languentium fratrum consulendi corporibus, et ecclesiastica negotia fidelius pertractandi, ad leges mundanas legendas, et confectiones physicas ponderandas, ut jurisprudentiae et medicinae dent operam, de claustris suis exire non formident, et ex eo ipso deficiant in interioribus, quando se putant aliis in exterioribus providere: ipsius concilii vestigiis inhaerentes, praecipimus, ut nisi infra duorum mensium spatium ad claustrum suum redierint, non obstante abbatis sui licentia, quam dare non potuit, sint excommunicati, et ab omnibus evitentur, et in nulla causa, si patrocinium praestare voluerint, admittantur.

This canon is included as document 19 in the cartularies of the University of Paris (n. 38).

42. See n. 32.

43. Tours is sometimes referred to as a general council (although it was not), even by leading canon scholars; e.g., by C.N.L. Brooke, "Canons of English Church Councils in the Early Decretal Collections," *Traditio* 13 (1957): 471.

44. The complete text is printed as document 32 in the cartularies of the University of Paris (n. 38). It is summarized as papal rescript 6165 of Honorius III in *Regesta Pontificum Romanorum inde ab anno post Christum natum MCXCVII ad annum MCCCIV,* ed. Augustus Potthast (1874; reprint, Graz: Akademische Druck- und Verlagsanstalt, 1957).

45. *Compilatio quinta* (see n. 16). These are, respectively, 5.2.1, 3.27.1, 5.12.3.

46. Gregory IX, *Decretales* 5.5.5, 3.50.10, and 5.33.28, respectively (see n. 18).

47. "Ad audiendum leges vel physicam."

48. Gregory IX, *Decretales* 3.50.10 (see n. 18).

Contra religiosas personas, de claustris exeuntes ad audiendum leges vel physicam, . . . Alexander praedecessor noster olim statuit in concilio Turonensi, ut, nisi infra duorum mensium spatium ad claustrum redierint, sicut excommunicati ab omnibus evitentur, et in nulla causa, si patrocinium praestare voluerint, audiantur. Reversi autem in choro, mensa, capitulo et ceteris ultimi fratrum exsistant, et, nisi forte ex misericordia sedis apostolicae, totius spem promotionis amittant. Verum, quia nonnulli ex talibus propter quorundam opiniones diversas excusationis aliquid assumebant, nos, volentes, ut . . . de cetero ipso facto sententiam excommunicationis incurrant, districte praecipiendo mandamus, quatenus tam a dioecesanis et capitulis ipsorum, quam . . . a ceteris episcopis, in quorum dioecesibus in huiusmodi student, tales . . . excommunicati . . . praedictis poenis obnoxii publice nuncientur. Quia vero theologiae studium cupimus ampliari, ut dilatato sui tentorii loco et funiculos suos faciat longiores, ut sit fides catholica circumcincta muro inexpugnabili bellatorum, quibus resistere valeat adscendentibus ex adverso: ad archidiaconos, decanos, plebanos, praepositos, cantores et alios clericos personatus habentes, nec non . . . presbyteros, nisi ab his infra spatium praescriptum destiterint, hoc extendi volumus et mandamus, et appellatione postposita firmiter observari.

49. Hastings Rashdall, *The Universities of Europe in the Middle Ages*, rev. ed., ed. F. M. Powicke and A. B. Emden (London: Oxford University Press, 1936), 1:322. On the *Super specula*, see Walter Ullmann, "Honorius III and the Prohibition of Legal Studies," *Juridical Rev.* 60 (1948): 177 ff.; and Stephan Kuttner, "Papst Honorius III und das Studium des Zivilrechts," *Festschrift für Martin Wolff*, ed. Ernst von Caemmerer et al. (Tübingen: Mohr, 1952), 79 ff.

50. Ibid., 2:29.

51. Rather, there is ample evidence of papal support. For example, the papal confirmation of the statutes of the medical faculty of the University of Montpellier (1239) lauds the study of medicine and contains such statements as "Medicine shines forth among the liberal arts." See Luke Demaitre, "Theory and Practice in Medical Education at the University of Montpellier in the Thirteenth and Fourteenth Centuries," *J. Hist. Med. Allied Sci.* 30 (1975): 107.

52. See n. 18, above. The *Decretales* was divided into five books; thus the title of Boniface VIII's supplement, the *Liber sextus*, i.e., the "sixth book."

53. The legislation of Clement IV referred to here does not seem to be extant. See, however, n. 2 to the text of the *Super specula* in the cartularies of the University of Paris, 1:93 (n. 38).

54. Boniface VIII, *Liber sextus* 3.24.1 (see n. 18).

Statutum felicis recordationis Honorii Papae III praedecessoris nostri, quod decanis, archidiaconis, praepositis, plebanis, cantoribus et aliis clericis, habentibus personatus, audire leges vel physicam interdicit, ad eos, qui parochiales ecclesias obtinere noscuntur, piae memoriae Clementis Papae IV praedecessoris nostri vestigiis inhaerentes, declaramus praesentis constitutionis oraculo ratione ecclesiarum huiusmodi non extendi, nisi eaedem ecclesiae fuerint plebaniae sub se capellas habentes, in quibus instituantur clerici perpetui, nequeuntes ab ipsis absque causa rationabili amoveri.

55. Ibid., 3.24.2.

Ut periculosa religiosis evagandi materia subtrahatur, districtius inhibemus, ne de cetero aliquis, quamcunque religionem tacite vel expresse professus, in scholis vel alibi temere habitum religionis suae dimittat, nec accedat ad quaevis studia literarum, nisi a suo praelato cum consilio sui conventus vel maioris partis eiusdem sibi eundi ad studium licentia primitus sit concessa. Si quis autem horum temerarius violator exstiterit: excommunicationis incurrat sententiam ipso facto. Doctores quoque sive magistri, qui religiosos, habitu suo dimisso, leges vel physicam audientes scienter docere, aut in scholis suis praesumpserint retinere, simili eo ipso sint sententia innodati.

56. Talbot, *Medicine in Medieval England* (n. 13), 96.

57. The whole question of privilege deserves much study, and until such is done on the question of medical studies, it is not safe to make any broad statements on the degree to which such dispensations were given. Rashdall, *Universities of Europe* (n. 49), 1:235 n. 4, writes that "the prohibition of the study [of medicine] to the priests, monks, and beneficed clergy . . . shows its growing importance, but did little to check the practice denounced, since dispensations were freely granted." He says the same about the study of secular law (1:260).

58. *Compilatio secunda* 1.8.2 (see n. 16).
59. Gregory IX, *Decretales* 1.14.7 (see n. 18).

Ad aures nostras te significante pervenit, quod, quum in arte physica eruditus sis, pluribus iuxta ipsius artis traditionem exhibuisti cum diligentia medicinam, licet pluries in contrarium successerit, et quibus putabas adhibere medelam, medicinis perceptis mortis periculum incurrerunt. Verum quia, ad sacros ordines desideras promoveri, super eo nos consulere voluisti. Tibi breviter respondemus, quod, si super praemissis conscientia tua te remordeat, ad maiores ordines de nostro consilio non ascendas.

60. *Compilatio quarta* 5.6.3 (see n. 16).
61. Gregory IX, *Decretales* 5.12.19 (see n. 18).
62. Sections italicized in the translation and in the text given below, although part of the original rescript, are not included in the *Decretales*.

Tua nos duxit fraternitas consulendos. Quaesivisti *per sedem apostolicam explicari,* quod sit de quodam monacho sentiendum, qui, credens, se quandam mulierem a gutturis tumore curare, ut chirurgicus cum ferro tumorem illum aperuit, et, quum tumor aliquantulum resedisset, ipse mulieri praecepit, ne se vento exponeret ullo modo, ne forte ventus, subintrans gutturis apertionem, sibi causam mortis inferret; sed mulier, eius mandato contempto, dum messes colligeret, vento se exposuit incaute, et sic per apertionem gutturis sanguis multus effluxit, et mulier diem ultimum sic finivit, *quae tamen confessa est, quod, quia vento exposuit semetipsam, sibi dederat causam mortis;* utrum videlicet, quum praedictus monachus sit sacerdos, liceat ei sacerdotale officium exercere. Nos igitur fraternitati tuae respondemus, quod, licet ipse monachus multum deliquerit alienum officium usurpando, quod sibi minime congruebat, si tamen causa pietatis, et non cupiditatis id egerit, et peritus erat in exercitio chirurgiae, omnemque studuit, quam debuit, diligentiam adhibere, non est ex eo, quod per culpam mulieris contra consilium eius accidit, adeo reprobandus, quod non post satisfactionem condignam cum eo misericorditer agi possit, ut divina valeat celebrare; alioquin interdicenda est ei sacerdotalis ordinis exsecutio de rigore.

63. Schroeder, *Disciplinary Decrees* (n. 22), 258 n. 16, explains: "Also Ruptarii and Ruptuarii, bands of robbers and plunderers, drawn chiefly from the peasant class."

64. Some texts read *artem,* others *partem.* It should be noted that medieval surgery included within its functional purview not only cautery and cutting but also the external, medicinal treatment of wounds and sores, the setting of fractures, the treatment of dislocations, etc. Hence I incline toward reading *partem.* Clark, *History of Royal College* (n. 15), 1:17 n. 3, writes: "The reading *artem* for *partem* would extend the prohibition to all surgery, but does not seem so satisfactory from the point of view of language."

65. Lateran IV 18. I have used Schroder's translation. Schroder, *Disciplinary Decrees* (n. 22), 258. The text given below is that of Alberigo (244), although I have substituted *partem* for *artem.*

Sententiam sanguinis nullus clericus dictet aut proferat, sed nec sanguinis vindictam exerceat aut ubi exercetur intersit. Si quis autem huiusmodi occasione statuti ecclesiis vel personis ecclesiasticis aliquod praesumpserit inferre dispendium, per censuram ecclesiasticam compescatur, nec quisquam clericus literas scribat aut dictet pro vindicta sanguinis destinandas, unde in curiis principum haec solicitudo non clericis sed laicis committatur. Nullus quoque clericus rottariis aut balistariis aut huiusmodi viris sanguinum praeponatur, nec illam chirurgiae artem subdiaconus, diaconus vel sacerdos exerceant, quae ad ustionem vel incisionem inducit, nec quisquam purgationi aquae ferventis vel frigidae seu ferri candentis ritum cuiuslibet benedictionis aut consecrationis impendat, salvis nihilominus prohibitionibus de monomachiis sive duellis antea promulgatis.

66. *Compilatio quarta* 3.19.2 (see n. 16).

67. Gregory IX, *Decretales* 3.50.9 (see n. 18).

68. Talbot, *Medicine in Medieval England* (n. 13), 55. I am indebted to both E. A. Hammond and Ruth Friedlander for bringing to my attention Talbot's treatment of this maxim.

·69. Philip Hughes, *The Church in Crisis: A History of the General Councils, 325–1870* (1961; reprint, Garden City, N.Y.: Doubleday–Image Books, 1964), 241.

70. Mansi, vol. 23, col. 756: "nec ullam partem chirurgiae subdiaconus vel diaconus vel sacerdos exerceat, quae adustionem vel incisionem inducit."

71. I.e., subdeacons, deacons and priests.

72. Mansi, vol. 24, col. 542. "Nullus quoque clericus in sacro ordine constitutus aliquam chirurgiae artem exerceat, quae ad ustionem, vel incisionem inducat."

73. I take "deacon, subdeacon or priest" to be partitive appositives to "cleric," since deacons, subdeacons and priests were clerics, but not all clerics were deacons, subdeacons or priests.

74. Mansi, vol. 24, col. 1190: "Nullus clericus, diaconus, subdiaconus, aut sacerdos artem chyrurgicam exerceat, aut, ubi exerceatur, intersit."

75. Ibid., vol. 25, col. 67: "nec ullam partem chirurgiae subdiaconus, diaconus, sacerdos exerceant, quae adustionem inducit vel incisionem."

76. Some scholars maintain that the proportion of clerical to lay physicians declined considerably as a result of the legislation discussed. Others say that it had little effect. Prosopographical research on this matter could provide a fairly definite answer.

NINE

Casuistry and Professional Obligations: The Regulation of Physicians by the Court of Conscience in the Late Middle Ages

During the late Middle Ages moral theologians and casuists directed much attention to defining the moral responsibilities (sins both of commission and of omission) of Christians generally. They also considered the moral responsibilities attached to those in various walks of life. Many of these sources discuss the sins of physicians and surgeons. It is to a sampling of such writings that this study is directed, with a view to analyzing the ethical standards that ecclesiastical authorities defined as essential for the Christian physician.

In the twelfth century, with the development of medical and surgical guilds and university faculties and, in some areas, with the imposition of licensure requirements, the practice of medicine was changed from a right to a privilege. This was a period marked by profound changes in the fabric of medieval society. Western Europe was changing from an almost exclusively agrarian to a more urban society. The corporate structure typified by guilds and universities began to constitute the norm of social, economic, and often political organization for an increasingly large proportion of the population. The time was one of great social and economic change, during which a wide variety of new commercial and professional activities arose. The church was engaged in an internal ideological struggle regarding the spiritual aspects of commercial activity, and the attitudes of canonists and the stipulations of church councils evidence an attempt at adaptation designed to cope with socioeconomic change. This is reflected in the fact that while in the *Decretum* of Gratian (ca. 1140) all commercial profit seems to have been condemned, even Gratian's earliest commentators did not sustain his views on the activities of merchants.[1] It is especially during the twelfth century that there was a "shift in values within the traditional scheme of the cardinal vices."[2] The primacy of pride as the supreme vice was being displaced by the sin of avarice in theological and popular conceptions. Indeed, as new roles rose and old ones became more complicated, as society itself became infinitely more complex, and as diverse circumstances and situations, which a century earlier could not have been imagined, were encountered either generally or as a consequence of one's calling, canonists and theologians were forced to wrestle with the religious implications of an environment significantly different from that of earlier eras.

As decretists (commentators on Gratian's *Decretum*) sought to apply the old verities to new exigencies, some theologians began to evaluate the vagaries of the contemporary scene in terms of both abstract and practical moral application. The theologians thus engaged during the twelfth century were the founding fathers of what is now known as moral theology. While their discussions were often on an abstract level, their designs were eminently practical. Peter the Chanter, a Parisian theologian of the twelfth century,[3] may be taken as an example. His *Summa de sacramentis et animae consiliis*[4] consists of three parts, the first dealing with the sacraments, the second with penance and excommunication, and the third, entitled *Liber casuum conscientiae,* with circumstances for resolving cases of conscience. This work was designed in part to aid confessors in the increasingly difficult task of determining what constituted sin in a society fraught with situations and circumstances not anticipated by the authors or compilers of earlier penitential literature.

Beginning in the sixth century, compilations of canons relevant to sin and penance had been made. The most notable of these are the Celtic or Irish penitentials.[5] The penitentials are stark lists of sins, with appropriate penances given for each offence.[6] Although they recognize levels of responsibility within various categories of sins, they are mechanical, rigid, and inflexible, and their penalties are usually severe. By the late twelfth century they appear hopelessly outdated and discordant with the spirit of the age. Additionally, during the tenth, eleventh, and twelfth centuries there was a shift from a public system of penance to a private system, the latter becoming universal and compulsory in the thirteenth century.[7] With this shift from public to private penance, the office of confessor inevitably became very prominent. The confessor's task now was also much more complex than earlier. He was "no longer the administrator of a hard and fast penal code. He had become a judge in the full sense with the obligation to base his decisions on the principles of the newborn theology."[8] This "newborn theology" was written in great part as a response to the needs of the confessor, whose role had greatly increased in significance and demand in a society in which new and puzzling moral problems were constantly arising.

The literature designed to help the confessor begins to appear in the late twelfth century and assumes a wide variety of forms; it does not lend itself to precise genre classifications. Works retrospectively grouped together under the rubric *summae confessorum* or *summae de casibus conscientiae* were written specifically to aid confessors in all aspects of their confessional responsibilities.[9] Scholars disagree as to which works should be thus classified[10]—the primary sources that are relevant to resolving problems encountered in the confessional fall into several categories that sometimes overlap, for instance general literature on moral theology (perhaps including specific sections on cases of conscience, e.g., Peter the Chanter's *Summa*), systematic treatments of confession and penance addressed precisely to the needs of the confessor, and short confessional manuals designed as handy reference works for the confessor.[11] All prove valuable as documents illustrating a serious and concerted effort to subject the broadest spectrum of human activities to Christian moral principles. The result was the birth of Catholic casuistic literature.

In 1215 Pope Innocent III presided over a general church council, the Fourth Lateran, at which various canons with far-reaching and significant consequences were adopted. One canon, which Henry Charles Lea called "perhaps the most important legislative act in the history of the Church,"[12] had been precipitated by a century of theological discussion of the nature of penance.[13] This canon, number 21 of Lateran IV, sometimes referred to by its incipit, *Omnes utriusque sexus*, was incorporated into *Compilatio quarta*[14] and, most important, was included in the *Decretales* of Gregory IX,[15] thus becoming part of officially codified canon law. This canon, which imposed on all Christians who had arrived at the age of discretion the obligation of confessing and receiving the Eucharist at least once a year, warrants quoting in full:

Every *fidelis* of either sex shall after the attainment of years of discretion separately confess his sins with all fidelity to his own priest at least once in the year: and shall endeavour to fulfil the penance imposed upon him to the best of his ability, reverently receiving the sacrament of the Eucharist at least at Easter: unless it happen that by the counsel of his own priest for some reasonable cause, he hold that he should abstain for a time from the reception of the sacrament: otherwise let him during life be repelled from entering the church, and when dead let him lack Christian burial. Wherefore let this salutary statute be frequently published in the churches, lest any assume a veil of excuse in the blindness of ignorance. But if any desire to confess his sins to an outside priest for some just reason, let him first ask and obtain permission from his own priest, since otherwise he [the outside priest] cannot loose or bind him. But let the priest be discreet and cautious, and let him after the manner of skilled physicians pour wine and oil upon the wounds of the injured man, diligently inquiring the circumstances alike of the sinner and of the sin, by which [circumstances] he may judiciously understand what counsel he ought to give him, and what sort of remedy to apply, making use of various means [*experimentis*] for the healing of the sick man. But let him give strict heed not at all to betray the sinner by word or sign or in any other way, but if he need more prudent counsel let him seek it cautiously without any indication of the person: since we decree that he who shall presume to reveal a sin discovered to him in the penitential tribunal is not only to be deposed from the priestly office, but also to be thrust into a strict monastery to do perpetual penance.[16]

This decree obviously did not institute the practice of confession. Nevertheless, at a time when a concerted effort was being made to establish and enforce uniformity of law and practice within Latin Christendom, such a canon, issued by pope and general council, included in codified canon law, and backed up by the authority to impose the disciplinary sanctions stipulated in its text, had momentous consequences. The decree was thoroughly publicized, reaching every level of medieval churchmen.[17] While it made annual confession mandatory on pain of excommunication, it also required that the confessor be discreet and cautious, "diligently inquiring the circumstances alike of the sinner and of the sin" so that he would know what counsel he should give; and if he needed more insight, he was to seek advice. Although before 1215 literature designed to aid the confessor had been written, it was in great part as a response to the demands of this canon that such writings began to be produced in much greater quantity and addressed most specifically to the thorough education of the confessor in the requirements of the confessional and its diversities and subtleties.

The literature under discussion was written by those who "were considered experts, with special knowledge about penitents, confessors, and confessing."[18] It was written for the priests, for the ordinary diocesan clergy, who did not have at their disposal the great commentaries and specialized writings of the major scholastics. In this literature the com-

plexities of legal and moral prescriptions could filter down in an easily understandable form to those who needed immediate answers. As Thomas
Tentler said, they were "reference books designed to give answers, not
philosophical inquiries designed to evoke debate."[19] They were intended
to simplify doctrine for practical application and were organized so that
the confessor could locate answers easily. And the answers he would be
seeking centered on sin. Sin, after all, is the subject of confession, and
the focus of literature designed to aid confessors was the definition, clas-
sification, and scrutiny of sins. As one examines this literature, one sees
sins identified everywhere, and articles on vices, activities, and obligations follow any of a number of systems of categorization.

The *Astesana* (ca. 1317) exhorts the confessor to "scrutinize the conscience of the sinner in confession as a physician scrutinizes wounds and
a judge a case."[20] Since the completeness of a confession was an absolute
necessity for the efficacy of absolution, a thorough examination of the
penitent was essential. To such an end the summae confessorum, confessional manuals, and related writings were an indispensable guide.
Confessional examination must penetrate into every area of life; nothing is outside its purview: birth, marriage, sex, the rearing of children—
indeed, every aspect of domestic, social, and economic life. Under the latter fall the special areas of sin that are attached to various occupations.

Early moral theologians recognized the importance of dealing with
moral implications of various occupations. The initial concern was with
identifying those which were patently sinful (e.g., public prostitutes,
usurers). The theologians then sought to single out those which were
morally hazardous and hence required special comment. Robert of
Courson in his *Summa* (ca. 1208–13) so designated surgeons, physicians,
lawyers, procurers, mimes, courtiers, mongers, cooks, and merchants of
dubious wares.[21] Taking a different slant on occupations in the light of
Genesis 3:19 and 2 Thessalonians 3:10,[22] which stated that earnings must
be commensurate with labor, Robert of Courson devoted one book of
his *Summa* to the "hiring of services" *(De locatione operarum)*. Here he first
discussed those professions whose practitioners seemed to perform no
labor and yet demanded exorbitant remuneration, centering his attention on lawyers, physicians, theologians, masters of arts, and notaries.
After these relatively respectable professions, he turned to more dubious
livelihoods, for instance, those of prostitutes, actors, mimes, retail merchants, and manufacturers of doubtful wares.[23] Robert of Courson's analyses were very detailed and lengthy. His colleague Thomas of Chob-

ham in his *Summa* (ca. 1215) first attempted to deal with the moral problems peculiar to various professions in a way that could be conveniently consulted and used by the confessor. Thomas instructed the confessor, as a preliminary to the interrogation, to determine whether the penitent's vocation fell into any of four categories: those completely sinful (e.g., prostitutes and actors), those highly susceptible to sin (e.g., mongers and merchants), those that were useless (e.g., manufacturers of dice, floral wreaths, etc.), and those that were useful but were seldom exercised faithfully (e.g., teachers and those who hired themselves out for wages). He then subjects eleven occupations to a detailed discussion. These vocations include among others, actors, prostitutes, beggars, teachers, priests, and judges.[24] Thomas gives no indication why he chose to treat these occupations in such detail and ignored, for example, lawyers, physicians, and soldiers. It was not until the early fourteenth century that the list of occupations singled out for special attention in the literature devoted to the confessional became stabilized to include all those occupations whose exercise posed special problems for hamartiology. Among these the rubric *medicus*[25] appears with regularity.

The pieces of confessional literature used in the preparation of this chapter sometimes differ from one another significantly in length, form, and emphasis. Some are short and refer the reader to no authorities for the opinions given, although they might list an abundance of sins with little or no comment. Others are longer, even very long, citing the *Decretum* and *Decretales* and numerous commentators (decretists on the former, decretalists on the latter)[26] to give weight to their opinions, but discuss a limited number of sins at quite great length. The order in which sins are given also differs from summa to summa. In most instances the sins mentioned are classified as mortal sins.

Practice and Competency

Several summae stress the responsibility not to practice medicine unless one is competent. The *Astesana* (ca. 1317) considers various ways in which a physician can be at fault. One is *ante factum:* "when he introduces himself into the practice of medicine although he is ignorant [*cum sit idiota*]."[27] The *Angelica* (ca. 1486) is similar, designating as *culpa ante factum* when a physician injects himself into a situation where he is ignorant and not able to manage it.[28] Antoninus, in his short *Confessionale* (1473), states simply that if one practices without adequate skill and has studied little or nothing, "he has sinned mortally and has exposed himself to the danger of killing men."[29] In his much longer *Summa theologica* (1477), Antoninus elaborates that the physician must be expert in the art as expertness is defined by known experts in the art. Simply having a doctorate is not sufficient, "since many unworthy men today in every faculty are masters and doctors to the detriment of themselves and of those promoting them." When from "exceptional ignorance" they harm their patient, they sin. "Nor are they excused . . . because they did not intend to do that, because they voluntarily placed themselves in that position." Even if health should follow their ministrations they have sinned, "because they placed themselves in danger of mortal sin."[30]

Chaimis (ca. 1474) maintains that if one has taken up the practice of medicine without adequate skill and on that account has given harmful medicine or treatment to a patient, he has sinned mortally, "because it was not permitted for him to usurp what was alien to him."[31] Chaimis here refers to the authority of the papal rescript *Tua nos,* written by Innocent III in 1212, included in *Compilatio quarta*[32] and later in the *Decretales* of Gregory IX.[33] This rescript, although it is addressed to the peculiar problems involved in medical practice by clerics[34] and contains little that pertains directly to the discussion at hand, lays down certain relevant principles and, as it is frequently cited by the summists when dealing with the medical profession, must be quoted in full:

Your brotherhood said that we should be consulted. You asked *to be advised by the Apostolic See* what must be decided concerning a certain monk who, believing that he could cure a certain woman of a tumor of the throat, acting as a surgeon, opened the tumor with a knife. When the tumor had healed somewhat, he ordered the woman not to expose herself to the wind at all lest the wind, stealing into the incision in her throat, bring about her death. But the woman, defying his order, rashly exposed herself to the wind while gathering crops, and thus much blood flowed out through the incision in her throat, and the woman died. *She, nevertheless, confessed that she was responsible because she had exposed herself to the wind.* The question is whether this monk, since he is also a priest, may lawfully exercise his priestly office. We therefore reply to your brotherhood that, although the monk himself was very much at fault for usurping an alien function which very little suited him, nevertheless, if he did it from piety and not from cupidity, and was expert in the exercise of surgery and was zealous to employ every diligence which he ought to have done, he must not be condemned for that which happened through the fault of the woman against his advice. Then, with no penance being required, he may be permitted to celebrate divine service. Otherwise, the fulfilling of the sacerdotal office must be strictly forbidden him.[35]

We have seen that the *Astesana* and the *Angelica* had designated ignorance as *culpa ante factum*. Both include the categories *in facto* and *post
factum* as well. The *Astesana* labels it "culpa in facto" when the physician,
"although he is skilled in the art, nevertheless does not follow the traditions of the art but the fancies of his own head."[36] The *Angelica* is nearly
identical, adding "or new experiments—unless they were reasonable."[37]
"Culpa post factum" is described in the *Astesana* as when the physician,
although skilled in the art and following procedures consistent with the
traditions of the art, "nevertheless does not apply diligence so that the
patient be preserved."[38] The *Angelica* classifies as "culpa post factum"
any instance in which the physician is negligent about the care of a patient, citing various commentators on the rescript *Tua nos*.[39]

Antoninus, in his *Confessionale*, simply says that a physician sins mortally if, in spite of having adequate skill, he negligently fails to do what
he ought to have done and "great detriment to the patient occurs or
could have occurred."[40] Antoninus enlarges on this in his *Summa theologica*, saying that when a physician is an expert, he sins mortally if he
should commit an act of "exceptional negligence in reviewing the literature, in visiting the patient, [or] in the quality of his medical materials, "
if death or great aggravation of the illness results. He cites Antonius de
Butrio's commentary on *Tua nos* to the effect that the physician "must
employ every diligence . . . following the traditions of the art; he should
visit the patient and personally prescribe diet and regimen."[41] He also
writes that the physician sins mortally "when he does not employ diligence in preparing medicines, unless he is definitely certain about the
adroitness and honesty of the apothecaries since they sometimes put
much adulterated material" in their medicines.[42] He sums up their responsibility by saying that they sin if they do not "diligently provide for
those things for which provision must be made."[43]

The *Baptistina* (ca. 1480) stresses that the physician ought to consult
with other physicians. The physician sins mortally if, owing to his *imperitia*,[44] the patient dies or is disabled. Baptista gives the example of a
patient with a broken shinbone or arm who is disabled because of the
physician's *imperitia*. The physician is to be held responsible for the damage. In the case of a patient with a family, the physician must make up the
equivalent of lost wages for support of the man's family. "The same applies
if it results from his negligence in not visiting the patient at the necessary
time as he should have." This responsibility applies to anyone who "pro-

claims himself to be skilled by words or by a doctorate." But damages should not be imputed to one who calls himself unskilled and, owing to a dearth of good physicians, does what he can in good faith. Rather, it should be imputed "to the one who chooses such a man."[45]

Cajetan (1525) attributes some of the gravest sins of physicians to rashness: rashly treating a disease without having adequately examined it, or rashly exploring the nature of the disease and thus exposing the patient to the risk of death or grave injury. "If, motivated by gain or fearing that he might appear ignorant, the physician who is ignorant or negligent in study attempts to treat a case, he sins mortally."[46] He also sins by treating rashly, that is, by neglecting either to study or visit, or to take counsel or examine the quality of the medicine if it is brought into doubt. "Or what is worse, he is ashamed to change his opinion and by his obstinancy he casts doubt on the correct cure, which he ought to follow, which was suggested by another."[47]

Fumus (ca. 1538) considered as guilty of mortal sin physicians who are able to know but are not willing to study or to consult experts. "They sin mortally whenever they are acquainted with an ailment and neglect to strive for remedies or to visit, or to give the appropriate medicines if they are able, or whenever they are using one medicine and seeing that it is not effective, continue using it lest they be thought ignorant."[48]

Treatments

Six of the summae used in this study deal with the question of whether a physician should administer a medicine if he is in doubt whether it will help or harm.[49] All answer the question in the negative and emphasize that it is safer to leave the patient in the hands of God[50] than to expose him to the danger of the medicine.[51] Where disagreement arises among the summists is over the question of what constitutes the doubt that should deter the physician from administering the medicine. The *Pisanella* (ca. 1338) states that even if he strongly *(vehementer)* believes it would be useful, if he has any doubts at all, he should not give it. Antoninus, in his *Summa theologica* (1477), and the *Baptistina* (ca. 1480) qualify the physician's doubt by classifying the medicine as one about which the physician is not certain, "following the art." Chaimis (ca. 1474) writes that "in no way ought he to give it unless it is, in accordance with the art, based on knowledge that it ought to be of help." Here he cites commentators on *Tua nos*. The *Angelica* (ca. 1486) is more liberal in its advice, suggesting that if the medicine "has any probability of helping rather than harming, he thus can give it, as long as he has applied necessary diligence and attention: hence he properly *(proprie)* is not in doubt."

Four of our summae go on to ask whether a physician is at fault if he administers a medicine that, owing to a defect or corruption or adulteration of the materials mixed with the drug, harms the patient.[52] All answer that the physician is not culpable if he employed the diligence that he ought in choosing the materials.

The attention of four of the summae is directed to the problems peculiar to surgery.[53] In the *Pisanella* the question of a surgeon's responsibility in the event of his patient's death is raised. As long as the surgeon performing the operation or the phlebotomy was expert and exercised the necessary diligence he is not held responsible, "because death is presumed to have resulted from chance [*casu*] rather than from his fault." Then these questions are raised: "What if the one who must be operated on does not have the usual arrangement of sinews and veins? Or if an unexpected and unusual fear or shaking seizes him and . . . he dies?" As long as the surgeon has not erred owing to inexperience, he has not sinned. If there is any doubt about anything, the surgeon should forgo operating rather than to proceed. The discussion in the *Angelica* is shorter but nearly identical to the above, and *Tua nos* is cited as the authority. Chaimis writes that as long as the surgeon operates in accordance with the art and performs only operations that are clearly useful, he has not sinned. But if he is in doubt about the operation or about his own ability to perform it, he should refrain and dismiss the patient into God's hands without the operation. Antoninus, in his *Summa theologica,* merely stipulates that the surgeon has not sinned if his patient dies, as long as he was skilled and applied proper diligence and did not err owing to inexperience. He cites the rescript *Ad aures* as his authority.

Between 1187 and 1191 Pope Clement III had received an inquiry from a *canonicus* who was in minor orders and wished to be advanced to major (sacred) orders but was concerned that his having practiced as a physician might be an impediment. Clement's reply, which bears the incipit *Ad aures,* reads:

You have brought to our attention that, since you are skilled in the art of physic, you have diligently treated many by the medical tradition of this art, although frequently it had happened to the contrary and those, to whom you thought you were applying a remedy, after taking the medicine, incurred the danger of death. But, because you desire to be advanced to sacred orders, you wished to consult us on this. We reply to you briefly that, if your conscience troubles you on account of those things said above, in our opinion you should not advance to major orders.[54]

Although both *Ad aures* and *Tua nos* were addressed to clerics practicing a healing art—in the one case, medicine, and in the other, surgery—nevertheless canonists extended their principles to cover the responsibilities of secular physicians. These two rescripts are the only decretals in medieval canon law addressed specifically to the general responsibilities of physicians, and the two are complementary. *Tua nos* contains the principle that one is obligated to refrain from usurping offices alien to him. The case in question there is that of a monk or priest usurping the role of surgeon—an alien role for which he was little suited as a monk or priest—but he is not held responsible, in this case, because he was expert in the exercise of surgery and had been zealous to employ all the necessary diligence. The principle is applied by commentators to anyone exercising a specialized role: one must be expert in the field and employ the necessary diligence. The concern is primarily with errors of omission (either in training and/or experience, or in diligence). *Ad aures,* by contrast, raises the question of whether the physician was responsible for harm to anyone owing to his treatments. The matter is left up to his conscience here, and this particular rescript places squarely on this cleric's shoulders the onus of searching his own heart to determine whether he was responsible for any harm having come to his patients. And the concern here is with error of commission, providing the commentators (and summists as well) with a fitting balance for the issues raised by *Tua nos.*

Faithfulness

An area in which the distinction between an error of omission and an error of commission can be easily blurred is in neglecting to give the appropriate medicines. The *Pisanella* (1338) laconically states that the physician sins "if he omits medicines which he ought to have given,"[55] while the *Angelica* (1486), with equal brevity, asserts that the physician is held at fault for prolonging a patient's illness.[56] Both of these leave the question of intent open. Antoninus (1477) approaches the problem in greater depth, insisting that the physician is obligated to cure the patient as quickly as he can. "If he diligently omits a useful medicine that cures quickly so that he might leave him in his illness so as to make more money, he sins gravely and is a thief."[57] Chaimis (ca. 1474) says that the physician sins if, for any reason, he neglects to give the patient appropriate medicine. But if he "zealously aggravates an ailment in any way for the sake of making a greater profit and causes the patient to relapse, he must be punished gravely beyond a mortal sin."[58] Fumus (ca. 1538) is in accord, saying that physicians sin whenever they are able to cure quickly but draw the illness out for a long time because as long as it hangs on they continue making money.[59]

We have seen above that several of the summists condemn a physician for following his own fancies rather than the traditions of the art, if harm results for the patient. Inherent in the idea of following one's own fancies is the possibility of experimentation. Although experimentation is not specifically mentioned by our earlier summists, three of our later sources include it. That these later sources, from the late fifteenth and early sixteenth centuries, specify experimentation is not surprising given the increased experimentation in medical and especially surgical circles during that period. Fumus writes that physicians sin "if they supply a doubtful medicine for a certain one, or do not practice in accord with the art, but desire to practice following their own stupid fancy, or make experiments, and such like, by which the patient is exposed to grave danger."[60] Two summists are especially condemnatory of physicians experimenting on the poor: Chaimis says that a physician sinned mortally "if he gave to the poor or to religious[61] or to any other whatsoever anything deceitfully or for experimentation."[62] Cajetan (1525) likewise castigates the physician who, when he has recognized the disease and knows how to treat it, "puts a poor patient in danger of life or grave injury in order to experiment with a medicine of doubtful efficacy."[63]

We have seen thus far that the summists stressed the physician's responsibility for errors both of omission and of commission in practice. There is a strong insistence that one be competent before assuming the position of physician or surgeon. Practicing without the necessary skill was considered a serious sin. The physician was held responsible for his diligence, for instance, in visiting his patients and in reviewing the literature, and for the quality of medical materials that he used. He was expected to practice in accordance with the traditions of the art, not endangering his patients by following his own fancies or experimenting or using doubtful medicines. He was also held responsible for curing as quickly as possible and castigated for intentionally prolonging an illness for the sake of gain. Expertise, diligence, and faithfulness to the traditions of the art are absolutely expected of both physicians and surgeons by the moral theologians surveyed.

Relations with Colleagues

While all our summists have much to say on competence and diligence, only a small minority are concerned with intra- and inter-professional conduct. Both in classical antiquity and in the Middle Ages, frequent references are made to physicians' envy of and strife with one another. The writings of physicians on medical etiquette and ethics sometimes stress the importance of amicable relations among colleagues, especially in the presence of laymen. This is also a theme of university and guild regulations. It was not, however, a subject that seems to have excited the interest of the summists. Only two of our authors speak of it. Antoninus, in his *Confessionale* (1473), in his closing statement on physicians, urges the confessor to "interrogate as often as it seems best to you about the envy and slander that physicians bear against each other."[64] In his *Summa theologica* (1477), he speaks of "their mutual envy from which they boast about cures, by being proud, and disparage their colleagues by vituperating their cures."[65] Chaimis (ca. 1474) holds the physician guilty of mortal sin "if owing to envy he disparages other physicians or causes them damage." The small interest shown by the summists in physicians' mutual envy and slander does not indicate that the subject was taken lightly. Envy and slander were regarded as serious sins in the casuistic literature but as sins to which everyone is susceptible and on which everyone should be interrogated during confession. Hence, the summists were interested in envy and slander as personal rather than professional matters. After briefly mentioning envy and slander, Chaimis goes on to make the only comment found in our summists on the physician's responsibility to abide by the codes of his professional organization: "If he has sworn to observe the statutes of his *universitas*[66] and afterwards was a violator of them, now as often as he has violated them, he has sinned mortally."[67]

Another matter about which medical guilds were concerned is the relations of physicians with apothecaries. Here again the summists take little interest, and once more only Antoninus and Chaimis comment. We have already noted that Antoninus, in his *Summa theologica*, says that a physician sins mortally if he administers medicines made by apothecaries "unless he is definitely certain about the adroitness and honesty of the apothecaries since they sometimes put much adulterated material" in their medicines. Elsewhere in the same work he writes that the physician sins mortally if he permits a dealer in spices *(aromatarius)* to use old drugs that accomplish little or nothing so that the dealer will not lose money. Here Antoninus gives the same advice we saw earlier, that a physician must not rely on an apothecary in compounding medicines "unless he knows him to be of devout conscience and well trained and practical in such matters," but instead he ought to compound his own drugs.[68] This advice, however, is complicated by as great a moral issue, an issue that was the basis for the nearly consistent requirement in the late Middle Ages that physicians not compound their own drugs. It is the potential for serious conflict of interest that arises here, with its consequent temptations, that Antoninus ignores.[69] It is not a matter that escaped the notice of Chaimis, who writes that if the physician had an apothecary shop and directly or indirectly compelled his patients to buy medicines from him or from another with whom he associated in practice and he did this for the sake of gain, he sinned. If on account of this the patients incurred any physical harm because they could have obtained better or more useful medicines elsewhere, or financial disadvantage because they could have obtained them for less elsewhere, the physician "is held for the price in respect to the entire loss."[70]

Fees

Our summists were, however, much more concerned with the physician's fees and his obligations to give treatment. The problems surrounding physicians' salaries or fees are varied. In the late twelfth and early thirteenth centuries, the question of whether knowledge could be sold was discussed at great length.[71] Stephen Langton dealt with the problem of whether a master of arts who collected fees was selling spiritual knowledge and thus committing simony. He concluded "that such fees were licit. Similarly, Peter the Chanter maintained that physicians, lawyers, and teachers were not selling the grace of God by accepting moderate salaries if they were in need."[72] Thomas Aquinas maintains that one may justly receive a fee for what one is not bound to do gratuitously, provided that they have "regard to their clients' position, profession and work, and also the customs of the country." If, however, one wickedly extorts an immoderate fee, he sins against justice.[73] Once it was generally agreed that members of professions could rightly receive remuneration for their services, a great debate ensued among theologians and canonists on how the "just price" for services should be defined. The summists surveyed here do not contribute to such discussions, at least not when dealing with physicians' sins. Even the most theoretical of our summists, Antoninus, in his *Summa theologica* (1477), does not become involved with previous scholastic analysis. Early in his section on physicians, he engages in an extensive analysis of the nature of medicine. During the course of his discussion he says that "a physician, because he demands and receives compensation, cannot be said to sell his knowledge or health, which are spiritual matters, but he hires out his services, and he seeks wages for his labor that was expended then [i.e., while rendering the service] or previously in his studying. For no one is constrained to give his service *de suo*."[74] Later, when he is ready to address the subject of physicians' remuneration, he begins by merely saying that they "can demand a salary or wage justly for their labor, as Luke 10 makes clear: 'A workman is worthy of his hire.'" He then distinguishes three different categories of physicians according to their income: (1) those paid by the community; (2) those who are not salaried but whose discretion in setting fees is limited by statute of the community or lord; and (3) those neither salaried nor limited in anything. The first are not able to receive anything besides their salary. "If their salary is not sufficient for them, let them credit themselves with having agreed to it." The second ought not to accept more than what is specified, "unless the statute has been invalidated by opposing custom." The third "can accept and ought to demand a reasonable [*moderatum*] fee, and what is 'reasonable' is determined by the quality of care, the labor of the physician, his diligence and conscientiousness, the means of the patient, and the custom of the place."[75] Chaimis (ca. 1474) simply states that the physician sinned "if he extorted an immoderate fee from the rich."[76] Fumus (ca. 1538) labels as sin the action of physicians who demand an exorbitant fee "contrary to justice, or whenever they cause exceedingly excessive expenses to arise, especially from the poor, so that either they themselves or the apothecaries might make a greater profit."[77]

Three of the summists were intrigued with the question of whether a physician is obligated to treat an illness that recurs for the fee he was paid for treating it in the first instance. Antoninus considers the case in which a contract had been drawn up specifying that the fee was to be paid after completion of the service. He maintains that if the illness returned to the man who was still "unwell," then the physician is obligated, "for the illness does not seem to have disappeared, nor is he fully freed who is not freed from the whole." The physician is not obligated, however, if the illness returned "after an interval of time" or if it returned "by the fault of the patient."[78] When the *Baptistina* (ca. 1480) addresses the same question, the decision is based on the interval of time between the disappearance of the illness and its return, unless other factors intervene. An extensive discussion is then presented involving the hypothetical case of Titius (the "John Doe" of classical and medieval Roman law), whom a physician had promised to free from gout. Titius seemed to have been freed, but after a time the gout returned. Titius then took the physician to court on the grounds that he had not eradicated the disease but only made it inactive. Since in this case the physician had promised to cure him entirely, he was obligated.[79] The *Angelica* (ca. 1486) presents us with Titius again, this time suffering from quartan fever. A physician agrees to free him from the disease and succeeds, but only for a brief time; the physician is held responsible because he did not extinguish the illess, although he had caused the distress of the man to cease.[80]

The Obligation to Provide Care

It is well known that in classical antiquity physicians were generally loath to take on hopeless cases. There were various reasons for this, which I have discussed elsewhere.[81] With the advent of medical licensure requirements and medico-surgical guild monopolies, the physician's option of simply refusing to treat or deserting a terminally ill patient certainly became more circumscribed. Antoninus, in his introductory discussion of the nature of medicine in his *Summa theologica* (1477), asserts that "desperate cases which, according to the judgements of men, are held to be fatal, sometimes the diligent physician is able to cure, but rarely. . . . Therefore, clear to the end the physician ought to do what he can to cure the patient."[82] The question, however, still remained as to whether physicians should receive a fee for treating incurable cases. Antoninus' opinion was that "because the physician was created as an instrument of nature, the instrument of medicine should not be entirely withdrawn from the patient as long as nature does not succumb. Therefore, the physician does not sin by accepting a stipend for the treatment of an illness which, following the principles of the art of medicine, he believes is incurable." The physician must not hide that knowledge from those who have the immediate care of the patient, or cause unnecessary expenses, or promise entirely to cure him. He thus can justly receive his stipend "as he displays in the care of his patient faithful attendance and true counsel . . . because the physician does not know what God has arranged concerning the patient, whether he will recover or die, although, according to the art of medicine, he ought to die. Therefore it is licit for the physician to pursue a cure and to accept a stipend clear up to the end or nearly."[83]

There is a statement attributed to Pope Symmachus, quoted in the *Decretum* of Gratian, to the effect that "there is not a great difference whether you inflict something fatal or allow it. He is proved to inflict death on the weak who does not prevent this when he is able to."[84] Although this says nothing directly concerning physicians, Joannes Teutonicus, in what became known as the *Glossa ordinaria* to the *Decretum* (ca. 1216–17), commented on this passage that the physician is obligated to treat both the poor and the rich gratis rather than to allow them to die. This gloss is the *locus classicus* for the summists' discussion of the question of whether a physician is obligated to cure gratis rather than to allow a sick person to die. Thomas Aquinas considered the problem of the extent to which the physician is morally obligated to treat the poor gratuitously. Beginning with the remark "Nobody can possibly help out all those in need," he then writes that kindness ought first to be shown to those with whom one is united in any way *(propinqui)*. In respect to others, if a man "is in such dire straits that it is not immediately obvious how else he is to be helped [then] one is bound to come to his assistance." Thus a lawyer is not always obligated to defend the destitute, "Otherwise he would have to give up all other work and devote himself exclusively to the cases of the poor. And the same considerations apply to the doctor in connexion with the care of the poor."[85] The *Astesana* (ca. 1317) follows Aquinas closely when discussing lawyers' obligations to defend the poor gratis, adding that "the same must be said concerning a physician as to the care of paupers."[86] The other summists rely also on Joannes Teutonicus' gloss on the passage from the *Decretum* quoted at the beginning of this paragraph, considering the obligation especially to exist if the alternative to free care is the death of the patient. This distinction, however, is not seen in Antoninus' short *Confessionale* (1473), in which he simply says that a physician has sinned "if he has not freely visited poor patients who he knew were not able to pay, because he is obligated to do that and even to pay for the medicines if he is able."[87] Such a bald statement disregards the principles laid down both by Aquinas and Joannes Teutonicus, and may well have sent the perplexed confessor to Antoninus' more extensive treatment in his *Summa theologica*, where he addresses the problem in different places. In his discussion of the nature of medicine, he says that the physician must treat gratis paupers who are unable to pay, and must not withdraw himself from their care "because this may be killing them indirectly."[88] Later, when dealing with the question in greater detail, he says that the physician "is not obligated to provide for all the poor ill simply and indiscriminately, but according to the place and time presenting itself, just as it was said above concerning lawyers and as it is said concerning other works of mercy."[89]

Generally the treatment of our summists[90] is along the following lines, with slight variations: A physician is obligated to give care and counsel gratis to a sick pauper, "for he is proved to inflict death on the weak who does not prevent it when he is able to." He ought to give care and medicines gratis rather than to allow a patient to die. This applies not only to the pauper but also to the rich. The physician should not only give care gratis but should even provide the medicines at his own expense for a sick rich man who is not willing to pay him anything, rather than to allow him to die. Antoninus here stipulates that the physician is thus obligated only if the patient or his relatives have called him. If the patient recovers, the physician can then demand his fee from him; if the patient dies, from his heirs. In the former case, the grounds are that he has rightly managed the patient's affair; in the latter, that he had rightly begun to conduct the affair, although the outcome did not follow. Nor may it be objected that the physician did it for charity *(causa pietatis)*, unless he is united in some way *(propinquus)* to the patient. He is both able and obligated to treat such a man and can afterwards demand a fee, even if the patient refuses to allow himself to be treated, just as we can drag one against his will from a building that is about to collapse and confer a benefit on one against his will. It must be assumed that the patient who refuses treatment is insane.

Sexual Impropriety

While our summists were vitally concerned with the physician's fee and his obligations to render treatment, they virtually ignored the possibility of sexual impropriety in the physician-patient relation. Only Chaimis (ca. 1474) addressed the subject; he wrote that the physician has sinned mortally "if in the course of visiting women and because of their ailment has handled them intentionally and with libidinous intent and has proceeded on to anything dishonorable."[91] That most of our summists ignore the subject simply indicates that, as with envy and slander, the problem was subsumed not under professional but rather under personal morality.

Spiritual Obligations

The summists, however, were not at all reticent about the physician's spiritual obligations, for it is here that the greatest concerns of the casuists, moral theologians, and canonists arose when considering the physician's responsibilities and sins, as well as potential harm to the patient. While there was a fair degree of concern to protect the patient from physical and financial harm at the hands of the incompetent, negligent, or unscrupulous physician, it was infinitely more important to consider the well-being of the patient's soul. There was in early Christianity and in the early Middle Ages a tension between medicine and Christianity. This tension remained, however latent. It sometimes rose to the surface when the physician's goals and procedures obviously conflicted with spiritual priorities as defined by medieval Catholicism. In the *Decretum* Gratian quotes Ambrose's statement that "the precepts of medicine are contrary to the divine position." The passage goes on to say that physicians lure people away from fasts and vigils and meditation.[92] Yet the physician, according to Scripture, is to be honored with the honor due him, for God created him, and so on.[93] An uneasy modus vivendi existed between medicine and theology, the potential for conflict being maximal when the physician's interest in the health of the body appeared at variance with the church's interest in the health of the soul.

At the Fourth Lateran Council of 1215 a canon was enacted that soon became part of Gregory IX's official codification of canon law.[94] This canon, number 22 of the council, coming immediately after *Omnes utriusque sexus,* and bearing the incipit *Cum infirmitas* (or *Quum infirmitas*), is the only official canon from the Middle Ages that deals directly with the responsibilities of the secular physician. Its text reads:

Since bodily infirmity is sometimes caused by sin, the Lord saying to the sick man whom he had healed: "Go and sin no more, lest some worse thing happen to thee" [John 5:14], we declare in the present decree and strictly command that when physicians of the body are called to the bedside of the sick, before all else they admonish them to call for the physician of souls, so that after spiritual health has been restored to them, the application of bodily medicine may be of greater benefit, for the cause being removed the effect will pass away. We publish this decree for the reason that some, when they are sick and are advised by the physician in the course of the sickness to attend to the salvation of their soul, give up all hope and yield more easily to the danger of death. If any physician shall transgress this decree after it has been published by the bishops, let him be cut off from the church till he has made suitable satisfaction for his transgression. And since the soul is far more precious than the body, we forbid under penalty of anathema that a physician advise a patient to have recourse to sinful means for the recovery of bodily health.[95]

This canon raises several important points. Since sickness is sometimes caused by sin, a physician, when called to a patient, must admonish him to call a priest before all else. Note that the interest expressed here is in the curative effect of confession, not in the desirability of ensuring that confession be made before a patient dies. Physicians who violate this requirement are to be strictly punished. The final stipulation in the canon is that physicians will be anathematized who "advise a patient to have recourse to sinful means for the recovery of bodily health." It is the summists' concern with this last stipulation that I shall consider first.

The *Astesana* (ca. 1317) simply states that "since the soul is worth much more than the body, under the threat of anathema, we forbid any physician to recommend for physical health anything that results in danger to the soul."[96] The statements in the *Pisanella* (ca. 1338),[97] the *Baptistina* (ca. 1480),[98] and the *Angelica* (ca. 1486)[99] are just as laconic, indeed even more so. All cite *Cum infirmitas.*[100] The treatments by Antoninus (1473 and 1477), Chaimis (ca. 1474), and Fumus (ca. 1538) are more involved, listing specific matters that a physician is forbidden to advise to a patient. All three begin their short lists by forbidding the physician to advise fornicating.[101] Fumus alone mentions masturbation *(pollutio)* and incantation, Antoninus and Chaimis forbid physicians to advise their patients to drink intoxicating beverages, and all three include the open category "and such things." Antoninus is the only one of our summists who discusses the circumstances of illicit counsel, maintaining that "a physician who says to a patient, 'I do not advise, but if you have intercourse with a woman, you will get well,' transgresses this regulation. . . . Therefore, the physician ought to beware in speaking, lest from concern for the situation of the illness he be aroused to doing something wrong."

Both Antoninus[102] and Chaimis[103] regarded it as a mortal sin for a physician to advise the sick to break the church's fasts or to eat meat on forbidden days "without reasonable cause," or to encourage the healthy to break fast days, "saying that they are harmful and such like."

Abortion

If one now were asked what aspect of medical ethics has historically excited the most interest on the part of the Catholic Church, abortion would be a reasonable reply. Surprisingly, of all the summists surveyed, only two mention abortion in their discussions of physicians' sins.

The history of the treatment of abortion by the church through the end of the Middle Ages is complex and diverse, fraught with inconsistencies of interpretation.[104] The practice of abortion is condemned in early Christian literature, for example, in the *Didache*[105] and the *Epistle of Barabas*,[106] and in works by Clement of Alexandria,[107] Minucius Felix,[108] and Tertullian.[109] In the fourth century the practice is denounced by one church council in the West[110] and by another in the East.[111] Jerome[112] and Augustine[113] make the distinction that abortion was not counted as homicide unless the fetus was "formed." The statements by Jerome and Augustine "were to be the *loci classici* on abortion in the West,"[114] and were transmitted by clerical writers and incorporated into penitentials through the mid–twelfth century. In the *Decretum* of Gratian, abortion is classified as homicide only when the fetus is formed ("vivified" or "ensouled").[115] In the *Decretales* of Gregory IX, two canons deal with the subject, one being in agreement with Gratian's interpretation,[116] the other applying the penalty for homicide to contraception and to the induced abortion of a fetus at any stage of development.[117] Considerable differences in interpretation of these two conflicting canons exist among various commentators on canon law, with one of the most influential, Hostiensis, arguing in favor of the stricter application. Among theologians, Thomas Aquinas held that the sin of abortion was a matter of degree that depended on the different stages of fetal development.[118] The subject of therapeutic abortion had not been directly addressed. Antoninus' contribution to the subject "may be taken to mark the beginning of a new era of thought on abortion."[119]

Antoninus makes only a passing and indiscriminate reference to abortion when treating the sins of physicians in his *Confessionale*. He says that a physician sins mortally "if he gives medicine to a pregnant woman to

kill the fetus even for the preservation of the mother."[120] Antoninus
wrote his *Confessionale* in 1473. Four years later, in his *Summa theologica,*
we find him making distinctions that conflict with his earlier statement
in his *Confessionale.* In his *Summa* he deals with abortion first in a general
discussion of homicide. John Connery writes:

There he deals with it under the question whether homicide can be justified
when necessary to avoid some evil. By way of example he speaks of women who
have committed fornication, adultery, or incest and try to hide their crime by
abortion or infanticide. They do this to preserve their reputation or even their
lives. Antoninus says that none of these reasons excuses them from a very serious
sin. . . . He admits, however, that there will be no question of homicide in causing
an abortion unless the fetus is already formed. He says that this occurs after 40
days in the male fetus, 80 days in the female fetus, thus following in general the
Aristotelian time distinction between male and female formation. He goes on to
say that it is not permissible for a woman, who is going to die anyhow, to shorten
her life to save the fetus, nor on the contrary is it permitted to take the life of the
fetus to save the mother. Anyone who does this, and all who cooperate with such
a person, will be guilty of homicide.[121]

It is in his section dealing with the sins of physicians that he makes
a distinction "vital to the future discussion of abortion."[122] The contribution of Antoninus here lies not in his originality but in his adopting
a distinction made a century earlier by an obscure theologian, John of
Naples, whose *Quodlibeta* never saw print. Antoninus writes:

physicians indeed sin mortally in giving medicines to pregnant women for producing abortion and for the death of the fetus [*mortem eius*], in order to cover up
a sin. But if they do this to preserve the pregnant woman from the danger of
death caused by the fetus [*in quo est ex puerperio*],[123] then, following John of
Naples, a distinction must be made concerning this fetus, whether it is ensouled
[*animatum*] or not ensouled with a rational soul. And if indeed it has been
ensouled, the physician sins mortally by giving such medicine.

He goes on to argue that if the fetus is ensouled, the physician has
caused both the physical and the spiritual death of the fetus. The physician who thus allows the mother to die by not giving her the abortifa-
cient is not the cause of her death directly, because the disease from
which she suffered is the direct cause. Nor has he caused her death
indirectly, "because even if he had been able to preserve the mother
from death by giving the medicine . . . he would have been the cause of
the death of the fetus." On the other hand,

if the fetus is not yet ensouled with a rational soul, he would then be able and
ought to give such medicine [*posset tunc et deberet dare talem medicinam*], because

even if it prevents the animation of such a fetus, nevertheless, it would not be the cause of the death of any person [*causa mortis alicuius hominis*]. And this good follows, that it frees the mother from death. Therefore he ought to give it in such a case. . . . But if there is doubt concerning the fetus, whether it is ensouled with a rational soul or not, he seems by giving such medicine to sin mortally, because he exposed himself to the danger of mortal sin, that is, of homicide.[124]

John Connery's comments here bear quoting:

Since Antoninus was one of the great moral theologians of all times, acceptance by him of this opinion undoubtedly assured it a hearing. In fact, it is only through him that we know of this exception since the *Quodlibeta* of John of Naples were never published. Discussion of the exception will occupy the attention of moral theologians for the next three or four centuries, that is, until theories of delayed animation on which it was based begin to give way. Although Antoninus and John of Naples will have a respectable following, there will not be unanimous agreement with their opinion about this case.[125]

Only one of our summists besides Antoninus mentions abortion under the rubric of the sins of physicians, and this is Chaimis (ca. 1474), who writes that a physician sins mortally if "he gives medicine to a pregnant woman for killing the child [*puerum*] in order to preserve the mother."[126] He apparently was unaffected by the distinction that John of Naples and Antoninus had set forth.

It is surprising that only two of the summists surveyed include any reference to abortion when discussing the sins of physicians, especially since the summists were provided with such an opportunity by the prohibition, in *Cum infirmitas,* of physicians' advising anything sinful, although this constraint did inspire several summists to list such offences as advising a patient to fornicate or to drink an intoxicating beverage. It is not that the rest of our summists were uninterested in the problem, since several include a discussion of abortion under *homicidium* or have a separate rubric *aborsus,* or both.[127] Any argument to the effect that abortion was not considered a grave enough sin to warrant their attention cannot be entertained seriously. Nor is it reasonable to say that the interpretive dilemma presented by the issue scared them away, lest they be forced to come down on one side of a question or on the other, since they demonstrate no such qualms about other difficult issues. The only even moderately appealing explanation that presents itself is that the majority of our summists simply did not regard the decision as something that physicians or surgeons had to face. It is probable that during the period under consideration a woman would have turned not to a male physician or surgeon for her obstetrical or gynecological needs, but rather to another woman, such as a midwife or one of the variety of female practitioners of the time. The inclusion of physicians in the discussions of abortion by John of Naples, Antoninus, and Chaimis may have been primarily for its theoretical value. Regardless of who should be involved, physician or midwife, by the early sixteenth century no theoretical defense or even definition of therapeutic abortion had yet been formulated. This fact left the conscientious physician or midwife in a moral quandary.

Euthanasia

The question was posed above as to what medico-ethical issue has historically been the greatest stimulus to discussion by Catholic theologians. Abortion was suggested as a reasonable response. A second would certainly be euthanasia. What we would call passive euthanasia, although never so considered in the Middle Ages, must be subsumed under the broader subject of the obligation to treat and to attempt to cure hopeless cases. But what we would call active euthanasia is a different matter and is a subject never raised by our summists when discussing the sins of physicians. Active euthanasia, which we now regard as a moral category unto itself, was regarded throughout our period as simply homicide on the physician's part and suicide on the patient's, assuming willing involvement by the latter. Martin Aspilcuetta, better known as Navarrus, the leading canonist of the sixteenth century and a post-Tridentine summist, writes in his summa (1568) that the physician sins who gives any medicine that he knows is harmful, "even if he administers it out of pity or in order to please the patient."[128] Navarrus' statement seems clear and unambiguous: active euthanasia, whether motivated by pity or by the wish of the patient, is sinful. This must be one of the earliest articulations regarding active euthanasia in such precise terms. Navarrus gives as authority for his statement the commentary of Panormitanus (after 1421) on the decretal *Tua nos* (which itself, of course, says nothing on the subject of euthanasia). Panormitanus had simply given the opinion that those having custody of or serving a sick person sin greatly if, motivated by "a sort of pity," they obey or indulge the "corrupted desire" of the ill man. Before active euthanasia was seen as a separate category, the closest the summists could have come to including relevant comments in their sections on physicians' sins would have been to have stated that it was a sin for a physician to kill or poison his patient intentionally, a statement as unlikely to be made as that it was a sin for a physician to steal a patient's property, rape his wife, or burn down his house, since it would be a sin not considered peculiar to the vocation under discussion.

Informing the Terminally Ill Patient

Throughout the history of medicine, a prerogative that physicians have usually guarded jealously is whether to inform the terminally ill patient of his condition. Although having no direct authority to cite on this matter from canon law, several of our summists made pronouncements on the question of whether a physician who foresees the impending death of one of his patients is obligated to tell him. Antoninus is the earliest of our summists to ask that question and, as in the case of abortion, it is to the *Quodlibeta* of the fourteenth-century theologian John of Naples, that he turns for an answer. John of Naples had distinguished as follows: Either the physician believes that it is very likely that such a prediction would be very useful for the patient, with a view toward his putting both his spiritual and his temporal affairs in order, or he believes the opposite, namely that it would not be useful, or he is in doubt about both. When the physician believes that the patient is in a state of mortal sin and has made no provision for the disposal of his material possessions, thus producing grave dissension among his heirs, and that the patient, if he hears that death is imminent, will prepare himself for dying well and will put his affairs in order, then the physician is obligated to inform the patient, either directly or through another. If he does not do so, he sins mortally. But when the physician believes that in all likelihood the announcement would profit the patient little or nothing, because he believes that the patient is in a good spiritual state and that his temporal affairs are in order, then he is not obligated to inform him. But he would do better by doing so, because any patient, regardless of how well his spiritual and temporal affairs might have been arranged, would set himself more in order having heard that death is near. If the physician is in doubt about the patient's spiritual and temporal state, he is obligated to inform him of impending death. This is especially important since both the condemnation of the patient's soul and harm to his temporal affairs can follow.[129] John of Naples, perhaps *via* Antoninus, is followed in these assessments by the *Baptistina* (ca. 1480),[130] the *Angelica* (ca. 1486),[131] and Fumus (ca. 1538).[132]

Antoninus pursues the matter further than these three summists. He cites Galen as saying that however much the physician despairs of the health of a patient he should always strengthen him and tell him that he will recover. Antoninus writes that John of Naples reacts to Galen's statement with the assertion that it is not necessary to follow this precept, citing in contrast Gratian's quotation from Ambrose that "the precepts of medicine are contrary to the divine position."[133] Antoninus seems to appreciate both sides of the question, saying that "by predicting death much harm is done, and by being silent no damage is done. Nevertheless, in no case ought one to lie, as they are wont to do."[134] His final assessment, as given in his recapitulation at the end of the section on physicians, is that a physician sins mortally if, "recognizing the impending death of a patient according to the art of medicine, he does not advise him or those caring for him or his confessor, so that they might make provision for him concerning the sacraments or concerning a will, if it is useful, and such like; fearing lest he get worse on account of this, or be in bad humor, or displease his family; following John of Naples in *Quodlibeta*."[135] Whether or not to inform the patient thus remained, for the conscientious physician, an onus requiring that he be certain of his terminal patient's spiritual condition and the state of his arrangements for disposing of his affairs.

Requiring the Patient to Call a Confessor

While the stipulation that pertained to informing the terminal patient has no direct basis in canon law, *Cum infirmitas* appears quite specific in requiring that "before all else" physicians, when called to the bedside of the sick, "advise and persuade[136] them to call for the physician of souls." Two reasons are given for this requirement. The first is that confession had a curative effect. Since much illness was caused by sin, the confession of sin would remove the cause, thus making the physician's attendance either superfluous or more effective. Second, if it was popularly believed that physicians advised the patient to call a confessor only if the hope of recovery was absent, patients thus advised would "give up all hope and yield more easily to the danger of death."

To anyone who attempts to understand how this canon should be applied, any of the following questions might arise: (1) Does this apply to every new case a physician undertakes? (2) Since the physician must "advise and persuade" *(moneant et inducant)* the patient to call a confessor, is he also responsible to ensure that the patient both agrees and complies? (3) If the patient is unwilling to call a confessor, may the physician treat him anyway, or must he withdraw from the case? (4) May the physician "advise and persuade" through others, such as relatives, friends, or attendants of the patient, or must he do so himself? (5) If physicians simply refuse to comply on the grounds that it is contrary to the established precepts of their art, can this canon be abrogated through non-use and prescribed by contrary custom? (Cf. the discussion of non-use and contrary custom, below.)

All our summists who wrote after Lateran IV include a discussion of *Cum infirmitas,* although their discussions vary widely in length, detail, and sensitivity to the problems posed by this canon. It should be noted that none of the summists surveyed dealt with all the questions posed above. Several give basically a short, rigid, and dogmatic demand that the physician persuade the patient to confess, without discussing the possibility of exceptions.[137] Even Antoninus, although he discusses the problems at some length in his *Summa theologica* (1477), simply makes the bald statement in his short *Confessionale* (1473) that a physician has sinned "if he has not abided by the precept made for physicians, namely that they should persuade their patients when they first are called to them that they must make confession, because, following the authorities [*doctores*], it is a mortal sin."[138]

Among those who considered the question of whether physicians are obligated in all cases to advise the patient to call a confessor, opinions vary. Antoninus, in his *Summa,* notes that some physicians comply with *Cum infirmitas* only when dealing with patients who they think are mortally ill, and not under other circumstances. "But such physicians do not fulfil this constitution and that is clear from the text of the decretal itself. There it is stated: 'for the reason that some, when they are sick and are advised by the physician in the course of the sickness to attend to the salvation of their soul, give up all hope and yield more easily to the danger of death.'" He then quotes the commentary of Joannes Andreas on this section of *Cum infirmitas,* to the effect that "from this patients will truly know that physicians say this in every illness, in mortal illnesses and also in those not judged fatal; then fear and danger will cease."[139] Andreas' interpretation appears consonant with the stated intent of the decretal, since if physicians generally advised only terminal patients or those suffering from dangerous illnesses to confess, the effect of such advice on patients could well be deleterious. But the other summists who consider this question seem to move away from the intent of the canon. The *Baptistina* (ca. 1480) lays it down that "the safe judgement always being the better judgement," this constitution applies only to dangerous or doubtful ailments. The *Baptistina* gives as examples "any accident or any pain of the head" and any ailment that is "dangerous in the physician's opinion, for instance continuous fevers, pleurisy, quinsy, colic pain of the kidneys, and such like." By contrast, the physician is not obligated to advise the patient to confess if he has "an ephemeral fever and such like."[140] The *Angelica* (ca. 1486) states that in any sudden accident that requires immediate treatment the physician is excused. "Although it is best that he persuade in every illness," he is not obligated except in dangerous illnesses. "And I call it 'dangerous' when one can credibly demonstrate a danger of death."[141] Fumus (ca. 1538) holds the physician obligated whenever the patient is in a serious illness, "even if not in imminent danger of death."[142] Cajetan (1525) feels that it must be an illness "from which a man truly lies ill. A physician is not held to this in every illness without distinction, lest the advice come into derision." He advises taking a middle road between extremely dangerous cases and ailments such as gout.[143]

Of the summists surveyed, only one addressed the question of whether a physician is obligated to ensure the patient's compliance in making a confession, but did not consider the obviously correlative question of whether the physician must withdraw from the case if the patient does not call for a confessor. Chaimis (ca. 1474) simply writes that physicians' advice and persuasion must be *cum effectu*, that is, with result, before they are permitted to undertake care. As authority for this he cites the commentaries of Hostiensis, Joannes Andreas, and Antonius de Butrio on *Cum infirmitas*.[144] Antoninus (1477) instructs his readers to "note that physicians must observe this rule 'before all things.'" This he takes to mean "before they raise a hand to treat, or before they come to an agreement on a fee," citing Joannes Andreas. But must the physician ensure his patient's compliance? Antoninus says that Hostiensis, interpreting *inducant* to be *cum effectu*, insists that the physician not undertake the case otherwise. "But such an opinion as this," writes Antoninus, "seems harsh, since succor must be given *secundum ordinem caritatis*, to those who are in danger, however stubborn they may be." He maintains that the text itself does not specifically require that the physician's advice be followed, and cites the opinion of Petrus de Palude that physicians are only obligated to admonish.[145] When the question is discussed in the *Baptistina,* Panormitanus is cited as having interpreted *moneant et inducant* as *cum effectu,* "namely that they [sc., the patients] call a priest: otherwise it does not satisfy this precept." Noting that others say "not unreasonably that when a physician does as much as he can to persuade the patient, even by threatening to abandon him," and still the patient absolutely refuses, the physician can proceed with the case, the *Baptistina* concurs. The reasoning is that if the physician withdrew, the patient might give up hope and die. But if he is cured, he might be able to be persuaded to tend to his spiritual needs.[146] The *Angelica* is in agreement with the *Baptistina* here, holding that an interpretation that required a physician to desert the recalcitrant patient would make "the precept of the church seem against the precept of God."[147] Fumus writes that if the patient "is not willing to confess, he ought not to be abandoned on that account, lest perhaps he despair and die, for this seems to be contrary to charity by which we are held to do good even to the bad and to the unjust, and this seems to me to be a good conclusion and sufficiently discreet."[148]

Three of the summists speak directly or indirectly to the question of whether the physician may advise and persuade through another. The *Pisanella* (ca. 1338) flatly states that it is a rule that the physicians "themselves advise and order" that patients call the confessor.[149] Cajetan, however, tells his reader: "Stop! lest you too quickly judge a physician guilty of mortal sin, because physicians are accustomed to do this not through themselves but through relatives or others."[150] And Fumus simply says that it is sufficient for them to have those near the patient urge the patient to call a confessor.[151]

Seven of our summists consider the question of whether *Cum infirmitas* can be abrogated through non-use and prescribed by contrary custom. A general principle in late medieval canon law was that any *reasonable* custom that prevailed throughout Christendom abrogated the written law. The classic doctrine was that the custom must be in accord with reason and that no custom could claim to be reasonable if it was prejudicial to ecclesiastical liberty and discipline. Gregory IX admitted this doctrine in the decretal *Cum tanto (Quum tanto).*[152] A clear definition of what was and what was not "prejudicial to ecclesiastical liberty and discipline," of course, could not be achieved with the inclusiveness necessary to cover every exigency. The *Astesana,*[153] the *Pisanella,*[154] and Antoninus in his *Summa theologica,*[155] simply say that it cannot be abrogated by any custom, the former two adding, "since it was introduced for the health of souls." The *Baptistina* says the same, citing Panormitanus, and maintaining that "such a custom does not have in itself any reason [*ratio*]. On the contrary, from it many evils result, as in the text."[156] The *Angelica* states forcefully that "it cannot be said to be abrogated on account of contrary custom, for it is not custom but is corruption and against good morals and therefore does not have strength."[157] Fumus says the same, nearly verbatim, but then concedes that considering that the requirement of *Cum infirmitas* "opposes their art which always predicts good hope, they do not sin mortally" if they merely advise those near the patient to urge him to confess.[158] In this he is close to Cajetan's development of the question. After mentioning that physicians are accustomed to advise patients through relatives or others, Cajetan writes:

For if this constitution has been thus accepted by consensus of those practicing, and the prelates, who have the authority to discipline such physicians, ignore those who violate it, physicians are excused from mortal sin, since it is established that decretals of substantive law [*ius positivum*] are abrogated by non-use, especially those never having been received accurately, as seems to be the case here. And this decree seems reasonable so far as it was written, but never affirmed by the consensus of those practicing, because it is opposed to the role [*officium*] of physicians and on account of this they always seem to have withstood it. Physicians indeed are bound by the precept of their art always to present pleasant things which are of health and hope for the patient. On that account they say not to look to them to bring in sorrowful tidings of such a kind if there is danger; and if there is no danger, they ought not to expose themselves or their words to ridicule. Understand these things to excuse the custom of good physicians.[159]

It is obvious that by the early sixteenth century there was no uniformity either of practice or of interpretation of the major provisions of *Cum infirmitas*. In 1566, a very few decades after Cajetan wrote his *Summula peccatorum,* and three years after the adjournment of the Council of Trent, Pope Pius V renewed *Cum infirmitas* in his constitution *Super gregem*. There it was declared that physicians were to discontinue their treatment of a patient after the third day if the patient failed to produce a document signed by a confessor certifying that he had duly confessed. Physicians violating this rule were to be declared infamous, denied the privilege of practicing, and ejected from their university or medical and surgical associations.[160]

Conclusions

We have seen that many of the summists were thorough in detailing and analyzing the sins to which physicians were considered most susceptible. They impressed upon physicians that failure to have the requisite expertness, failure to exercise the necessary diligence, and failure to maintain the traditions of the art are mortal sins. The obligation to extend charity to the poor was important to most of our summists, as was the treatment of the rich miser. Also, the physician's obligations to the spiritual well-being of the patient weighed heavily on the minds of the summists.

Now that we have seen the scope of the summists' interests and the details of their analyses, an obvious question must be posed: What if any effect might all this have had on the shaping of late medieval medical ethics and on actual practice? As we consider the question just posed, it is absolutely necessary to bear in mind that medieval society was, with the exception of a small number of Jews and heretics, exclusively Christian. There was only one church, and everyone was a member of it. The allegiance, willing or otherwise, of virtually the entire population of western Europe, coupled with the prestige of ecclesiastical institutions, enabled the church to exercise coercive jurisdiction over areas of life that now would be the concern either of secular authority or of the individual conscience. The church promulgated laws and expected obedience. Its coercive jurisdiction was exercised through ecclesiastical courts where penalties ranging from penance to imprisonment to excommunication were imposed. Church courts were of two different but complementary kinds, the *forum externum* and the *forum internum*. The former, the external, also called the *ius fori*, "represented the right of the Church to judge her members in relation to the social body of Christendom. . . . The external forum was simply the jurisdiction of the Canonical courts. On the other hand, the internal forum, termed the *ius poli* in the Middle Ages, represented the right of the Church to judge her members in view of their personal and intimate relationship to God. This forum was simply the confessional in which the believer confessed his sins to his priest and received moral and spiritual guidance."[161]

The extent to which the confessional influenced ethics and conduct cannot be gauged with certainty. A few observations, however, can be made legitimately. Thomas Tentler, whose studies of the *summae confes-*

sorum qualify him as a leading authority on the historical significance of the genre, likes to speak of the confessional as an instrument of social control. While he concedes that he "cannot prove the importance of confession quantitatively," nevertheless he "can say a great deal about the teachings that religious authorities wanted the Christian community to believe and put into practice."[162] It cannot reasonably be denied that the confessional literature was written for the purpose of educating the clergy to the end that they, in turn, should educate the laity as part of the confessional objective. For the goal of confession was not only to forgive known sins committed but also (1) to educate laypersons so that they might be able to identify previously unknown sins, both of commission and of omission, in their lives, and (2) to correct sinful practices. The best confession was one that led to a changed life, and a changed life should be one in as close conformity to the expectations and standards of the church as possible. Were the expectations and standards expressed in this literature unrealistic products of ascetic theologians far removed from the realities of life? Tentler writes that "it would have been impractical and self-defeating" for these authors "to appeal to ideas and expectations that were novel, irrelevant, or unintelligible." For what he sees in this body of literature "is the practicality of men who understood the inherent power of the system placed at the disposal of every rank of ecclesiastical authority."[163] For men in the forum internum—the forum of conscience—were responsible not only to God but also, and quite directly, to men who had the authority "to loose and to bind." And this authority "to loose and to bind," although ultimately of eternal consequence, was applicable to the present life in that it included the authority, indeed the responsibility, to grant forgiveness only to those who satisfied the requirements of the confessional and to impose sanctions upon those who refused. And the ultimate sanction, excommunication, when imposed upon anyone who exercised his vocation by license, would deprive that person of his livelihood.

There was a strong tradition in the church, from Augustine through Gratian, in canon law and conciliar legislation, that whatever was gained through dishonest practices had to be restored in full before remission of sin could be given, before *ego te absolvo* could be pronounced efficaciously.[164] Restitution was an absolute condition of forgiveness, and the confessor had considerable freedom of discretion in determining situations in which restitution must be made. The principle of restitution was applied to much besides ill-gotten gain, indeed to damages generally. The *Angelica* defines the nature of the obligation as "any satisfaction that must be done to someone else."[165]

Tentler considers the confessional system of the late Middle Ages a "most effective means of social control" because of its "clear and explicit expectations, clear and direct accountability," and in the same context he says of the summae confessorum that "they are, if any books ever were, devoted to the clarification, definition, and publication of expectations, as well as to the assertion of the legitimacy of the authority of priest over penitents and the hierarchy over the church."[166]

Medieval economic historians have commented on the possible effects of the forum internum on merchants' activities in the late Middle Ages. Their conclusions are generally expressed thus: "Although undoubtedly of influence, [the evidence i.e., the available primary sources] gives no assurance that the penitent merchant followed the ideals of his confessor."[167] "Unfortunately, we have no direct indication of what the merchant thought. He was not a moralist and he did not write moral treatises. Nor did the confessor assess the effects of his work quantitatively. The connective doubtless was there, but the historian has no means of accurately charting it."[168]

The medical historian also cannot "accurately chart" the influence of the confessional on medical ethics and practice, if "accurately chart" means to subject a problem to anything that even approaches statistical certainty. But the medical historian has at his disposal various types of medical and surgical literature that directly or indirectly shed some light on the state of medical deontology in the late Middle Ages. Writings of this kind should be investigated thoroughly, with such an objective in view, after a more extensive and comprehensive study of late medieval casuistic literature shall have been made than was possible in the present essay.

NOTES

All translations in this chapter are my own unless otherwise indicated.

1. The subject is complex. As a beginning one should see J. Gilchrist's discussion of the economic doctrines of the canonists: *The Church and Economic Activity in the Middle Ages* (London: Macmillan, 1969), 53 ff. On the special problem of usury, see John T. Noonan, Jr., *The Scholastic Analysis of Usury* (Cambridge: Harvard University Press, 1957).

2. L. K. Little, "Pride Goes before Avarice: Social Change and the Vices in Latin Christendom," *Am. Hist. Rev.* 76 (1971): 16.

3. On whom see John W. Baldwin, *Masters, Princes, and Merchants: The Social Views of Peter the Chanter and His Circle* (Princeton: Princeton University Press, 1970).

4. In process of publication in Analecta Mediaevalia Namurcensia (Louvain: Editions Nauwelaerts).

5. On the history of penance before the thirteenth century, see Oscar D. Watkins, *A History of Penance* (London: Longmans, Green, 1920); and Paul Anciaux, *La théologie du sacrement de pénitence au XIIe siècle*, Universitas Catholica Lovaniensis, Dissertationes in facultate theologica vel in facultate iuris canonici, 2d ser., no. 41 (Louvaine, 1949).

6. For examples of this literature, see John T. McNeill and Helena M. Gamer, *Medieval Handbooks of Penance: A Translation of the Principal Libri Poenitentiales and Selections from Related Documents*, Columbia Records of Civilization: Sources and Studies, no. 29 (New York: Columbia University Press, 1938).

7. Watkins, *History of Penance* (n. 5), 2:735.

8. F. Broomfield, ed., in his preface to Thomas of Chobham, *Summa confessorum*, Analecta Mediaevalia Namurcensia, no. 25 (Louvain: Editions Nauwelaerts, 1968), xv.

9. On the genre, see Pierre Michaud-Quantin, *Sommes de casuistique et manuels de confession au moyen âge (XII–XVI siècles)*, Analecta Mediaevalia Namurcensia, no. 13 (Louvain: Editions Nauwelaerts, 1962).

10. When F. Broomfield edited the *Summa* (ca. 1215) of Thomas of Chobham (n. 8), he gave Thomas' work the title *Summa confessorum*, and in his preface he referred to Bartholomew of Exeter (latter half of the twelfth century) as having composed essentially the first recognizable summa confessorum. Leonard E. Boyle, in "The *Summa Confessorum* of John of Freiburg and the Popularization of the Moral Teaching of St. Thomas and Some of His Contemporaries," in *St. Thomas Aquinas, 1274–1974: Commemorative Studies*, ed. A. A. Maurer et al. (Toronto: Pontifical Institute of Mediaeval Studies, 1974), 2:245–68, writes that John of Freiburg's *Summa* (ca. 1297–98) was the first to be called a summa confessorum, and comments that "the use of this title in editions of pre-1300 works for confessors is anachronistic, as in F. Broomfield, Thomas de Chobham, *Summa confessorum*" (248 n. 18). However, whereas Thomas N. Tentler, "The *Summa* for Confessors as an Instrument of Social Control," in *The Pursuit of Holiness in Late Medieval and Renaissance Religion*, ed. Charles Trinkaus (Leiden: Brill, 1974), 105, refers to Raymond of Peñafort's *Summa de casibus poenitentiae* (ca. 1220) as the first summa for confessors, Leonard E. Boyle, "The *Summa* for Confessors as a Genre, and Its Religious Intent," in ibid., 126 f., writes that the genre was in existence earlier, "as will be clear to anyone who has had to study the manuals of Robert Flamborough (c. 1210) and Thomas Chobham (c. 1215)."

11. The primary sources I have located that have yielded material for this discussion are here listed in order of composition:

—Peter the Chanter, *Summa de sacramentis: Liber casuum conscientiae* (1197), ed. Jean-Albert Dugauquier, Analecta Mediaevalia Namurcensia, no. 16 (Louvain: Editions Nauwelaerts, 1963).

—Robert of Courson, *Summa* (ca. 1208–13), as quoted by Baldwin, *Masters, Princes, and Merchants* (n. 3).

—Thomas of Chobham, *Summa confessorum* (ca. 1215; see n. 8, above).

—Astesanus de Asti, *Summa de casibus conscientiae* (ca. 1317; Venice, 1478), copy at Free Library of Philadelphia; generally cited as *Astesana*.

—Bartholomaeus de Sancto Concordia, *Summa casuum* (ca. 1338; Venice, 1473), copy at University of Pennsylvania; generally cited as *Pisanella*.

—Antoninus of Florence, *Confessionale-defecerunt* (1473; Esslingen, 1474[?]), copy at College of Physicians of Philadelphia.

—Bartholomaeus de Chaimis, *Interrogatorium sive confessionale* (ca. 1474; Nuremberg, n.d.), copy at Free Library of Philadelphia.

—Antoninus of Florence, *Summa theologica* (or *Summa moralis*) (1477; 1740; reprint, Graz: Akademische Druck- und Verlagsanstalt, 1959).

—Baptista Trovamala de Salis, *Summa de casibus conscientiae* (ca. 1480; Venice, 1495), copy at College of Physicians of Philadelphia; generally cited as *Baptistina*.

—Angelus Carletus de Clavasio, *Summa Angelica de casibus conscientiae* (ca. 1486; Lyons, 1494), copy at Free Library of Philadelphia; generally cited as *Angelica*.

—Cajetan (Tommaso de Vio), *Summula peccatorum* (Florence, 1525), copy at University of Pennsylvania.

—Bartholomaeus Fumus, *Summa armilla* (ca. 1538; Cologne, 1627), copy at Catholic University of America.

12. Henry Charles Lea, *A History of Auricular Confession and Indulgences in the Latin Church* (Philadelphia: Lea Brothers, 1896), 1:230.

13. See Baldwin, *Masters, Princes, and Merchants* (n. 3), 1:50.

14. *Compilatio quarta* 5.14.3. This is one of the *Quinque compilationes antiquae*, the five most famous decretal collections between ca. 1187 and 1226. The actual sequence of composition was *prima, tertia, secunda, quarta*, and *quinta*. All were unofficial collections except for *tertia* (1210) and *quinta* (1226). The entire collection was published as *Quinque compilationes antiquae*, ed. E. Friedberg (1882; reprint, Graz: Akademische Druck- und Verlagsanstalt, 1956).

15. Gregory IX, *Decretales* 5.38.12. The most important collection of canons in the Middle Ages having the force of law is the *Decretales* of Gregory IX. This, the first official collection of a universal character, rendered all previous official or unofficial collections obsolete excepting the *Decretum* of Gratian, which the official collections did not supplant but rather supplemented. The *Decretales* is part of what became known as the *Corpus iuris canonici*, a title that was first used in 1580 by Gregory XIII and refers to the *Decretum* of Gratian (ca. 1140), the *Decretales* of Gregory IX (1234), the *Liber sextus* of Boniface VIII (1298), the *Clementinae* (1317; named after Clement V), the *Extravagantes* of John XXII (1325); and the *Extravagantes communes* (1500 and 1503). These were edited by E. Friedberg under the title *Corpus iuris canonici*, 2 vols. (1879; reprint, Graz: Akademische Druck- und Verlagsanstalt, 1959).

16. As translated by Watkins, *History of Penance* (n. 5), 2:748 f.

17. Thomas N. Tentler, "Response and Retractatio," in Trinkaus, ed., *Pursuit of Holiness* (n. 10), 134.

18. Thomas N. Tentler, *Sin and Confession on the Eve of the Reformation* (Princeton: Princeton University Press, 1977), xiv.

19. Tentler, "Summa for Confessors" (n. 10), 108.

20. *Astesana,* as quoted in ibid., 115.

21. Baldwin, *Masters, Princes, and Merchants* (n. 3), 57.

22. Gen. 3:19—"In the sweat of your face you shall eat bread." 2 Thess. 3:10—"If any one will not work, let him not eat" (Revised Standard Version, National Council of Churches [1946 and 1952]).

23. Baldwin, *Masters, Princes, and Merchants* (n. 3), 57 ff.

24. Thomas of Chobham, *Summa confessorum,* ed. Broomfield (n. 8), 290 ff.

25. There are no separate entries for surgeons in the summae that I have seen. Indexed versions send the seeker after *chirurgus* to *medicus.* Some summae label the relevant section simply *medicus,* while others give *medicus et chirurgus* and others *medicus, phisicus et chirurgus* (with orthographical variations).

26. Usually the citations given are to sources dealing with principles that the summist then applies to the medical profession. I do not mention such sources. Occasionally a summist will refer to an authority who speaks directly to a medico-ethical issue. In such an instance I shall sometimes comment on the content of the source.

27. *Astesana* 6.14.

28. *Angelica,* s.v. "Medicus," pr.

29. Antoninus, *Confessionale,* s.v. "Circa medicos."

30. Antoninus, *Summa theologica,* 281 f. The page numbers I give when citing this work refer to the edition cited in n. 11, above.

31. Chaimis, *Interrogatorium,* s.v. "Medicis, phisicis, et cirogicis."

32. *Compilatio quarta* 5.6.3 (see n. 14).

33. Gregory IX, *Decretales* 5.12.19.

34. On which see Darrel W. Amundsen, "Medieval Canon Law on Medical and Surgical Practice by the Clergy," *Bull. Hist. Med.* 52 (1978): 22–44; reprinted with minor changes as chap. 8, above.

35. Innocent III, *Tua nos.* Italicized sections, although part of the original rescript, are not included in the text as it appears in the *Decretales* (see n. 15).

36. *Astesana* 6.16. The idea that the physician sins who, instead of following the traditions of the art, follows his own inclinations and thus causes harm, appears in several of the sources: e.g., in the *Baptistina* (ca. 1480), s.v. "Medicus vel cirugicus," 5; in Bartholomaeus de Chaimis (ca. 1474), *Interrogatorium,* s.v. "Medicis, phisicis, et cirogicis"; and in the *Angelica* (c. 1486), s.v. "Medicus," 1.

37. *Angelica,* s.v. "Medicus," pr.

38. *Astesana* 6.14.

39. *Angelica,* s.v. "Medicus," pr.

40. Antoninus, *Confessionale,* s.v. "Circa medicos."

41. Antoninus, *Summa theologica,* 282. Cf. Chaimis, *Interrogatorium,* s.v. "Medi-

cis, phisicis, et cirogicis": "If he does not apply necessary diligence about the care of the patient personally when visiting, by observing the internal signs, by regulating medicines, diet, and regimen of life, he is at fault and has sinned."

42. Antoninus, *Summa theologica*, 291 f.

43. Ibid., 290.

44. *Imperitia* basically means inexperience, and signifies the ignorance or incompetence that results from inexperience.

45. *Baptistina*, s.v. "Medicus vel cirugicus," 5. Similarly *Angelica*, s.v. "Medicus," 1: "He accuses himself who chooses one who says that he is incompetent."

46. Compare Fumus, *Summa armilla* (ca. 1538), s.v. "De medico," 1: "when ignorant of the ailment but from rashness or lest they be thought to be ignorant, or for the sake of gain, they undertake to treat the patient, exposing him to the danger of death, or of notable harm, this is a mortal sin."

47. Cajetan, *Summula peccatorum*, s.v. "Peccata medicorum."

48. Fumus, *Summa armilla*, s.v. "De medico," 1.

49. *Pisanella*, s.v. "Medicus vel cirurgicus"; Antoninus, *Confessionale*, s.v. "Circa medicos"; Antoninus, *Summa theologica*, 282; *Baptistina*, s.v. "Medicus vel cirugicus," 5; *Angelica*, s.v. "Medicus," 2; Chaimis, *Interrogatorium*, s.v. "Medicis, phisicis, et cirogicis."

50. Some have "Creator"; the *Baptistina* reads, "It is safer to leave the patient to nature."

51. Here the *Baptistina* reads: "than to commit him to an unskilled physician."

52. *Pisanella*, s.v. "Medicus vel circurgicus"; *Baptistina*, s.v. "Medicus vel cirugicus," 11; *Angelica*, s.v. "Medicus," 3; Chaimis, *Interrogatorium*, s.v. "Medicis, phisicis, et cirogicis."

53. *Pisanella*, s.v. "Medicus vel circurgicus"; Antoninus, *Summa theologica*, 287; *Angelica*, s.v. "Medicus," 4; Chaimis, *Interrogatorium*, s.v. "Medicis, phisicis, et cirogicis."

54. Clement III, *Ad aures*. This rescript was included in the *Compilatio secunda* (1.8.2) and later in the *Decretales* of Gregory IX (1.14.7).

55. *Pisanella*, s.v. "Medicus vel cirurgicus."

56. *Angelica*, s.v. "Medicus," 1.

57. Antoninus, *Summa theologica*, 282. Later in the same work, he writes that physicians sin "when they detain the patient in his illness a long while so that they might make more money by seeing him frequently" (292).

58. Chaimis, *Interrogatorium*, s.v. "Medicis, phisicis, et cirogicis."

59. Fumus, *Summa armilla*, s.v. "De medico," 3.

60. Ibid., 1.

61. A term designating those clerics living under a rule (often including a vow of poverty). They are also called regular (from *regula*—rule) to distinguish them from secular clergy (i.e., those not living under a rule).

62. Chaimis, *Interrogatorium*, s.v. "Medicis, phisicis, et cirogicis."

63. Cajetan, *Summula peccatorum*, s.v. "Peccata medicorum."

64. Antoninus, *Confessionale*, s.v. "Circa medicos."

65. Antoninus, *Summa theologica*, 292.

66. *Universitas* has a different meaning from simply "university." Although it

is applied to the organization of faculty, it also can be applied to corporate entities such as guilds, "universities" themselves being guilds.

67. Chaimis, *Interrogatorium*, s.v. "Medicis, phisicis, et cirogicis."

68. Antoninus, *Summa theologica*, 282.

69. Antoninus lived in Florence, the only city, to my knowledge, where physicians and apothecaries were in the same guild.

70. Chaimis, *Interrogatorium*, s.v. "Medicis, phisicis, et cirogicis."

71. There is extensive secondary literature on the subject. See, in particular, Gaines Post, Kimon Giocarinis, and Richard Kay, "The Medieval Heritage of a Humanistic Ideal: '*Scientia Donum Dei Est, Unde Vendi Non Potest*'" *Traditio* 2 (1955): 196–234.

72. Baldwin, *Masters, Princes, and Merchants* (n. 3), 1:125.

73. Thomas Aquinas, *Summa theologiae* 2–2, 71, 4, various translators (Westminster: Blackfriars, 1964–84), 38:153.

74. Antoninus, *Summa theologica*, 277.

75. Ibid., 283 f.

76. Chaimis, *Interrogatorium*, s.v. "Medicis, phisicis, et cirogicis."

77. Fumus, *Summa armilla*, s.v. "De medico," 3.

78. Antoninus, *Summa theologica*, 284.

79. *Baptistina*, s.v. "Medicus vel cirugicus," 6.

80. *Angelica*, s.v. "Medicus," 14.

81. Darrel W. Amundsen, "The Liability of the Physician in Classical Greek Legal Theory and Practice," *J. Hist. Med. Allied Sci.* 32 (1977): 202 f.; idem, "The Physician's Obligation to Prolong Life: A Medical Duty without Classical Roots," *Hastings Center Rep.* 8, no. 4 (1978): 23 ff.; reprinted with minor changes as chap. 2, above.

82. Antoninus, *Summa theologica*, 281.

83. Ibid., 289 f.

84. Gratian, *Decretum* D. 83, 1. *Pars*.

85. Thomas Aquinas, *Summa theologiae*, 2–2, 71, 1, vol. 38, p. 145 in the edition cited in n. 73.

86. *Astesana* 1.39.

87. Antoninus, *Confessionale*, s.v. "Circa medicos."

88. Antoninus, *Summa theologica*, 277.

89. Ibid., 285.

90. *Pisanella*, s.v. "Medicus vel cirurgicus"; Antoninus, *Summa theologica*, 284 f.; *Baptistina*, s.v. "Medicus vel cirugicus," 7; *Angelica*, s.v. "Medicus," 5 and 6; Chaimis, *Interrogatorium*, s.v. "Medicis, phisicis, et cirogicis"; Fumus, *Summa armilla*, s.v. "De medico," 1 and 2.

91. Chaimis, *Interrogatorium*, s.v. "Medicis, phisicis, et cirogicis."

92. Gratian, *Decretum, De cons*. D. 5. c. 21.

93. Ecclus. 38.

94. This canon was included in the *Compilatio quarta* (5.14.4; see n. 14) and then in the *Decretales* (5.38.13; see n. 15).

95. As translated by R. J. Schroeder, *Disciplinary Decrees of the General Councils* (St. Louis: Herder, 1957), 236.

96. *Astesana* 5.16. The Latin text here is nearly identical to the last sentence

of *Cum infirmitas*. My translation of this passage from the *Astesana* is strictly literal, unlike Schroeder's of *Cum infirmitas*.

97. *Pisanella*, s.v. "Medicus vel cirurgicus."

98. *Baptistina*, s.v. "Medicus vel cirugicus," 1.

99. *Angelica*, s.v. "Medicus," 7.

100. Cajetan, *Summula peccatorum* (1525), s.v. "Peccata medicorum," makes only a brief comment on this subject, follows a different format, and does not cite *Cum infirmitas*, referring to the action as a sin against divine, as opposed to canon, law, when physicians "advise to do anything against the safety of the soul, whatever mortal sin they advise. For according to the Apostle, evil must not be done that good of health or of life result."

101. Antoninus, *Confessionale*, s.v. "Circa medicos"; idem, *Summa theologica*, 282; Chaimis, *Interrogatorium*, s.v. "Medicis, phisicis, et cirogicis"; Fumus, *Summa armilla*, s.v. "De medico," 1.

102. Antoninus, *Confessionale*, s.v. "Circa medicos"; idem, *Summa theologica*, 281 f. and 292.

103. Chaimis, *Interrogatorium*, s.v. "Medicis, phisicis, et cirogicis."

104. Two excellent discussions are John T. Noonan, Jr., "An Almost Absolute Value in History," in *The Morality of Abortion: Legal and Historical Perspectives*, ed. John T. Noonan, Jr. (Cambridge: Harvard University Press, 1970), 1–59; and John Connery, *Abortion: The Development of the Roman Catholic Perspective* (Chicago: Loyola University Press, 1977).

105. *Didache* 2.2.

106. *Epistle of Barnabas* 19.5.

107. Clement, *Pedagogus* 2.10.96.1.

108. Minucius Felix, *Octavius* 2.43.

109. Tertullian, *Apologeticum ad nationes* 1.15; idem, *De anima* 25.5 f.

110. Elvira (A.D. 305), canon 63, in *Sacrorum conciliorum nova et amplissima collectio*, ed. J. D. Mansi et al., new ed. (Florence and Venice, 1795–98), vol. 2, col. 16.

111. Ancyra (A.D. 314), canon 21, in ibid., vol. 2, col. 514.

112. Jerome, *Letters* 121.4.

113. Augustine, *On Exodus*, 21.80.

114. Noonan, "An Almost Absolute Value" (n. 104), 17.

115. Gratian, *Decretum* C. 32 q. 2 c. 7 *(Aliquando)*.

116. Gregory IX, *Decretales* 5.12.20 *(Sicut ex)*.

117. Ibid., 5.12.5 *(Si aliquis)*.

118. Thomas Aquinas, *Summa theologiae*, 2–2, 64, 8, 2.

119. Noonan, "An Almost Absolute Value" (n. 104), 26. Connery is slightly less emphatic, saying "considerable impetus was given to the theological discussion in the work of Antoninus." Connery, *Abortion* (n. 104), 114.

120. Antoninus, *Confessionale*, s.v. "Circa medicos."

121. Connery, *Abortion* (n. 104), 114 f.

122. Ibid., 115.

123. Antoninus uses the word *puerperium* to designate the fetus whether *animatum* (ensouled) or not.

124. Antoninus, *Summa theologica*, 283.

125. Connery, *Abortion* (n. 104), 116.

126. Chaimis, *Interrogatorium*, s.v. "Medicis, phisicis, et cirogicis."

127. The *Baptistina* (ca. 1480) discusses abortion under *homicidium,* Fumus (ca. 1538) includes a separate section labeled *aborsus,* and the *Angelica* (ca. 1486) does both.

128. Navarrus, *Manuale sive Enchiridion confessariorum at poenitentium* (Lyons, 1574; copy at Gonzaga University), 25.60.2, s.v. "De peccatis medici et chirurgi."

129. Antoninus, *Summa theologica,* 285 f.

130. *Baptistina,* s.v. "Medicus vel cirugicus," 4.

131. *Angelica,* s.v. "Medicus," 12.

132. Fumus, *Summa armilla,* s.v. "De medico," 5.

133. Gratian, *Decretum, De cons.* D. 5. c. 21.

134. Antoninus, *Summa theologica,* 286.

135. Ibid., 291.

136. The Latin here reads "moneant et inducant," literally "let them advise and persuade," considerably stronger than Schroeder's translation, "admonish."

137. *Astesana* (ca. 1317), 5.16; *Pisanella* (ca. 1338), s.v. "Medicus vel cirurgicus"; Chaimis (ca. 1474), *Interrogatorium,* s.v. "Medicis, phisicis, et cirogicis."

138. Antoninus, *Confessionale,* s.v. "Circa medicos."

139. Antoninus, *Summa theologica,* 285.

140. *Baptistina,* s.v. "Medicus vel cirugicus," 3.

141. *Angelica,* s.v. "Medicus," 8 and 9.

142. Fumus, *Summa armilla,* s.v. "De medico," 4.

143. Cajetan, *Summula peccatorum,* s.v. "Peccata medicorum."

144. Chaimis, *Interrogatorium,* s.v. "Medicis, phisicis, et cirogicis."

145. Antoninus, *Summa theologica,* 285.

146. *Baptistina,* s.v. "Medicus vel cirugicus," 1.

147. *Angelica,* s.v. "Medicus," 8.

148. Fumus, *Summa armilla,* s.v. "De medico," 4.

149. *Pisanella,* s.v. "Medicus vel cirurgicus."

150. Cajetan, *Summula peccatorum,* s.v. "Peccata medicorum."

151. Fumus, *Summa armilla,* s.v. "De medico," 4.

152. Gregory IX, *Decretales* 1.4.11 (see n. 15).

153. *Astesana* 5.16.

154. *Pisanella,* s.v. "Medicus vel cirurgicus."

155. Antoninus, *Summa theologica,* 285.

156. *Baptistina,* s.v. "Medicus vel cirugicus," pr.

157. *Angelica,* s.v. "Medicus," 8.

158. Fumus, *Summa armilla,* s.v. "De medico," 4.

159. Cajetan, *Summula peccatorum,* s.v. "Peccata medicorum."

160. See Schroeder, *Disciplinary Decrees* (n. 95), 263 f. When the *Cum infirmitas* was promulgated, it applied to all physicians, and any physician who attempted to live in accord with the dictates of the church would have endeavored to achieve some modus operandi consistent with at least a liberal interpretation of its provisions. By the time that the post-Tridentine *Super gregem* was promulgated, many physicians were at least nominally within the ranks of Protestantism

and thus no longer subject either under canon law or in conscience to the regulations of Roman Catholicism. Catholics receiving doctorates in medicine were apparently obligated to swear that they would honor the provisions of *Super gregem*. For an example, see Martha Teach Gnudi and Jerome Pierce Webster, *The Life and Times of Gaspare Tagliacozzi, Surgeon of Bologna, 1545–1599* (New York: Herbert Reichner, 1950), 55 f., 388 f., for a translation and the Latin text of such an oath.

161. J. W. Baldwin, *The Medieval Theories of the Just Price: Romanists, Canonists, and Theologians in the Twelfth and Thirteenth Centuries,* Transactions of the American Philosophical Society, n.s., vol. 49, pt. 4 (Philadelphia, 1959), 57.

162. Tentler, *Sin and Confession* (n. 18), xv.

163. Ibid.

164. The classic study of the doctrine of restitution is Karl Weinzierl, *Die Restitutionslehre der Frühscholastik* (Munich: M. Hueber, 1936). Tentler treats the subject in *Sin and Confession* (n. 18), 340 ff.

165. As quoted by Tentler, *Sin and Confession* (n. 18), 341.

166. Tentler, "Response and Retractatio" (n. 17), 137.

167. Baldwin, *Just Price* (n. 161), 10.

168. Gilchrist, *Church and Economic Activity* (n. 1), 50.

TEN

Medical Deontology and Pestilential Disease in the Late Middle Ages

Although the scholarly literature on the plagues of the late Middle Ages is voluminous, there has been a remarkable lack of concern with the place of pestilential diesease in the history of medical ethics. Only one separate article has been written on the subject, and that a three-page survey covering the period from Hippocrates to Sydenham.[1] What then were the ethial principles of the late medieval medical profession when faced with pestilential disease of unprecedented magnitude that subjected the physician to an extremely trying test of fortitude and conscience? During plague epidemics the ethics of the medieval physician were taxed by conditions much more extreme than those normally encountered in practice. Although the available sources do not supply any quantifiable data, they do provide observations on the conduct of some physicians and their responses to the plague.[2]

With few exceptions the contemporary sources, medical and lay, that discuss the various outbreaks of pestilential disease in the late Middle Ages reveal a strong belief in the extremely contagious nature of the "pest." Many assert that, merely by being in the vicinity of the sick, one was doomed to become infected with diseases from which there was no hope of recovery. Numerous sources describe in chilling detail fathers and mothers who deserted their dying children, sons and daughters who deserted their parents, husbands who fled from their sick wives, and wives who fled from their husbands. Fear of contagion and death set at nought every moral value: love and compassion were destroyed, every sense of obligation was forgotten. All who could, nobles, magistrates, merchants, physicians, and clerics, fled the towns and cities and sought refuge in rural areas. Not only were the sick deserted by their families but also the physicians would not approach them. As a final blow, even the priests would not minister to their ultimate spiritual needs. Such accounts abound.[3] If not exaggerated in specifics they are undoubtedly so in the pervasiveness of the actions described. They must be balanced by the equally plentiful documentation of responsible action by, for example, magistrates, physicians, and clerics. For every account of a magistrate fleeing his office, of a physician hiding in terror, and of a priest refusing to tend to the spiritual needs of his suffering parishioners, there are descriptions of magistrates seeking to do all in their power to serve the public good, of physicians trying desperately to help their patients, and of priests administering the sacraments to the dying. Richard W. Emery has performed a valuable service by investigating the notarial records of Perpignan for the period of the Black Death. His conclusion is that "the evidence for panic, terror, and general demoralization is entirely lacking; the evidence for a considerable resiliency, and for people simply carrying on, is, after the initial two-week period, reasonably strong. The social organization would seem to have remained cohesive, intact, and functioning."[4] Similar studies of individual cities or regions may indeed require a drastic revision of opinions now popularly held.[5]

The question is how the physician's responsibility in such circumstances was conceived both by physicians and by those outside the profession. Did the physician who fled, or who refused to diagnose those perhaps afflicted with pestilence or to treat patients actually suffering from plague, thereby violate responsibilities inherent in his profession *as conceived at that time?* Such questions must be explored in historical perspective. It is well known that Galen fled Rome during the great plague of the second century. He readily admitted having done so.[6] Later in life he gave other reasons for his hasty departure from Rome and glossed over the impetus provided by the plague.[7] Probably in any period physicians, as they are at least ostensibly devoted to healing and ideally motivated by compassion, may have been viewed with a degree of disdain if they fled from possible contagion. If, however, as in Galen's time, the title of physician might be claimed by anyone, if the practice of medicine were a right and the "physician" might exercise his art completely at his own discretion on whomsoever, whenever, and wherever he might wish, bound to his fellow men by no obligation, however ill-defined, other than whatever ethical principles he might choose to adopt, would it then be meaningful to speak of a deontological basis for the practice of his art? There were in classical antiquity no professional standards enforceable by sanctions against physicians who violated the ethics of the profession. Even to speak of "ethics of the profession" is misleading. At no time were physicians *required* to swear any oath or to accept and abide by any formal or informal code of ethics. Moreover, the physician sold his services at his own discretion to those who asked and paid for treatment; he exercised his art as he wished. Although, during the early Middle Ages, Christian charity and moral principles effected some significant changes in the perception of medical ethics, yet it is not until the late Middle Ages that we can speak of the development of a clearly defined medical deontology and professional ethics, appreciated (at least in theory) by both those within and those outside the profession.

The Medical Profession and Medical Ethics in the Late Middle Ages

The first and foremost obligation of a magistrate was to serve the public interest. For king or elected official, political theory of the late Middle Ages clearly defined the responsibility of office as directed toward the common good. A magistrate who fled his obligations in order to preserve his personal interests and failed to perform his duties was considered to have violated his office. That efforts were made by governments to combat and contain the plague shows that some people acting in a public capacity not only continued to fulfill their functions during times of plague but also enlarged their obligations in the face of a common danger to the community.[8] A priest's duties included as a vital obligation the spiritual care of his flock, and a priest who refused to administer the sacraments to a dying man, owing to fear for his own safety, clearly violated his office in denying to a man that which was viewed as an absolute necessity for spiritual well-being. There were many priests who thus abused their office, and considerable attention was given by ecclesiastical authorities to this problem.[9] Do the roles and responsibilities of the magistrate and the priest serve as analogues to those of the physician as they were viewed at that time?

The structure of the medical profession during the period under consideration reflected one of the most striking features of late medieval city life, namely, its corporate aspect, particularly in its guild organization. By the end of the twelfth century, most towns had at least one guild consisting, in the aggregate, of several trades. Large towns or cities usually had a merchant guild and a variety of craft guilds. The guilds had their earliest and most precocious development in Italy. During the thirteenth century they proliferated rapidly throughout Europe, in a variety of forms, but having some common features. The guilds were fraternal, political, and commercial in purpose. In the defense of their commercial interests, the guilds, in obtaining municipal or royal charters, secured the right to exercise a monopoly of their product or service in a particular geographical area. Typically they had the right to enforce standards of quality in their products or services, to control hours and working conditions, to limit competition among members, to limit entry into the craft or profession, and to ensure the proper treatment of customers. Part of the monopoly was the right to train and, essentially, to license new members, thereby eliminating competition from outside the guild. Although one of the major aims of such measures was economic, the guilds frequently claimed that such restrictions were necessary to maintain a high level of competence and ethics in the trade or profession. Distinct from the merchant and craft guilds, the medieval universities were essentially educational guilds, corporations either of students (as at Bologna) or of teachers (as at Paris). Some universities gained charters, beginning in the late twelfth century, and thus became corporate bodies designed to further educational interests and to protect their members. The *collegium* of teachers who examined the candidates for a degree was, at some universities, vested with the authority to license those who were successful or, at others, to recommend to municipal, royal, or ecclesiastical authorities that a license be granted.

So great was the diversity of conditions that generalities are often misleading. But, in great part, surgeons (or barber-surgeons) were organized in craft guilds, and physicians, at least in cities having a university, were not members of a craft guild but were part of, affiliated with, or under the supervision of the medical faculty of the university. In university cities the institution of medical licensure requirements generally occurred earlier than in those without a university but, from the early fourteenth century, many cities and towns required those who wished to practice medicine within their jurisdiction to have a degree and license from an acceptable university. Physicians practicing in such cities or towns often organized themselves into collegia or guilds and, in some instances, obtained the authority to examine and license physicians seeking the right to practice within the community, regardless of the degrees held by the applicants.

When guilds sought official recognition they commonly justified the restrictive measures they wished to apply by appealing to the need to ensure a high standard of competence and ethics in the trade or profession. This was true of medical or surgical guilds, including collegia and university medical faculties. Accusations that the monopolistic measures of guilds reflected self-interest were frequently made. Such accusations were also made against medical and surgical guilds and faculties, particularly by those who tesitifed on behalf of practitioners who were brought to trial for practicing without a license.[10] In restrictions on medical and surgical practice, the same justifying terms were employed whether the restrictive measures were imposed by authorities, either secular[11] or ecclesiastical,[12] or were requested by medical faculties or medical or surgical guilds. Emphasis was consistently placed on the common good, and the grave dangers to the people if charlatans and quacks were permitted to undertake medical or surgical care. At Paris, the medical faculty of the university initiated medical licensure provisions and, in seeking ecclesiastical and royal support to enforce these regulations, appealed to the "public interest." The same appeal was made in the medical faculty's attempts to establish a right to oversee the activities of apothecaries, herbalists, and surgeons and to prosecute unlicensed practitioners, whether before ecclesiastical or secular courts.[13]

With the beginning of medical licensure requirements in the late Middle Ages, whether imposed by authorities or granted by them at the request of guilds or faculties, there was a fundamental change in the basis for practicing medicine. Earlier (and throughout Western civilization) anyone might claim the right to practice medicine. When the practice of medicine became limited to a select group of individuals and their exclusive right to practice was enforced, physicians and surgeons began to feel a previously unknown collective and individual sense of responsibility to the community (municipal or regional) in which they were permitted to practice by virtue of their membership in the appropriate guild or faculty. It was not unusual for the individual, before being admitted to the exclusive circle of practitioners, to be required to swear that he would, for example, faithfully care for the ill of the city or region.[14]

Hence, while the magistrate had a definite duty to the common good and the priest to the common spiritual welfare, so also did guilds and collegia of physicians and surgeons then speak of serving the public interest when they sought the right to adopt and enforce requirements for licensure.

A Duty Not to Flee during Plague Epidemics?

From the tone of various historical sources, physicians who fled during the plague seem to have been viewed as acting shamefully, both by the public and by colleagues. When writers commented on instances of physicians who fled from the plague, their tone was condemnatory.[15] The extent to which physicians did flee cannot be determined from the evidence with any certainty. The number of physicians who did flee from plague-ridden cities may have been relatively small. I have not found, in the pest tractates, any allusion to physicians who fled from areas infected by pestilence. Physicians might have avoided such a topic, but medieval physicians were not at all timid in criticizing their colleagues in writing. Vehement condemnations of fellow physicians occur frequently in the medical literature of the Middle Ages, untempered by humility. The authors of pest tractates frequently condemned the theories and techniques of their colleagues. If the flight of physicians were as extensive as some modern scholars suggest, then among the pest tractates one might expect to find many statements like "While many physicians fled in terror, I, however, remained." Even if some such statements were found, they would be proportionally so few as to prove little concerning the conduct of the majority of physicians.

Many physicians advised flight from plague-infected areas as the most effective means of prophylaxis.[16] Such advise was often followed by the statement that since flight "rarely is easy even for the few, I advise that, while remaining, you. . . ."[17] Although only a minority of the plague tractates do, in fact, advise flight, all are at least partially addressed to prophylaxis, and prophylaxis is indeed the major concern of most of the tractates. Even if the tractates were unanimous in urging flight, it would not follow that the physicians who wrote them thereby intended to justify flight for themselves and their colleagues. Many of the authors of the pest tractates seem to have assumed that their readers would have access to the services of physicians during a time of plague. The physician Jacme d'Agramont (writing at Lerida in 1348, shortly before the city was invaded by the Black Death) did not discuss the regimen of treatment which "properly belongs to the physician, since in this anybody without the art of medicine could easily err."[18] Johannes Widman (second half of the fifteenth century) included only prophylaxis in his pest tractate, leaving the curative side "to the skill and industry of the physicians at hand."[19] Johannes Hartmann (also in the second half of the fifteenth century) likewise dealt only with prevention in his tractate, saying, "I entrust the cure to the faithful physician."[20] Gentile da Foligno in 1348 recommended that those afflicted follow their doctors' orders,[21] Matthaeus Genevensis (near the end of the fifteenth century) stressed the importance of following the advice of one's physician,[22] and the author of an anonymous pest tractate of the first half of the fifteenth century urged the sick to "follow the advice of a 'good physician.'"[23] Thomas fforestier (1485) devotes part of his tractate to "teaching the poor how to choose to which physician they ought to have recourse . . . so that they may follow good and sound advice without falsity or deception."[24] The author of an anonymous pest tractate composed early in the fifteenth century pleaded that those afflicted should not forsake the advice of their physicians.[25] Nicolo de Burgo (1382) wrote that "all things should always be done with the advice of a physician." Especially since the unexpected may occur, and since there are many differences between individuals, "all must be left for the physician who is handling the case."[26] An anonymous tractate written before 1400 and another from the first half of the fifteenth century recommend consulting one's physician for certain types of procedures.[27]

Undoubtedly some physicians did flee. Venice in 1382 forbade physicians to leave the city during epidemics "under pain of loss of citizenship."[28] Similar action was taken during the sixteenth century at, for instance, Barcelona and Cologne.[29] Ilza Veith writes that Thomas Sydenham, in the seventeenth century, "behaved entirely within the framework of acceptable ethics when in 1666 he left plague-stricken London and joined his well-to-do patients who had sought refuge in their country places. The possibility that he might have stayed in the city and helped the unfortunate sufferers of the plague who had not previously been his patients never entered his mind."[30] It is doubtful, however, that Sydenham did act "entirely within the framework of acceptable ethics." Compare the comments made by the physician and surgeon Guy de Chauliac concerning his own activities during the Black Death: "It was so contagious . . . that even by looking at one another people caught it. . . . And I, to avoid infamy, dared not absent myself but with continual fear preserved myself as best I could."[31]

The ethical quandary of the physician when faced with both extreme peril to himself and the knowledge of his own inability to be of any real help is mentioned by Chauliac: "It was useless and shameful for the doctors the more so as they dared not visit the sick, for fear of being infected. And when they did visit them, they did hardly anything for them, and were paid nothing."[32] Chauliac is saying that physicians feared to visit those suffering from the plague, but nevertheless did so, although they could accomplish little. Various contemporary lay accounts from the time of the Black Death remark that some physicians shut themselves up in their houses and would not visit the sick for fear of infection.[33] The authors of many pest tractates did advise the general public to avoid contact with those afflicted with plague. For example, Johannes Jacobi (ca. 1373)[34] writes that "one must flee from those who are infected";[35] an anonymous tractate written before 1400 advises that "you should not leave your home . . . or visit the sick";[36] Sigmund Albichs (1406) urges people to beware of contact with the infected;[37] and two anonymous tractates written during the first half of the fifteenth century include the recommendation to beware of visiting the sick[38] and to abstain from contact with the infected.[39]

A Duty to Treat Plague Victims?

That the authors of the plague tractates did not direct such advice to their colleagues is clear from the extent of comments in the tractates on special prophylaxis that should be employed by physicians when visiting plague victims. Johannes Jacobi was just quoted above as writing that "one must flee from those who are infected."[40] He then observes that "on this account, prudent physicians, since they must [*debent*] treat the ill, on visits to the sick stand at a distance from the patients, holding their face toward the window. . . . I was not able to avoid contact because I went from home to home in order to treat the ill for the sake of my poverty[41] and then I kept in my hand a piece of bread, or a sponge or a cloth, dipped in vinegar, and held it to my mouth and nose and thus escaped such pestilence, though my friends did not believe that I would survive."[42] The author of an anonymous pest tractate composed during the first half of the fifteenth century echoes some of Johannes Jacobi's advice. After speaking of the highly contagious nature of the plague, he wrote: "And therefore prudent physicians, since they must [*debent*] treat or visit the ill, stand at a distance from the patients and keep their face toward the door or window."[43] Some tractates simply stressed the dangers and the need for precautions. For example, Sigmund Albichs, in 1406, writes: "You should take care, physician, because this [i.e., the pest] takes hold of the young physician just as it does the old."[44] But the majority of those that acknowledge the dangers faced by physicians have specific recommendations for protection. According to an anonymous tractate of the second half of the fourteenth century, "physicians, before they enter the rooms of the ill, first ought to have the windows opened and remove all superfluities and sputum. The room ought to be fumigated with frankincense and juniper and then the physician may enter the patient's room and take his pulse. The physician should not examine him with his face close to the patient's, lest he be infected by breathing in fetid air; [otherwise] it would be better not to visit him at all."[45] One short tractate (ca. 1400), written for physicians, was devoted exclusively to the subject of precautions "to be followed when you visit a plague victim." It contained sixteen points:

1. The physician should bring a urinal covered with three or four layers of linen so that the fumes of the urine could not escape.

2. He should note whether the home had sufficient air space. If it did not, the urine should be examined in the street.

3. The urinal should be held by a member of the patient's household. If the physician did hold it himself, he should wear gloves.

4. Any voided matter should be viewed at a distance and in the open air.

5. If the patient's room was small and poorly ventilated, the physician should not enter it but should have the patient carried outside the room and held higher than the physician, if possible. The pulse should be taken without the physician's touching the patient's clothes or anything around him.

6. In taking the pulse, the physician should use whichever wrist was more easily reached.

7. The physician should order the windows and door of the patient's room to be left open, at least from sunrise to sunset. If this bothered the patient, it should be done at least for a certain time before the physician's arrival. Otherwise the physician should not enter the room.

8. All voided matter should immediately be removed from the room and "be kept in a suitable and remote place."

9. The patient's linen and bedclothes should be changed daily.

10. Rose water mixed with vinegar should be sprinkled often through-

out the room, "and perhaps it would be good for some vases to be filled with equal amounts of heated rose water and vinegar, so that, by means of their vapors, they might mix better with the air."

11. As long as the physician was present in the home of the patient, he should hold to his nose a sponge soaked in vinegar and other substances. The physician should do this whenever he was with the patient but should not remain with him long.

12. The physician should enter the patient's home slowly, "lest the necessity of attracting air be increased."

13. The physician should wear under his clothes, extending clear up to his head and also in his hood, many odoriferous things.

14. The patient's room should frequently be fanned with the windows and door open, both during the day and in the middle of the night.

15. In the patient's room various cold, odoriferous substances should be hung, and the patient should have various precious stones around and on him.

16. The physician should always carry with him some of the above-named stones.[46]

Regardless of how ineffective such precautions may have been, the frequency with which they are encountered in the pest tractates shows the extent to which they were thought to be effective. Prophylaxis in general was one of the major concerns of the authors of the pest tractates. Most of the tractates were written for the general public. While their authors advocated flight from an infected area as the best means of protection, they were aware that for most people it was not a real alternative. Thus they recommended a wide variety of protective measures for the general public. Although it was considered important to avoid contact with the sick, physicians necessarily came into frequent contact with patients suffering from pestilence. Various prophylactic techniques were developed and adopted by physicians to protect themselves from contagion. The tractates reveal a high degree of faith in these methods, and in most instances where they mention such techniques it is with the intention of sharing them with those outside the medical profession who might have occasion to visit or tend the sick.[47]

Johannes Jacobi wrote that physicians "must treat the ill,"[48] and the author of an anonymous pest tractate of the first half of the fifteenth century declares that "they must treat or visit the ill."[49] The difference between these two statements may seem slight, but the distinction was of considerable importance. While Jacobi holds that the physician must treat the plague victim, the author of the anonymous tractate feels that the physician must treat *or* visit the afflicted. The physician who fled from a plague-infected area or hid in fear, refusing to expose himself to possible contagion, failed in his primary duty to diagnose the illness. But if the sick person were afflicted with the plague (since not everyone who became ill during a time of plague was necessarily afflicted with the plague), and if the variety of pestilence with which he suffered was thought by the physician to render the patient incurable, did the physician have an ethical obligation to attempt treatment? There was in medieval medical ethics a strong tradition of refusing to treat those whom the art of medicine could not help.[50] This had also been a *nearly* constant feature of ancient medicine, both Near Eastern[51] and classical.[52] To take on hopeless cases was considered by many to be the mark of a charlatan, and the motive for doing so was thought to be avarice. Jacme d'Agramont stressed the highly contagious nature of the plague, mentioning cases where "the master and the servants died of the same disease, and even the physician and the confessor." He then wrote: "Therefore all physicians should guard in times of pestilence, against financial cupidity, because he, who has such a motive, may bring about his own death and that of his friends. Unless he be the son of avarice and greed he would have given all the treasures of the world to avoid such a result."[53] The conscientious physician was in a delicate position in relation to public opinion, which impugned his actions with charges of avarice if he seemed too eager to take on cases (especially if they terminated with death) and with charges of cowardice or irresponsibility if he were not willing to undertake the care of those ill with contagious disease. Some chroniclers living at the time of the Black Death complained that no amount of money could get physicians to treat the sick.[54] Other physicians attempted to treat the sick without thought of remuneration. One physician, for example, wrote in his diary—concerning a female patient who "died of the worst and most contagious kind of plague, that of blood spitting"—that he treated her "out of compassion as I would not have done it for money."[55] Quacks appeared to thrive during outbreaks of pestilence, moved by greed to promise recovery to the hopeless.[56]

The extent to which medical practitioners during different outbreaks of pestilence viewed the plague as untreatable cannot be determined with certainty. When the Black Death struck, it was, to the physicians of the time, a new disease, and so also were the various other pestilences that beset Europe in the ensuing centuries. They felt acutely the need to investigate such diseases, to seek ways both to prevent and to cure them. Although many authors of pest tractates tried desperately to find the answers in the writings of classical and Arabic medical authorities, some dismissed the ancient writings as useless in the existing circumstances and called for experimentation and experience.[57] Many of the authors of pest tractates discuss treatment, distinguishing among different varieties of pestilence. The majority of them stress their faith in the efficacy of their curative methods.

That some physicians considered plague to be incurable is manifest in a statement made by Theobaldus Loneti in his pest tractate written in the second half of the fifteenth century: "When . . . there was a debate among physicians over incurable diseases such as leprosy, paralysis, pestilence, and the like, they finally came to the conclusion that no remedy for the pestilence could be found, especially since Galen and Hippocrates and other ancient physicians made no mention of one. But after much discussion, it was I alone who maintained that many remedies against this plague could easily be employed."[58]

It was considered necessary to visit the patient to determine whether or not he was suffering from pestilence. If the condition was diagnosed as plague, some physicians would then seek to determine whether or not the patient was curable. The author of an anonymous plague tractate composed in 1411 gives some interesting advice: "If it is certain from the symptoms[59] that it is actually pestilence that has afflicted the patient, the physician first must [*debet*] advise the patient to set himself right with God by making a will[60] [and] by making a confession of his sins, as is set forth according to the Decretals: since a corporal illness comes not only from a fault of the body but also from a spiritual failing[61] as the Lord declares in the gospel and the priests also tell us. Next the physician should examine the patient's urine and feces and take his pulse. If the patient is curable, the physician will undertake treatment in God's name. If he is incurable, the physician should leave him to die,[62] in accord with the commentary on the second of the aphorisms.[63] Those who are going to die must be distinguished by prognostic signs and then you should flee from them. He labors in vain who attempts to treat such as these."[64] The physician acted totally within the strictures of accepted ethics by refusing to treat a patient for whom the physician had no hope of recovery. The only criticism that contemporaries could make would be that he was in error to regard the condition as untreatable.

Some Obstacles to Treating Plague Victims

While there was some disagreement on the efficacy of treatment for plague victims, there was on the part of the authors of pest tractates virtual unanimity on the importance and efficiency of prophylactic measures. The frustrations of physicians generated by a sometimes unresponsive public are illustrated by the comments of Johannes de Saxonia in his pest tractate written during the first half of the fifteenth century. Johannes lists various reasons why "so few attempt the recommended prophylaxis":

1. Some people feel that the length of every individual's life and the time of his death are established and fixed.

2. Some lack faith in medicine and have confidence that is bred of good health.

3. Some have hope in their own virtue.

4. Some desire death. He writes that during one plague episode in Montpellier, "when many men desired to die, the pope gave to the dying absolution from punishment and guilt and thus they hoped immediately to be translated to heaven; for this reason they did not want physicians to prolong their lives."

5. Many men are extremely parsimonious and loath to spend on medicines and "will not do so unless the physician guarantees them a certain and healthy state of preservation, for they fear that otherwise they are squandering their fortunes, but they are not afraid to lose life, body, and possessions."

6. Many are debilitated by the use of laxative medicines "by which they hoped to be able to preserve themselves."

7. Some use their wild imaginations about wells and water poisoned by the Jews and others.[65]

8. There is a lack of faithful helpers for the sick (because of parents' deserting children, etc.), which causes the ill to provide for their own necessities.

9. The problem is complicated by the immense folly of physicians' diverse theories, which makes them "objects of derision and mockery."[66]

The Significance of the Plague Tractates

But in spite of such obstacles, many physicians composed pest tractates in what appears to have been a sincere effort to do all in their power to help in such crises. Many authors stated their reasons for composing their tractates, and for the most part they were motivated *pro bono publico*. Jacme d'Agramont wrote: "As I am a native of this city and have received my being in it, and am constantly receiving, and have received, divers honors and great profits from the whole city and from its notables, I want . . . to render some service and save from damage the city aforementioned and its notables, and to save all men and women from becoming sick in times of pestilence. Therefore I decided to prepare the following tract which . . . I present to you, honorable Aldermen and Councillors of the city of Lerida, as to all who represent the aforementioned city. . . . And as the said tractate, as already expressed above, is prepared for the common and public good, may it please you, my Lords, to give it to anybody who wishes to make a copy of it."[67] Johannes Jacobi composed his tractate in honor "of the trinity and the Virgin Mary and for the utility of the republic and for the preservation of the healthy and for the healing of the ill."[68] John of Burgundy (1365) began his tractate with the assertion that his intention was to ensure "that if someone lacks a physician, then each and everyone may be his own *phisicus, praeservator, curator et rector*."[69] He concluded the work with this statement: "Moved by piety and anguished by and feeling sorrow because of this calamity . . . I have composed and compiled this work not for a price but for your prayers, so that when anyone recovers from the diseases discussed above, he will effectively pray for me to our Lord God."[70] Francischino de Collignano (1382) wrote that he was moved "by pure love, by affection and charity for all the citizens and especially for friends,"[71] while Michael Boeti (ca. 1400–20) wrote "in response to the requests of certain of my friends, for the service of God and for the common good."[72] The author of an anonymous tractate of 1411 wrote because he was sorely troubled that "many near to me and, as it were, the majority of the population are devoured by the pestilence which, as if it were a stepmother of mankind, harasses and destroys the whole human race."[73] The author of an anonymous tractate, probably written during the fifteenth century, composed his work "sorrowing for the destruction of men and devoting myself to the common good and . . . wishing health for all."[74] Not only did the authors of the pest tractates write them generally without thought of profit, but also they attempted to make their advice employable by the poor as well as by the well-to-do. Many of the tractates list for the various recommended substances, both prophylactic and curative, alternatives readily available to the poor.[75]

How many hundreds of these tractates were written is not known, but more than 280 are extant. Ziegler's overall appraisal is negative:

The plague literature as a whole, drawn from some half-dozen countries, was voluminous, repetitous and of little value to the unfortunate victims of the epidemic. . . . It seems unlikely that the intelligent and enlightened men who worked out these preventive measures had any great faith in their efficacy. Essentially they were a morale-building exercise: the morale of the physician, in that they made him feel at least remotely in control of the situation, and of the patient, in that they offered a slight hope of escape from death. But if the doctors lacked confidence in their capacity to keep the plague at bay, still more did they doubt their ability to cure it once it had struck. They knew too well how few of the sick recovered. But this knowledge of their helplessness did not stop them putting forward a host of remedies.[76]

If Ziegler's assessment is correct, the authors of these tractates were either deluded or dishonest. The evidence does not support the latter conclusion. The faith shown by these medical authors in the efficacy of the prophylactic measures that they took when visiting patients is demonstrated by the numerous artistic representations of physicians who employed such measures while visiting plague victims.[77] Many tractates were devoted exclusively to prophylaxis, on the ground that treatment had to be left to the individual physician handling the case. Of those tractates that do include a discussion of treatment, some distinguish cases thought to be curable from those considered incurable. But for the greater part, the tractates that discuss treatment show faith in the curative methods prescribed. Many of these were written from a strictly academic point of view, beginning with theories of etiology and ending with theories of treatment that are fully in accord with medical theory of the time. Many introduce new methods that are declared effective by physicians who claim to have employed them. We should be hesitant to question the honesty and integrity of such medical authors. It is easy to dismiss the cures recommended since from the perspective of modern science they are known to be ineffective. Such knowledge gives rise to assessments such as Ziegler's, quoted above, and to statements such as "Trained physicians tried any expedient, no matter how irrational, if it promised relief."[78] Although some of the medieval physician's methods are now assessed as irrational, they would not have been considered so by the physicians employing them. One might object that if the treatments were not effective, the physicians employing and recommending them could not have failed to recognize their ineffectiveness. But some people did recover from the plague, from some strains of the disease more than from others, and while it is now recognized that such cases of recovery may have been in spite of the curative methods employed, the physicians administering the treatment would have thought that their techniques had been effective. The success rate in medieval medicine was generally lower than in modern medicine, and accordingly the expectations both of physicians and of the general public were not nearly as high as those of the present day. Although the efforts of the medical profession to combat and cure the plague may be considered of little value in the history of medical science, such an assessment does not hold in the social history of medicine. Sylvia L. Thrupp's evaluation deserves to be quoted:

> The general effect of plague crises was to heighten individual concern about all diseases, and to make people deeply dependent on their doctors. . . . The prestige of doctors was not weakened by heavy plague mortality, for they could take credit for cases of recovery and by personal concern and courage they eased the atmosphere of fear. Popular devotion to a favorite doctor was expressed in terms of love and of the honor due a father by a son. This relationship was strengthened by the fact that medieval doctors were interested in advising people how to preserve their health.[79]

Although to the modern reader the plague tractates may seem at worst fraudulent and at best esoteric, they were in reality exoteric in the best sense of the word. While they provide sidelights on the ethics of medieval medical practice, they also illustrate a high degree of ethical motivation on the part of their authors, because almost all were written for the use of the public and represent a massive effort, in the aggregate, at popular health education.

During the various attacks of pestilence some physicians fled or refused to treat the ill, but many (probably most) remained and attempted to help the sick. Statements made by some physicians show that their treatment of plague victims was motivated by compassion, charity, and a sense of duty. The very fact that so many plague tractates were produced, in the attempt to explain the plague and educate people in prevention and treatment, is in itself evidence of a high degree of ethical and professional responsibility.

NOTES

All translations in this chapter are my own unless otherwise indicated.

1. G. Rath, "Ärztliche Ethik in Pestzeiten," *Münchener medizinische Wochenschrift* 99 (1957): 158–60.

2. The numerous plague tractates (the general significance of which will be discussed below) provide the major source material for this paper. Although several of the tractates have been published elsewhere, the majority of those written up to the beginning of the sixteenth century were published, in whole or in part, or summarized, by Karl Sudhoff in a series of articles entitled "Pestchriften aus den ersten 150 Jahren nach der Epidemie des 'schwarzen Todes' 1348," in *Archiv für Geschichte der Medizin* between 1910 and 1925: article I, in ibid., 4 (1910–11): 191–222; II, in ibid., 4 (1910–11): 389–424; III, in ibid., 5 (1911–12): 36–87; IV, in ibid., 5 (1911–12): 332–96; V, in ibid., 6 (1912–13): 313–79; VI, in ibid., 7 (1913–14): 57–114; VII, in ibid., 8 (1914–15): 175–215; VIII, in ibid., 8 (1914–15): 236–89; IX, in ibid., 9 (1915–16): 53–78; X, in ibid., 9 (1915–16): 117–67; XI, in ibid., 11 (1918–19): 44–89; XII, in ibid., 11 (1918–19): 121–78; XIII, in ibid., 14 (1922–23): 1–25; XIV, in ibid., 14 (1922–23): 79–105; XV, in ibid., 14 (1922–23): 127–68; XVI, in ibid., 16 (1924–25): 1–69; XVII, in ibid., 16 (1924–25): 77–188; XVIII, in ibid., 17 (1925): 12–139; XIX, ibid., 17 (1925): 241–91. These will be cited in this chapter as "Sudhoff," followed by the article number and page number(s).

3. The most famous and frequently quoted is in Boccaccio's "Preface to the Ladies," which introduces his *Decameron*. This mass hysteria and flight is often overemphasized in modern accounts, e.g., by William L. Langer, "The Black Death," *Sci. Am.* 210, no. 2 (1961): 114–21.

4. Richard W. Emery, "The Black Death of 1348 in Perpignan," *Speculum* 42 (1967): 620–21.

5. Cf. Elizabeth Carpentier, *Une ville devant la peste: Orvieto et la Peste Noire de 1348* (Paris: S.E.V.P.E.N, 1962).

6. Galen, *De libris propriis* 1.

7. Galen, *De praenotione ad Posthumum* 9.

8. For the role of public health boards during pestilence, see Carlo M. Cipolla, *Public Health and the Medical Profession in the Renaissance* (Cambridge: Cambridge University Press, 1976). Cipolla's greatest emphasis is on Italy, where the earliest developments occurred, some concurrent with the Black Death. For later developments in the Low Countries, see M. A. van Andel, "Plague Regulations in the Netherlands," *Janus* 21 (1916): 410–44.

9. See, e.g., G. G. Coulton, *Medieval Panorama: The English Scene from Conquest to Reformation* (New York: Macmillan, 1938), 497–502, 749; and Philip Ziegler, *The Black Death* (New York: John Day, 1971), 261–65. Dorothy M. Schullian, in "A Manuscript of Dominici in the Army Medical Library," *J. Hist. Med.* 3 (1948): 395–99, has published some revealing correspondence between a cardinal and a bishop during the 1360s on the question of whether it was a sin for a member of the clergy to flee from the plague.

10. See, e.g., Pearle Kibre, "The Faculty of Medicine at Paris, Charlatanism

and Unlicensed Medical Practices in the Later Middle Ages," *Bull. Hist. Med.* 27 (1953): 1–20.

11. E.g., medical licensure legislation from Sicily: "This is designed so that no subjects in our kingdom shall be endangered by the inexperience of doctors" (Roger II, 1140); "We secure advantage to the individual whenever we provide for the health of our faithful subjects. Accordingly, being mindful of the heavy loss and irreparable harm that can result from the inexperience of doctors . . ." (Frederick II, 1231). For the text and translation and a discussion of these regulations, see Edward F. Hartung, "Medical Regulations of Frederick the Second of Hohenstaufen," *Med. Life* 41 (1934): 587–601.

12. E.g., the statutes from the University of Montpellier, issued by papal legates in 1220: "Since it often happens that, on account of ignorance of the cause and lack of training, physicians cause the death of the patient when there was hope for his life . . ." Quoted by Helène Wieruszowski, *The Medieval University* (Princeton: Van Nostrand, 1966), 176.

13. See Kibre, "Faculty of Medicine" (n. 10), 2–14; Vern L. Bullough, *The Development of Medicine as a Profession: The Contribution of the Medieval University to Modern Medicine* (New York: Karger, 1966), 93, 99–103.

14. Madeleine Pelner Cosman, "Medieval Medical Malpractice: The Dicta and the Dockets," *Bull. N.Y. Acad. Med.* 49 (1973): 26; cf. Hartung, "Medical Regulations" (n. 11), 592.

15. Francis Aidan Gasquet, *The Black Death of 1348 and 1349*, 2d ed. (London: G. Bell and Sons, 1908), 31, 35; Anna M. Campbell, *The Black Death and Men of Learning* (New York: Columbia University Press, 1931), 98; Coulton, *Medieval Panorama* (n. 9), 749.

16. Nicolo de Burgo (1382), Sudhoff IV, 355; Nycolaus de Utino (1390), Sudhoff V, 361; anonymous tractate of 1405, Sudhoff XI, 79–80; Sigmund Albichs (1406), Sudhoff X, 132; Petrus de Kothobus (first half of the fifteenth century), Sudhoff XII, 126; Hermann Schedel (1453), Sudhoff XIV, 92; Hartmann Schedel (ca. 1463), Sudhoff XIV, 139–40.

17. Nicolo de Burgo (1382), Sudhoff IV, 355. Cf. Nycolaus de Utino (1390), Sudhoff V, 361: "Although flight from pestilence has been much praised by expert physicians, it cannot be conveniently done by some people; therefore . . ."

18. Jacme d'Agramont, "Regimen of Protection against Epidemics or Pestilence and Mortality," trans. M. L. Duran-Reynals and C.-E. A. Winslow, *Bull. Hist. Med.* 23 (1949): 58.

19. Sudhoff XVI, 10.

20. Sudhoff XVI, 48.

21. Sudhoff III, 85.

22. Sudhoff XVI, 67.

23. Sudhoff X, 164.

24. Sudhoff XVIII, 94. See also Dorothea Waley Singer, "Some Plague Tractates (Fourteenth and Fifteenth Centuries)," *Proc. Roy. Soc. Med. (Sect. Hist. Med.)* 9, no. 2 (1915–16): 197.

25. Sudhoff XII, 168.

26. Sudhoff IV, 365.

27. Sudhoff II, 393; and Sudhoff II, 43, 46.

28. Stephen D'Irsay, "Defense Reactions during the Black Death of 1348–1349," *Ann. Med. Hist.* 9 (1927): 176.

29. Rath, "Ärztliche Ethik" (n. 1), 159.

30. Ilza Veith, "Medical Ethics throughout the Ages," *Quart. Bull. Northwestern Univ. Med. School* 31 (1957): 355.

31. Quoted by Campbell, *Black Death* (n. 15), 3.

32. Ibid.

33. See, e.g., Gasquet, *Black Death* (n. 15), 31, 45, 71–72; and Campbell, *Black Death* (n. 15), 98.

34. Singer in "Some Plague Tractates" (n. 24), 179, gives ca. 1364.

35. Sudhoff III, 57.

36. Sudhoff II, 396.

37. Sudhoff X, 125.

38. Sudhoff X, 157.

39. Sudhoff X, 159.

40. Sudhoff III, 57.

41. "Causa paupertatis meae." This can mean "compelled by need," either in a purely material or in a spiritual sense. In the latter case it would have the force of "compelled by Christian charity."

42. Sudhoff III, 57.

43. Sudhoff XII, 135.

44. Sudhoff X, 125.

45. Sudhoff V, 338. Some other examples of prophylactic techniques of physicians: Johannes de Tornamira (ca. 1372), Sudhoff III, 50–51; Nicolo de Burgo (1382), Sudhoff IV, 365; Pietro di Tussignano (1398), Sudhoff IV, 394; Bartholomeus de Ferraria (near the end of the fourteenth century), Sudhoff XVII, 127–28; anonymous tractate of the early fifteenth century, Sudhoff XII, 175; Michael Boeti (ca. 1400–20), Sudhoff XVIII, 47; Johannes de Piscis (1431), Sudhoff XVIII, 52; Hermann Schedel (1453), Sudhoff XIV, 94.

46. Sudhoff II, 405–6.

47. One must then doubt the validity of the assertion made by Ziegler, *The Black Death* (n. 9), 131, that "the only defense against the plague in which the doctors had the slightest faith was flight from the afflicted area."

48. Sudhoff III, 57, "debent curare infirmos."

49. Sudhoff XII, 135, "debent curare infirmos seu visitare."

50. Mary Catherine Welborn, "The Long Tradition: A Study in Fourteenth-Century Medical Deontology," *Medieval and Historiographical Essays in Honor of James Westfall Thompson*, ed. J. L. Cate and E. N. Anderson (Chicago, 1938; reprint, Port Washington: Kennikat, 1966), 350–51.

51. James Henry Breasted, ed., *The Edwin Smith Surgical Papyrus* (Chicago: University of Chicago Press, 1930), contains the record of fifty-eight examinations, each followed either by treatment or by a decision not to treat. Sixteen patients are recommended to be left untreated. In three of these cases (nos. 6, 8a, and 20) some alleviative treatment is indicated. In the Ebers papyrus some cases were classified as untreatable. *The Papyrus Ebers*, trans. B. Ebbell (Copen-

hagen: Levin and Munksgaard, 1937), cols. 108–10. In Assyria-Babylonia the āšipu was a prognosticator who did not hesitate to withdraw from hopeless cases. See Edith K. Ritter, "Magical-Expert (= āšipu) and Physician (= asû): Notes on Two Complementary Professions in Babylonian Medicine," in *Studies in Honor of Benno Landsberger on His Seventy-fifth Birthday*, Assyriological Studies, no. 16 (Chicago: University of Chicago Press, 1965), 299–321.

52. See, e.g., in the Hippocratic corpus, *The Art* 3, *On Fractures* 36. For a brief discussion see Darrel W. Amundsen, "The Liability of the Physician in Classical Greek Legal Theory and Practice," *J. Hist. Med.* 32 (1977): 202–3.

53. D'Agramont, "Regimen of Protection" (n. 18), 71.

54. Gasquet, *Black Death* (n. 15), 45, 71–72.

55. Cipolla, *Public Health* (n. 8), 24.

56. See, e.g., Boccaccio, "Preface to the Ladies," introducing his *Decameron;* Charles F. Mullett, *The Bubonic Plague and England: An Essay in the History of Preventive Medicine* (Lexington: University of Kentucky Press, 1956), 16.

57. E.g., John of Burgundy (1365), Sudhoff III, 68–69. A translation of this passage is available in Campbell, *Black Death* (n. 15), 122. Johannes Jacobi (ca. 1364 or 1373), Sudhoff XVIII, 23. Cf. the recommendations for research made by Jacme d'Agramont (1348), "Regimen of Protection" (n. 18), 85.

58. Sudhoff XVIII, 54.

59. Many authors of plague tractates stress the extent to which physicians may be confused by the symptoms. See, e.g., Jacme d'Agramont (1348), "Regimen of Protection" (n. 18), 73; Johannes Jacobi (ca. 1364 or 1373), Sudhoff XVIII, 23; Johannes de Tornamira (ca. 1372), Sudhoff III, 48; Nicolaus Florentinus (first half of the fifteenth century), Sudhoff V, 340.

60. It was considered necessary for the patient to make a will in order "to set himself right with God." Navarrus, the leading canonist of the sixteenth century, in his *Enchiridion* (basically a book of moral guidance) includes a lengthy discussion of the sins to which members of different professions are most susceptible. In the section devoted to physicians, he writes that the physician sins who believes that his patient is about to die and does not advise him to make a will, as thereby "great quarrels among the heirs are prevented." Navarrus, *Enchiridion* 25, 5, 63. Navarrus cites as his authorities on this question John of Naples *(Quodlibeta)* and Antoninus of Florence *(Summa theologica)*.

61. This echoes the spirit of canon 22 of the Fourth Lateran Council (1215), a canon that was included in Gregory IX's officially promulgated codification of canon law (1234; *Decretales* 5.38.13).

62. Sigmund Albichs (1406) writes in his pest tractate that the physician should not immediately inform the patient if his condition is diagnosed as hopeless. He then writes that "the expert [*peritus*] physician should refrain from administering anything to the patient that will cause him to die quickly, for then he would be a murderer." Sudhoff X, 139.

63. Probably a medieval commentary on the second book of the *Aphorisms* in the Hippocratic Corpus.

64. Sudhoff XII, 160–61.

65. For an excellent discussion of this aspect of plague history, see Séraphine

Guerchberg, "The Controversy over the Alleged Sowers of the Black Death in the Contemporary Treatises on Plague," in *Change in Medieval Society*, ed. S. L. Thrupp (New York: Appleton-Century-Crofts, 1964), 208–24.

66. Sudhoff XVI, 26.

67. D'Agramont "*Regimen of Protection*" (n. 18), 57–58.

68. Sudhoff III, 56.

69. Sudhoff III, 62.

70. Sudhoff III, 69.

71. Sudhoff IV, 384.

72. Sudhoff XVIII, 46.

73. Sudhoff XII, 144.

74. Sudhoff XV, 162.

75. E.g., John of Burgundy (1365), Sudhoff III, 63; Bernhard of Frankfurt (1381), Sudhoff VIII, 248; Johannes de Noctho (1398), Sudhoff IV, 386; Magister Henricus (late fourteenth century), Sudhoff VI, 89; Bartholemeus de Ferraria (late fourteenth century), Sudhoff XVII, 128; anonymous tractate of the late fourteenth century, Sudhoff II, 411–12; anonymous tractate written sometime after 1400, Sudhoff XVIII, 135; anonymous tractate of the early fifteenth century, Sudhoff VI, 78; anonymous tractate of 1405, Sudhoff XI, 79–80; Sigmund Albichs (1406), Sudhoff X, 123, 131, 134, 149, 155–56; anonymous tractate of 1411, Sudhoff XII, 158; Johannes Hartmann (second half of the fifteenth century), Sudhoff XVI, 50.

76. Ziegler, *Black Death* (n. 9), 68, 75.

77. See, e.g., van Andel, "Plague Regulations" (n. 8), plate i, fig. 2.

78. Mullett, *Bubonic Plague* (n. 56), 3. Note the attitude of Singer in her discussion of the tractate of John of Burgundy (1365): "Having shown the exalted combination of learning and experience for successful treatment, John modestly proceeds to explain that he therefore has himself written a series of works on the plague, and that this, the latest flower of his wisdom, is especially designed for the plain man." Singer, "Some Plague Tractates" (n. 24), 164.

79. Sylvia L. Thrupp, "Plague Effects in Medieval Europe," *Comp. Stud. Soc. Hist.* 8 (1966): 480–81.

ELEVEN

The Moral Stance of the Earliest Syphilographers, 1495–1505

Questions that arose soon after the outbreak of a devastating disease that afflicted the soldiers of the French king Charles VIII during and following his siege of Naples in the winter and spring of 1494–95, and then seemingly spread rapidly throughout Europe, still remain to mock scholars from a variety of disciplines who seek to provide conclusive answers. Was this affliction, which was later to be called syphilis,[1] an old or a new disease? How and where did it originate? How is one to account for the spectacular change that the disease is reported to have undergone during its first five or six years? These and several related questions will never be answered conclusively. Some questions, however, were asked during the early decades of the syphilis "epidemic" that need no longer be asked. At that time no one knew of the treponema pallidum spirochete, and there was only a very limited observational awareness of what are now designated as the primary, secondary, latent, and tertiary stages of the disease. Hence there were numerous instances of supposed "cures" following upon therapeutic techniques that could have had little pernicious effect on the spirochetes. Consequently, a wide variety of questions about the nature of the disease and about the ostensible efficacy of various treatments continued to be asked until, quite recently, they were conclusively put to rest.[2]

One question that was asked then but that few if any would now venture to ask retrospectively about the syphilis "epidemic" of the late fourteenth and early fifteenth centuries (although some do pose it about, say, AIDS today) is, *Why* (not how) was this scourge afflicted upon the human race? In investigating the various responses that were made to this question, I shall address and explore the following questions: During the first decade of the syphilis "epidemic," what was the moral response of the authors of medical treatises both to the disease and to those suffering from it, especially as its primarily venereal mode of transmission became patent? And did these syphilographers feel a duty to treat those whose actions had brought the disease upon themselves, especially if the sufferers' actions were popularly or religiously perceived as immoral? It is not my intention to address any issues that do not contribute to answering these specific questions. Hence, for the purpose of the present study, I shall ignore, with a few notable exceptions, all nonmedical sources. The majority of the primary sources that I shall systematically review are treatises on syphilis that are contained in the three major syphilographic collections listed under "Abbreviations" immediately preceding the endnotes.

Our sources range from the outspokenly devout to those whose religious beliefs found no direct expression in their medical writings.[3] Nevertheless, they shared a common ethico-religious tradition, however much the extent of their conscious personal commitment to particular aspects of it may have varied. Any historian's appreciation and interpretation of many salient features of their writings will be, if not determined, at least considerably affected by his or her own understanding of their shared ethico-religious tradition. My own understanding of the nature and development of this tradition, which not only provides the conceptual context for my appreciation and interpretation of these authors but also encourages me to address the particular questions that I do, is articulated in those of my writings of the last eighteen years that appear as chapters 1 through 10 of this volume.

Numerous related themes, which are vital for an accurate picture of the ethico-religious ethos of those late medieval or Renaissance physicians who wrote on syphilis, were explored in the earlier chapters in this volume.[4] A theme immediately pertinent to the questions raised above is the perceived relationship of sin and sickness (see especially chaps. 5 and 7, above). Historians, especially recent ones, often show an incomplete, sometimes even a grossly distorted, grasp of the Christian idea of sin that prevailed at the time with which we are here concerned. Their discussions of several of our primary sources, especially the first, exemplify their misapprehensions of this issue, which is propaedeutic to our discovery and understanding of the moral stance of the earliest syphilographers.

The Blasphemy Edict of 1495

The earliest references to syphilis depict it in much the same way as plague was depicted. Hence it was regarded, of course, as a visitation of the wrath of God upon humanity for sin. That could be sin with a capital *S*, or specific sins. On August 7, 1495,[5] the Emperor Maximilian, at the Diet of Worms, issued what has become known as the blasphemy edict. It states that as a punishment for blasphemy, "previously famine and earthquakes and pestilence and other plagues were created and still in our time, as is evident, along with these and many other and diverse plagues and punishments, especially that new and most harsh disease of mankind has arisen in our day, which is popularly called the *malum Francicum*,[6] which never had been heard of before within human memory."[7] The edict specifies rigid punishment for those who were caught blaspheming.

Theodor Rosebury remarks, "The first explanations of syphilis . . . were made in terms of punishment for blasphemy rather than for sin. Yet as the venereal nature of the disease came to be understood, the result was merely to add sin to blasphemy among the crimes being punished."[8] The ambiguities of this quotation are less semantic than conceptual and illustrate, by extreme example, the danger of reading into the early history of syphilis some modern misperceptions of the nature of sin in the history of Christianity. Blasphemy was, of course, regarded as sin, arguably as a more serious sin than fornication. Furthermore, as we shall see, the venereal nature of the disease would not typically have caused those who contracted it to be regarded as guilty of an act of sexual immorality for which they were being punished. Hence one should approach with a degree of caution the following statement by Richard Palmer: "Although in an edict of 1495 the Emperor Maximilian pronounced syphilis to be God's punishment for the prevailing vice of blasphemy, it was soon evident that syphilis was at least primarily a venereal disease, and often the consequence of sexual immorality. The appearance of this new disease did much to provide factual support for the association of disease with sin."[9] It must be understood, however, that the venereal nature of syphilis would not, *eo ipso*, preclude the disease from being explained as punishment for sins that were unrelated to sexual activity.

Even greater circumspection must be used when reading Bruce Thomas Boehrer's assertion that because Maximilian's edict declares the *malum Francicum* to be God's punishment for the sin of blasphemy, "it promotes a moralized view of the illness that will prevail for the next century and more."[10] There was, of course, absolutely nothing novel or revolutionary in Maximilian's interpreting this scourge as divine punishment for sin. For more than the preceding millennium, epidemics had typically (but with some very important qualifications) been understood as visitations of God's wrath against prevailing sins (see chap. 7, above). Furthermore, Maximilian's edict did not set the tone, as it were, for future theological interpretations of syphilis. Once the disease was regarded as endemic, blasphemy was seldom if ever again mentioned as the sin against which God's wrath was directed.

Boehrer then observes that "the edict significantly ignores any notion of natural medical causality. Syphilis emerges here as purely and simply a judgment from God, and as such it supplies the perfect excuse to institute close censorship and surveillance of speech—which is, after all, the edict's declared purpose."[11] Contemporary and earlier sources' emphasis on ultimate causality of any disaster never precluded their identifying immediate and intermediate causes. Boehrer's conviction that Maximilian jumped at the opportunity to use the outbreak of syphilis as "the perfect excuse" to oppress his subjects reveals much more about the cynical ideology of the former than about the motives of the latter. Likewise, Anna Foa's conviction that Maximilian sought out "opportune scapegoats" upon whom he could place the blame for this new plague seems to have little to commend it. One of Foa's theses is that, in the early stages of the "epidemic" of syphilis, "European society did not activate its customary mechanism to preserve itself from mental disintegration in the face of calamity: it did not seek out opportune scapegoats. Certainly, there were attempts of this kind, such as Maximilian's edict against blasphemers, but they were rare."[12] There are, of course, numerous examples of singling out specific groups of people as causal agents of plague in the late Middle Ages. The example that comes most readily to mind is that of the Jews who, during the Black Death of 1348–49, were accused, by the residents of some communities, of having poisoned the wells. But blasphemers were hardly an identifiable minority group. Maximilian's motivation in suggesting that blasphemy was the cause of this new plague was the same as that which had encouraged many civil and ecclesiastical leaders and private citizens from a variety of vocations to specify as having precipitated God's righteous judgment those sins that they regarded as most rampant in the community. There is a fundamental, if fine, conceptual and categorical difference between this type of communal "soul searching"—which was intended to lead to conviction, repentance, reformation, and restoration—and finding a scapegoat, an "other" to blame for a natural disaster such as pestilence, famine, or earthquake.

Three German Reactions: Sebastian Brant, Jacob Wimpheling, and Konrad Schellig (1495–1496)

Three of Maximilian's subjects soon addressed this new plague. They were a physician, Konrad Schellig; a priest and humanist, Jacob Wimpheling; and a humanist poet, Sebastian Brant. Brant's fame had recently been assured by the publication of his *Das Narrenschiff*. His eulogium, entitled *De pestilentiali scorra sive impetigine anni XCVI*,[13] is a political manifesto, a plea to the German people to support their emperor so that this scourge, sent from heaven to punish them for their lack of patriotism, would be removed. The poem is illustrated by a woodcut by Dürer, which, as Claude Quétel describes it, "shows us the Virgin Mary, on a throne of clouds, with the Infant Jesus on her knee. With her right hand she is about to place the imperial crown on the head of Maximilian of Hapsburg, who is surrounded by his men-at-arms. On the other side a group of entreating pox-sufferers covered in pustules receive beams of light from the Infant's left hand." Quétel then remarks, "It is impossible to say for certain whether this is a punishment or a cure. (And why should it not be both, each in its turn?)"[14] Brant's motives in writing his eulogium were unabashedly political and entirely consistent with contemporary pro-imperial German patriotism. The same cannot reasonably be said of the second response to syphilis that was precipitated by the Diet of Worms, that of the physician Konrad Schellig.

Philip, Elector of the Palatinate, participated in the Diet of Worms, accompanied by his personal physician, Schellig, whom Philip instructed to compose a *consilium*, that is, a regimen, against this new disease. This treatise, entitled *In pustulas malas morbum, quem malum de Francia vulgus appellat, quae sunt de genere formicarum, salubre consilium*,[15] was published late in 1495 or early in 1496, with an introductory epistle by the German humanist, priest, and friend of both Brant and Schellig, Jacob Wimpheling,[16] who had also been present at the Diet of Worms. In this prefatory letter Wimpheling asserts,

The righteous severity of God, either because of terrible and sustained blasphemy or on account of adultery, which is rendered most vile because of its continual increase, or owing to other sins, and mediated through the motions of the heavenly bodies and other causes as well, has in our generation let loose in the lands, so that it would most appropriately attack wretched mortals on account of their iniquity, a certain disease, which, in our time, as the Insubrians[17] lament, the French have imported into their country. This is not a new disease, as the common people believe, but was well known in earlier times and is endured with the most excruciating pains imaginable. Nevertheless, by his characteristic love and infinite mercy, God gave to us the hidden virtues of natural properties.[18] These he has given by the very means that he established,[19] by which means human diligence in turn would be happily able to bring help to the sinner, who has experienced these just punishments, especially once the sinner has turned from his offences. In this way God's compassion will surpass his retributive justice, because whenever a blow has fallen, then a remedy will follow.

Wimpheling now commends to the reader the consilium of "Konrad Schellig of Heidelberg, eminent doctor of medicine," which he composed at the request of Prince Philip and *ex fraterna charitate*. Wimpheling concludes his epistle with a brief description of Schellig's understanding of the proximate causes of the disease and modes of prevention and cure.[20]

Schellig's consilium is very similar to the numerous pest tractates that physicians had composed in response to various epidemics, beginning with the Black Death of 1348–49. Roger French thus summarizes Schellig's treatise: "Schellig treats the matter in a purely medical way, explaining that the influence of the stars caused a disturbance in the humours of the body. Congruent causes were a qualitative equilibrium of the air, causing adustion and putrefaction of the humours; and the consumption of putrescible foods. Cure (and prevention) was a question of adjusting the non-naturals in a regimen that obviated these causes."[21] Schellig begins his treatise by saying, "I call these pustules evil [*malae*], for they are contagious at least through contact, immediate or mediate, and also because they are from evil [*malae*] humors." He then asserts that, following Avicenna, he regards them as *de genere formicarum*. Drawing primarily from Avicenna, but also citing other authorities, he enlarges on the nature of, and various names for, these pustules. Then he states that the "causes of these pustules are threefold, *primitiva* or *antecedens* and *coniuncta*." Under the heading *causa primitiva* Schellig gives, for example, excessively warm air, excessively cold air, excessively humid air, or excessively dry air, along with a description of the effect of each of these on the humors. He includes as a *causa primitiva* the influence of the stars that produces a disturbance of the humors. He proceeds then to list a variety of activities—for instance, excessive exercise—that can create humoral imbalances that render one more susceptible to contracting these pustules. The *causae antecedens et coniuncta* are various humoral irregularities that are present in some people.

Schellig's understanding of this disease was entirely consistent with prevailing humoral theory of health and disease. Hence he gives no special attention to sexual intercourse in his consilium, except such attention as was conventionally given to its role in the scheme of the non-naturals in humoral theory's conception of the prevention and treatment of disease. As distinct from the contra-naturals (pathological states) and the naturals (the essential anatomical and physiological components of the human organism), the non-naturals were those things without which one either cannot live well or cannot live at all. Typically there were six: air, food and drink, exercise and rest, sleep and waking, repletion and excretion, and emotions. Lists by individual authors vary a little and sometimes include more than six items.[22]

Schellig describes his *regimen praeservativum* as consisting of "the necessary management of the six things non-natural,"[23] and then produces nine separate rubrics: air, food, drink, movement and rest, bathing, sleep and waking, repletion and excretion, emotions, and sexual intercourse. His discussion of sexual intercourse is as follows:

Excessive and boisterous [*violentus*] sexual intercourse must especially be avoided because it diminishes the potencies [*vires*] of the body, and debilitates the most vital members, adversely affects the faculty of sight and all the joints and nerves, and finally it hastens the onset of old age. One must abstain from sexual intercourse when excessively hot, when excessively cold, hungry, full of food or drink, also when fatigued by labor, and after much evacuating either by a flux of blood or wind or vomit, or by much perspiration. Also, in the present situation, frequent and excessive sexual intercourse must be avoided because it moves the corrupt matters to the exterior regions of the body and it summons the warm and putrid vapors to the surface of the skin. From this a stench of the body, mouth, and gums arises, and an itch and roughness [*pruritus et scabies*] are multiplied [*multiplicatur*] on the body. Thereby conversely those who multiply [*multiplicantes*] sexual intercourse appear fetid and mangy. One who is healthy, married, and accustomed to sexual intercourse is able at this time to engage in it moderately, as long as his nature is aroused internally and not only stimulated externally. The best time for sexual intercourse is after the first and second digestions have taken place, that is, during the early morning around dawn. After sexual intercourse one must be quiet and sleep.[24]

So much for the role of sexual intercourse in the regimen of preservation from contracting this disease. In his regimen for the cure of the disease, Schellig devotes a section each to air, diet, food, drink, "other things non-natural," medications, and surgical applications and procedures. Among various matters under the rubric "other things non-natural" he includes the statement that "sexual intercourse should be entirely abandoned." He then concludes this section with the following sentence: "In short, those infected with pustules, at least in the beginning, ought to avoid all things that tend to heat their bodies, either from the outside or from the inside."[25]

We should note the following about this, the earliest in a long series of treatises devoted to what will retrospectively be called syphilis. First, Schellig and Wimpheling were adamant in their conviction that it was not a new disease, "as the common people believe," and this in spite of the equally adamant insistence of their emperor, Maximilian, that it was an entirely new plague, "never . . . heard of before within human memory." Second, Wimpheling, certainly with Schellig's concurrence, designated three levels of causality: final, "the righteous severity of God"; mediate, the motions of the heavenly bodies; and proximate, various features of humoral pathology. And third, they clearly did not regard this as a venereal disease. The role that they assigned to sexual intercourse in their regimens of both prophylaxis and treatment is entirely consistent with the humoral theory of health and disease, in spite of Wimpheling's adding to the sin of blasphemy that of an increase of adultery as a possible cause of God's sending this plague. Fourth, Schellig regarded avoiding contact with the infected as the most efficacious prophylaxis against this disease, a view that he emphasizes in both the section on air and that on bathing.

Joseph Grünpeck's First Treatise (1496)

The next treatise to be published on this disease was by yet another German, Joseph Grünpeck. At about age twenty-three, Grünpeck, who was liberally educated but not a physician, published, in November 1496, his *Tractatus de pestilentiali scorra sive mala de Franzos*.[26] Following a short dedicatory note to a fellow German humanist and prominent academician, Bernard of Walkirch, and a brief introduction, he quotes the entirety of Brant's eulogium. Grünpeck also reproduces the woodcut from the printing of Brant's poem, which, in Quétel's words, "has undergone slight modifications, although it would be rash to guess at the intentions behind this. The groups have drawn closer together; the emperor on the left and the pox-sufferers on the right are kneeling, whilst in the foreground lies a pox-victim who is undoubtedly either dead or in a very bad way. Are we to interpret this as a subtle attempt to link the group of victims with the great men of this world? Perhaps not. But it certainly indicates the desire to put the spotlight on the new disease, to dramatize it."[27]

Like Schellig's approach, Grünpeck's is similar to that of the numerous other authors who had been composing plague tractates since the inception of the Black Death a century and a half earlier. To Grünpeck this new plague was generically the same as previous plagues. His first chapter, concerning plagues (de plagis) or afflictions (flagellis) of men, "whether they come naturally or supernaturally by the will of God," acknowledges that life is filled with misery (e.g., old and new diseases, aging, floods, storms, shipwreck). "Nature is itself a cruel stepmother to man."[28] Now "we are threatened with a new kind of disease, hateful by the ferocity of its nature." Throughout the remainder of chapter 1 and all of chapter 2, Grünpeck wrestles with questions of ultimate, intermediate, and proximate causality of a multitude of ills that afflict humanity. In regard to the first, there are three kinds of sins that God hates most: pride, greed, and theft. These three are invariably punished by pestilence, wars, and famines. Clearly this new bane, the *mala de Franzos*, is divine vengeance. The stars, although they have no power in and of themselves, are the intermediate cause.

Chapters 3 through 9 are an elaborate explanation of astrally generated disease as explicated by humoral pathology. In the case of mala de Franzos, "a terrifying conjunction of Saturn and Jupiter" had occurred on November 25, 1484; and on March 26, 1485 a "terrible and dire eclipse of the sun." This "was followed by infinite disturbances," such as pestilential floods, tempests, wars, and this new disease that, "consuming like fire, inflaming, incinerating, and torturing . . . is so oppressive that . . . many long for death to relieve their pain." Grünpeck's awareness of the venereal nature of this disease was only slightly greater than Schellig's. At least he was aware that the genitals typically were the organs most dramatically affected by the pox, for he concludes chapter 9 with the assertion that "nature strives to expel by force this most sordid material and sends it down to the *pudenda* where the veins are collected," a view that will for some time be the dominant explanation for the involvement of the genitals in this disease.

In chapter 10 Grünpeck recommends the use, against this new disease, of a prophylaxis typical of the plague tractates: avoid contact with the afflicted, with public baths, and with latrines, and use various fumigations to purify the air of the miasma that causes the mala de Franzos (see chap. 10, above). He goes on to recommend for the afflicted a regimen, efficacious ways to evacuate the humors, and various medicines. But "in other matters, the most worthy doctors of medicine are to be consulted, who can advise more wisely than I." And "we should have recourse to the Heaven-governing Jehovah, the first and greatest physician, and to his Divine Mother, the Virgin Mary."

A German translation of Grünpeck's treatise was published in December 1496 and dedicated to the bürgermeister and council of the city of Augsburg. These two dedications aroused Boehrer's anxiety:

Grünpeck clearly wished to get as much mileage as possible out of his book. It is thus hard to avoid viewing these early texts as to some degree government documents, responsive to the needs and expectations of an aristocracy that claims its authority as God-given and immutable. In effect, when we read early texts like Grünpeck's, with their careful appeals to patronage and their oblique echoes of theological and imperial authority, we witness the elaborate mutual fondling whereby political orthodoxies are established and maintained.[29]

Boehrer sees this imaginary elitist conspiracy against the lower classes also in Grünpeck's recommendations for prophylaxis against the disease: "Grünpeck's notion of cleanliness extends well beyond the specifics of washing and diet to involve a more general notion of spiritual purity, to be reflected (of course) in the way one comports oneself and in the company one keeps. . . . One avoids syphilis, according to Grünpeck, by avoiding *people* [Boehrer's emphasis]; and this avoidance is an accurate marker of spiritual regeneration. . . . One contracts the disease by mingling with the wrong sort of people."[30] But who, according to Grünpeck, are the "wrong sort of people"? They are, of course, those infected with this disease. And how, in Grünpeck's opinion, did people contract it? In the same way in which people became infected with plague. Were those who were afflicted with plague or with this mala de Franzos worse sinners than those who were not? Definitely not, according to Grünpeck. Boehrer apparently assumed that Grünpeck clearly recognized the venereal nature of the disease and judgmentally castigated the infected for their sexual sins (of course, only if they were not fellow aristocratic elitists). Since Grünpeck did not recognize the venereal nature of the disease, such a conclusion is twice as unwarranted as it otherwise would be. But if he had known, how would he have reacted to those who suffered from it? We shall consider that question when we encounter Grünpeck again, after he has himself contracted syphilis.

Bartholomaus Steber's Treatise (ca. 1497)

Bartholomaus Steber, professor of medicine at the University of Vienna, had held the distinguished position of Rector Magnificus at that university around 1490. It was to the current Rector Magnificus that he addressed his treatise, *A malafranczos, morbo Gallorum, praeservatio ac cura,*[31] which was published in Vienna sometime around 1497, with no date indicated. The title page is graced by a woodcut showing a couple afflicted with syphilis. Both patients are entirely covered with pustules. "They are being treated by two physicians," writes Karl Sudhoff. "The woman lies in bed while a physician in a pointed cap stands by with a urine-flask in his hand performing a urinoscopy. By the side of the bed sits the man. A second physician in a biretta is treating him with ointment which he is applying with a spatula."[32]

Steber writes that he had been "asked by certain people most dear to me . . . to direct my attention to the disease that they call *morbus Gallicus.* I was thoroughly terrified by the newness and the magnitude of the affair (for I was convinced that something divine belonged to whatever is unusual,[33] which is not undeserved by this age of ours)." He laments that "the distinguished men, who were quite thoroughly versed in the causes of these things and about how much it was given to man to know about such matters, do not say anything about this affair." He would not have had the temerity to write on this disease

had it not been that the audacity of some thoroughly profligate, vile, and contemptible men compelled me to undertake this task. Those people, being completely ignorant of the first principles of philosophy, in fact being devoid of the requisite first elements of knowledge, not for the sake of peoples' health, but rather for the sake of gathering air and expending wind, presume to treat those poor folk who are afflicted with this *morbus Gallicus* with a single medication (perhaps somewhere acquired by stealth from physicians), uselessly boasting that they have something secret for the repelling of this foul sickness, the cause of which they maintain is completely unknown to physicians. These most worthless fellows impudently proclaim that we are unable to produce any work for those suffering from this sickness. Deeply grieved that so great a scandal must be so unfairly borne by professors of the art of medicine, coming as it is from these most filthy men, I resolved to proceed with this undertaking.[34]

Three matters warrant comment. First, Steber must have believed that he was the first physician, at least the first professor of medicine, to write on this disease. Second, his reaction to those who had come forward to treat the victims of *morbus Gallicus* is similar to the attacks of several other early syphilographers against those whom they regarded as rustics and charlatans. Steber's motivation for writing his treatise was in great part provided by insinuations of these "rustics and charlatans" that physicians were ignorant about the causes of the disease. Third, Steber gives deference to divine causality. This, however, is a subject to which he does not return in the main body of the treatise.

The treatise itself is disappointing. It is almost a stereotypical, generic treatment of illness along the standard lines of humoral pathology. He does not deal with sexual intercourse anywhere, not even in his discussion of the non-naturals, and his only mention of the involvement of the genitals is with reference to the supposed tendency *expellere inutiles humores a membris dignioribus ad loca ignobilia.*[35] He expatiates at some length on the importance of understanding the astral causality of morbus Gallicus[36] and by differential diagnosis distinguishes the disease from a variety of other conditions, including leprosy.

Hans Widmann's Treatise (1497)

Konrad Schellig was not the only physician to attend the Diet of Worms in 1495. A famous professor and personal physician of Count Eberhard V of Württemburg, Hans Widmann of Tübingen, was also present. On January 20, 1497, he sent to Johann Nell, municipal physician of Strassburg, for his criticism, a manuscript entitled *De pustulis quae vulgato nomine dicuntur mal de Franzos,*[37] which was published sometime later that year. In his introductory letter to Nell, Widmann remarks that he had frequently pondered the miseries of the human race and was "amazed by the new kinds [*genera*] of diseases that are arising at random." After remarking that "we are entirely overcome by evils," he quotes Pliny's statement "Nature offers nothing better to men than brevity of life,"[38] and then exclaims, "Also in our time a foul disease has seized humanity. It is difficult to determine whether this has happened by divine will, as our deeds justly merit, or by the influence of the stars and the unfavorable orbit of Saturn."[39] He returns to this subject in the section of the treatise devoted to causes of this disease. There he speaks of causes that are "far removed, one being divine vengeance [*ultio di-*

vina] for the punishment of men's sins and transgressions" and another the "determined aspects or arrangements of the heavenly bodies that cause a *dispositio* to occur in the air and on the earth through which this sickness is introduced in human bodies arranged to be thus assaulted." He then makes a most interesting observation: "But since the physician, as a physician, does not concern himself much with these causes [*Sed quoniam de his causis non multum curat medicus, ut medicus*], but rather with the cause that is within the body, by the removal of which the disease is removed, I shall therefore attend to this."[40]

Let us first note that Widmann does not deny that God and the heavenly bodies may be causally involved in the *mal de Franzos*. But both are remote causes, and the physician *qua* physician is not much concerned with them, according to Widmann. Does his statement accurately reflect the position of typical physicians of his time? To this question both a negative and an affirmative answer must be given. To say that the astrological aspect of disease causality was not a matter of much concern to physicians then was simply incorrect and places Widmann among a minority, albeit a growing minority, of contemporary physicians. The importance of astrology in prophylaxis, diagnosis, prognosis, and treatment was a matter of general belief, especially during the fourteenth, fifteenth, and sixteenth centuries, although its position seems to have become more controversial in the course of the sixteenth. Nevertheless, for the period under consideration, the sentiment was strong that the physician who was not versed in astrology was incompetent or imbecilic.[41] Such accusations were especially leveled against those physicians who were ignorant of astrology or who denied the salutary and pernicious influences of the heavenly bodies on the atmosphere and thence on the humors, or on the humors directly. Although Widmann's assertion that astral causality of this disease was not the concern of physicians did not necessarily place him in the category of those castigated for their ignorance of, or contempt for, astrology, nevertheless it did distinguish him from a significant number of his fellow physicians.

Widmann's remarks on divine causality are (by contrast, and as we shall see) typical of those members of the medical community of that time who had anything to say about final cause. He does not deny that there may be a divine purpose behind this new plague. Indeed he admits that "our deeds justly merit" God's punishing humanity in this manner. Nevertheless, such considerations are not the business of the physician when he is occupying the physician's role. That there were few if any physicians during the period under consideration who would have disagreed with him on this matter will become increasingly manifest as we proceed.

Widmann devotes no separate section to prophylaxis but recommends that for prevention one should follow the directions for regulating the non-naturals that he gives in his instructions for curing the disease. Widmann lists and discusses the standard six. Under the rubric "air" he suggests that if people must come in contact with the infected, they should use the same safeguards that he had described in his *Tractatus de pestilentia*.[42] In his discussion of emotions, he maintains that

all things are harmful that much arouse, inflame, and excite the humors. Hence anger, fighting, frenzy, and sustained idleness, as well as fear and sorrow, prolonged care and anxiety, are especially to be avoided. Indeed, it is more for the moral philosopher to correct such things than it is the business of the physician. Therefore, whoever would be the corrector and regulator of himself in these things, let him be diligent to hope optimistically, to live happily, to rejoice frequently, and to meet and talk with friends and loved ones.

He explains that such delightful things "conduce to the generation of *sanguis laudabilis*, which is hostile to the evil humors . . . from which the present sickness arises." Since sexual intercourse is closely connected with the emotions, Widmann felt that it was necessary to address the place of that activity in the regimen of morbus Gallicus. Widmann's next several sentences are similar to Schellig's discussion of the subject, supplemented by the tentatively expressed suggestion that this disease usually first manifests itself in the genitals because the evil humors are drawn there by the strong *concussio* that sexual intercourse causes in them. Then Widmann sets his own course beyond that of Schellig, by maintaining that nonetheless sexual intercourse is not entirely interdicted, *lege permittente*, for some categories of people, for instance, the young, and those who are accustomed to the act. In fact, it is salutary in some cases. But for the rest it is very harmful. "Nevertheless, the most extreme care must be taken lest one engage in sexual intercourse with a pustulous woman, or even with a healthy woman with whom a pustulous man has lain recently, in order to avoid the risk of contagion. For already it is known by experience that one following recently after a pustulous man is infected. Therefore one must especially beware of prostitutes at this time."[43]

Widmann's concern with sexual intercourse on the part of those wishing to avoid the mal de Franzos does not go beyond that which one would expect of humoral pathology, although he recognized sexual inter-course as one means of transmission, as the last three sentences quoted above demonstrate. From what source had he derived this insight? Wid-mann, in addition to being a professor of medicine and personal phy-sician to Count Eberhard, had long been the inspector of lepers for Tübingen. This led Sudhoff to suggest that "the experience he thus gained is reflected in his writings,"[44] and to comment that "among the regulations then in vogue for leprosy . . . was the avoidance of inter-course with a *mulier leprosa* and also with a woman with whom a leprous man had cohabited. Thus it does not surprise us when Widmann tells us that a man must be on his guard in the presence of a *mulier pustulata* and also in the presence of a woman with whom a *vir pustulatus* has lain."[45] We should note, however, that not only does Widmann clearly distin-guish the mal de Franzos from leprosy, a disease with which it was then sometimes confused, but he distinctly states that "already it is known by experience" *(iam enim cognitum est experientia)* when speaking of trans-mission of the mal de Franzos through sexual intercourse. This surely suggests that he did not simply transfer theories of transmission of lep-rosy over to this new disease.

Nicolo Leoniceno's Treatise (1497)

Public medical disputations, both in Leipzig and in Ferrara,[46] were raging about the question of whether the mal de Franzos was new or old. Nicolo Leoniceno, a highly respected professor at the University of Fer-rara, at nearly seventy years of age, published in 1497 the fruit of an academic disputation on the nature of the malady, entitled *Libellus de epidemia quam vulgo morbum Gallicum vocant.*[47] He begins his treatise by reminding his readers that, at other times in the past, supposedly new diseases had arisen. For instance, during the reign of Claudius, Pliny erroneously had believed that a particular condition, which actually was lichen, was new.

Likewise in our age now, in fact, a disease of an unusual nature has invaded Italy and many other regions. Pustules, which begin on the genitals, soon cover the whole body and especially the face itself, bringing, for the most part, besides the stench, a very severe pain. Nevertheless, the physicians of our time have not yet assigned an accurate name to this disease, but they call it by the commonly used name, *malum Gallicum,* as if its contagion had been imported by the French into Italy or, at one and the same time, Italy was attacked both by this disease and by the French army.[48]

But Leoniceno knew better. It was in reality an old disease. He was convinced that humanity had always been afflicted by the same diseases. "For if anyone believes differently than I, just what would he say that this is other than a punishment of the gods [*deorum vindicta*]? For if natural causes are examined [one would conclude] that the same conditions have repeated themselves thousands of times since the beginning of the world."[49] It would indeed appear that Leoniceno rejected out of hand the possibility of a divine causality of this disease and that consequently he insisted on a strictly natural causality. Both could be taken as the result (perhaps an inevitable result) of his unequivocal insistence on the impossibility of totally new diseases ever arising. Foa thus renders the passage just quoted: "And if someone thinks differently, I will clear up this point: Is one dealing with a revenge of the gods? In fact, if one considers natural causes, the same conditions repeat themselves thousands of times from the beginning of the world."[50] Foa then remarks on "the ease with which" Leoniceno "dismissed the hypothesis that syphilis was a divine punishment." Leoniceno, however, was not denying the possibility of divine purpose behind a disease's reappearing with devastating severity. He goes on to insist that if one were to examine the laws of nature, one must conclude that they have remained unchanged since the beginning. Old diseases reappear, sometimes taking on or manifesting some new characteristics. But a totally new disease? Impossible, unless the Creator himself were dramatically to have intervened supernaturally in nature. It is not necessary to resort to such explanations for this or any other disease, is what Leoniceno is saying. We need to bear in mind, however, that those physicians who did regard the morbus Gallicus as a new disease did not consequently need to explain its origin by recourse to an exclusively theological understanding. Rather, their view of nature allowed for new diseases to arise under certain circumstances. Leoniceno's did not. Foa should have read further in Leoniceno's treatise, since, when bringing his treatise at last to a conclusion, he asserts that this disease, "which the vulgar call morbus Gallicus, ought to be numbered among epidemics, that is, diseases that spread throughout the populace. These certainly happen either owing to divine wrath, as the theologians think, or by the power of the stars, as the astrologers suppose, or from a specific inclemency of the air just as the physicians judge. We, following the physicians in this respect, assign the proximate causes to nature."[51] These three are not mutually exclusive. They are complementary. Leoniceno does not deny the possibility of a divine final, or an astral intermediate, cause. In this he is typical of physicians of his time. He is also consistent with his medical contemporaries in focusing on proximate causality as the purview of the physician. Where he differs from many of his fellow physicians is in his conviction that it was impossible for any totally new disease to arise. Nevertheless, those who held Leoniceno's view did not *eo ipso* reject final and intermediate causes, especially of epidemics. Within both camps, however, there was considerable divergence regarding the extent to which individual physicians were inclined to discuss final and intermediate causes. Leoniceno's preference was to limit his concern to proximate causality. Hence he assigns "the proximate causes to nature," most specifically to telluric miasma caused by recent floods.

Near the end of the treatise, Leoniceno raises the question of why the pustules appear first on the genitals. His explanation is, as is to be expected, entirely consistent with humoral pathology. W.P.D. Wightman remarks:

This little book by Leoniceno, though conservative in outlook and adding nothing to scientific or medical knowledge, nevertheless provides us with an almost complete picture of contemporary views on this new problem. It is characteristic of the best type of humanistic medicine, showing both its strength—accurate, critical, comprehensive, free from superstition or quackery, even "scientific" in preferring proximate to remote causes—but also its weakness, namely that in consequence of its blind reverence for the classical writers the possibility of transfer of contagion in the sexual act is not even entertained: the appearance of pustules on the *pudenda* being "explained" *(ut inquit Galenus!)* as a result of the excessive "warmth and moisture" of those parts.[52]

Coradinus Gilinus' Treatise (1497)

Another Italian, Coradinus Gilinus, *artium et medicinae doctor,* probably also a resident of Ferrara or at least thoroughly familiar with the disputations there on morbus Gallicus, followed Leoniceno with his *De morbo quem Gallicum nuncupant* in the same year.[53] He begins his treatise, "In the past year, 1496, a certain most violent disease attacked a great many people both in Italy and beyond the Alps. . . . This malady is unknown to the moderns and various debates upon it have been and are being held among physicians."[54] So he had decided to write a brief study himself, addressing first the cause, next the essence, then the diagnosis, and finally the treatment of this disease, which he will identify with the ancient *ignis Persicus* (a theory that received no support from other members of the medical community until early in the nineteenth century).

Gilinus maintains that the causes of morbus Gallicus "can be reduced to the same as those of plague, namely the lower causes and certain higher ones." He will enumerate the astrological causes "because the lower causes are governed by the higher." After describing certain astrological factors, he quotes the sentiments of pagan, Jewish, and Islamic medical authorities (Galen, Isaac Judaeus, and Avicenna, respectively) that ultimate causality must be traced back to God. With this he concurs:

We see then that the Creator on high, being angered with us at this time for our impious deeds, is afflicting us with this most terrible distemper that is raging not only in Italy but throughout the whole of Christendom. Everywhere the blare of trumpets is sounding, everywhere is heard the clash of arms, everywhere are being constructed military weapons, bombards, instruments and a great many engines of war, moreover instead of the spherical stones, which have been in use up to the present time, they are now making iron balls, a hitherto unheard-of thing. The Turks are called into Italy, and would that I could deny how many conflagrations, how many depredations, how many massacres of wretched human beings we have already seen, how many and how great we are yet to see! Let us therefore say with the prophet in the sixth Psalm, "O Lord, rebuke me not in thine anger, neither chasten me in thy hot displeasure."[55]

Gilinus is by far the most theologically minded of the medical syphilographers that we have thus far encountered. To what degree does he differ from Widmann, who, as we have seen, says that the physician *qua* physician is not much concerned with such matters? We must recognize that Widmann was speaking specifically about the identification and discussion of nonimmediate causes of disease. The key word in Widmann's statement is *much*. A physician *qua* physician would be only minimally interested in ultimate causality. The level of causality with which the physician would be predominantly concerned was the immediate. Gilinus' interest in expatiating on ultimate causality is certainly greater than Widmann's and than that of most physicians who wrote on morbus Gallicus. Widmann, as we have seen, did not allow theological considerations to enter into his understanding of immediate causality and his formulation of a regimen. Nor did Gilinus.

When Gilinus turns to a consideration of the "lower causes," he asserts that there is no point in mentioning them because "they are the same as those which produce plague, alopecia, leprosy, scabies, and other pustules, and these have been investigated by our predecessors."[56]

In regard to prophylaxis, "those measures that protect against the above-named sicknesses, protect also against this one, the Divine aid being first invoked, as Moses did when he said, 'Lord, why doth thy wrath wax hot against thy people? Turn from thy fierce wrath,' for these measures were handed down by the most learned. Likewise in the control of this malady I deem we must have recourse to them." He then makes the same observation that Widmann had: "But one thing among others I will say, that this disease is contagious: Wherefore I again and again warn men on no account to lie with women who are suffering from this pernicious sickness or those who have had intercourse with men rendered dangerous thereby, for I have seen many infected from this cause who have suffered very great torments."[57]

After warning against treatment by "such practitioners as barbers, cobblers, journeyman laborers, and especially travelling mountebanks," he discusses therapy. He begins with the management of the six non-naturals, during which he refers to sexual intercourse under the rubric "sleep and waking": "Coitus is very harmful except in good-complexioned young patients fairly accustomed to it, in which case a little is not so injurious."[58] We have seen and shall continue to see that physicians typically recommended sexual abstinence or at least moderation for their syphilitic patients, not in order to avoid spreading the disease but owing to humoral pathology's principle of the supposedly deleterious effects of intercourse on certain categories of the ill who are undergoing certain kinds of therapy.

Gaspar Torrella's First Treatise (1497)

Gaspar Torrella, physician to Pope Alexander VI and his family, the Borgias, was himself a priest and had been the bishop of Saint Justa since 1494. He dedicated and addressed to the notorious Cesare Borgia, bastard son of Pope Alexander VI, then cardinal of Valencia, his *Tractatus cum consiliis contra pudendagram seu morbum Gallicum,*[59] which Karl Sudhoff calls "the most valuable and 'first hand' of all our tracts. It is the least prejudiced, the freshest, and the least academic."[60]

Torrella begins his treatise by listing a series of questions that Cesare Borgia had addressed to him: "What is this pestiferous sickness, popularly named *morbus Gallicus?* Have doctors of medicine written anything about it? Why, in the whole course of time, has no specific remedy been found and proved? And why do the pains attack more at night than during the day?"[61] Torrella then says that it is easy to ask such questions, but much more difficult to answer them. "Nevertheless, in order to comply with your request . . . I shall try to introduce in this brief compendium those things, insofar as they are pertinent, which I shall be able to find here and there in the books of both ancient and modern physicians." He then remarks that the challenge had been complicated by his having been occupied with ecclesiastical responsibilities for the previous ten years and hence able to devote only minimal time to the art of medicine.[62]

After emphasizing that a positive attitude and the "very hope of health itself" have "cured the infected and preserved the healthy,"[63] Torrella proceeds: "Astrologers say that this disease comes from a conjunction of superior bodies, for they say that a universal effect must be explained in reference to universal causes.[64] Others say that it is the *flagellum Dei*." Without any comment on either of these explanations, Torrella continues: "This malignant sickness, as they say, began in the year 1493 in France,[65] and from there, by way of contagion, it reached Spain, the islands, and Italy. At last, by its gradual spreading, it traveled through all Europe and, if it is possible to say, the whole world."

Torrella next engages in a prolonged discussion of the nature and identity of this disease. He dismisses a variety of seemingly possible ancient precedents and criticizes those physicians who maintained that if the identity of a disease was unknown, it was incurable. "But there is another sect of physicians with which I hold, who say that this disease is known along with its causes and manifestations, and will be curable." He then cites Avicenna's comment that often diseases receive their names from the bodily members in which they are located. "And therefore it will have to be christened with the name *pudendagra*, because it first begins on the *pudenda*. Thus it is able to be described. *Pudendagra* is a universal defilement of the skin of the body accompanied by pain and moderate loss of skin. And note that it does not always affect the whole body but most frequently it affects the extremities. But it is called universal because it can occupy the whole body or the greater part of it." He then asserts that it is curable, "which I prove by authority, reason, and experience."[66] Later he maintains that "although most frequently it comes by way of contagion, nevertheless also it otherwise can come from having a bad regimen."[67] A lengthy discussion of a wide variety of matters pertinent to humoral pathology then follows, in which he suggests that there are three species of *pudendagra*.

Torrella's recommendations for the cure of this disease are as conventional as are his explanations of its causes. He begins with a discussion of the non-naturals (although he does not employ that term) containing the only mention of sexual intercourse in the treatise, prior to the appended *consilia*. The patient "should forsake sexual intercourse, for sexual intercourse moves matter to the exterior and causes the warm vapor to come to the surface of the skin and then it putrefies there. On that account the sweat of the body of one who is engaging in sexual intercourse stinks."[68]

The main body of the treatise ends thus: "And I hope that, with the help of God omnipotent and the Virgin Mary, his most glorious mother, every species of *pudendagra* can be cured, if the adept physician apply and observe, in reference to place and time seriatim, those things that have been written above."[69]

Thus far Torrella has added nothing new to the understanding of morbus Gallicus. Although he would appear, by renaming it pudendagra, to have recognized that it was a venereal disease, his perception is entirely that of traditional humoral pathology. The disease may be contracted through bad regimen as well as by contact with the infected. Its appearance on the genitals is simply due to the bad humors' collecting in the weaker members. And for a physician who was also a priest and bishop, Torrella appears to be surprisingly uninterested in the theological significance of the disease. This is quite evident in the consilia that were appended to his treatise.

He writes that during September and October of 1497 he, as ordered by Cesare Borgia, had treated and cured seventeen patients who were suffering from pudendagra. The consilia are descriptions of five of these. This section begins thus: "And because I have written rather extensively not only about the understanding but also about the cure of this disease in general, it came to my mind to describe certain particular cases, so that greater faith might be placed in the dicta of physicians recorded in the treatise above,[70] for, as Seneca says in his tragedies, 'The greatest part of health is to believe oneself to be healthy.'"[71]

The first patient,[72] a twenty-four-year-old male, had had sexual relations in August with a woman who suffered from pudendagra "and therefore on the same day he himself was infected with the same disease, the infection beginning to appear on his penis." Torrella then describes other symptoms that appeared on the sixth and tenth days. The patient, a servant of the Borgia family, asked why, since he was infected by his first contact with an infected woman, he had not infected any of the numerous healthy women with whom he had subsequently had sexual intercourse. Torrella's response, typical of humoral pathology, was that this was not surprising "since men are warmer than women and they have open pores in their male member, and the fumes, corrupted by the matrix and weakened, corrupt it more quickly. But a woman, because she is colder, is not thus infected, except, perhaps, by frequent intercourse with an infected man. For the matrix is cold and dry, dense, and not at all open to harm. Also the semen of an infected man that is received by her is rather quickly ejected or, if retained, is quietly destroyed."

Before describing the cure of this patient, Torrella remarks that Cesare Borgia, "realizing that this servant of his had been seized by *pudendagra*, not only instructed me to cure him, but also said that he would allow himself to be cured, and with the greatest diligence he would observe and practice those things that I would prescribe. And so, beseeching God's help, I shall begin to write in the present *consilium* the method that I employed in his cure." The treatment began with the regulation of the non-naturals. In this section, Torrella says, "I forbade to him anger, quarreling, and sexual intercourse, by promising to him a quick return to health." The consilium ends with a description of the medications to be taken internally and applied externally, ending with the statement, "Thus with the help of almighty God and of the most glorious Virgin Mary, his mother, the patient was completely cured."

The second patient[73] was a forty-six-year-old man, a dock worker, who, according to Torrella's diagnosis, had contracted pudendagra in mid-August by exposing himself excessively to the rays of the sun and having an irregular regimen. Nevertheless, his penis was infected, and after thirty days other symptoms developed, including nonpustular sores over his whole body. Additional severe symptoms were soon evident. He was shunned by all owing to the extreme disfigurement of his face. "And therefore he came to me asking whether his sickness could be cured. He had no hope of recovery because he had been told that he was suffering from leprosy." After describing why this patient's symptoms could easily be confused with those of leprosy, Torrella writes, "Therefore, with good words, reasoning, and experience, I promised that man perfect health in a brief time, God permitting. And cure him I surely did." He next described the immediate treatment and then the regimen of the six non-naturals that he prescribed for this patient. In that context he remarks that "because there is a certain pleasure in sexual intercourse, for that reason, while I was talking about pleasure, I said that he should avoid sexual intercourse as much as possible for the time being, and if he were not able to abstain, he should at least be intimate with a woman who is not infected, and only after digestion is completed." The remainder of this consilium describes in detail the regimen and medications that Torrella prescribed.

The third patient[74] was a man thirty years of age. He, according to Torrella, "had been infected with *pudendagra* by contagion" ten months earlier. His night-pains were now so intense that he was unable to sleep. Torrella first turned his attention to a regimen of adustion of the patient's humors, which included the injunction to "rejoice and be joyful, flee from anger, sorrow, and anxiety, for before the month of October would pass he would be completely cured. And God is my witness that he related to me that the very same night he slept owing entirely to a firm belief and hope for health." Torrella continues with his description of this patient's regimen and concedes that the night-pains soon returned. The remainder of this consilium is devoted to a detailed account of the varied therapy that ostensibly proved effective for this patient.

The fourth patient[75] was a man of undisclosed age who had contracted the disease "by sleeping in the same bed with his infected brother." He came in much pain to Torrella. "And because it is an act of piety to succor the weak and especially the poor, by command of my most reverend Cardinal Valentinus [i.e., Cesare Borgia] and at his expense, with the patient's agreement, I cured him." Torrella arranged his regimen in accordance with the six non-naturals and prescribed a variety of medications. In addition a surgeon, a friend of the patient, treated his ulcerous sores. This consilium ends with the statement that he did not write these things for the sake of teaching but for the sake of remembrance. For all these things are commonplace and known to any educated physician. Nevertheless they may be corrected and emended in accordance with the judgment of doctors of medicine who should "entreat God, who is blessed for ever and ever, that by his mercy and love he would determine to purge the world of this plague."

The fifth and final patient[76] was a certain John of Toledo, a servant of the Borgias, fifty-five years of age. He had become infected with pudendagra during October, had been treated unsuccessfully by various physicians as well as quacks, "and after considerable trials, he had grown worse. And so, although with the greatest effort (for he was hardly able to move), he came to me saying, 'I am crushed, tortured, dying, and every night my mind begs for death.'" At this point the case history takes a very different turn from the previous four. Ernest L. Zimmermann remarks, "To him Torrella read a lengthy sermon (a digression well left out by Luisinus [a late-sixteenth-century editor of earlier syphilography])."[77] One could naturally assume that this "sermon" was a verbal chastening of the patient for his immorality. After all, the physician was also a bishop. But the "sermon" is a stern admonition not to listen to those who maintain that, if the *flagellum* was sent by God, then it is only to God himself that one should go for healing. This would be to put God to the test. Torrella recounts that years earlier he had "learned from a certain priest, a theologian who feared God, that I would sin if I were to hold this view." For God created physicians and herbs and other medicines for the succor of humanity's ills. Nevertheless, "I advise all to remember that they are both mortals and sinners, and that first of all it is proper that they seek divine help, but that they also should consult physicians, for the Almighty himself is kind and loving and merciful. He has already permitted physicians to understand this disease." Rather than a rebuke of the sinner, this "sermon" is simply a theological justification of the use of medicine and physicians in the face of what appear to have been some strong objections raised in various quarters.[78]

After this "sermon," Torrella informed the patient that he was suffering from a particular form of pudendagra that he then distinguished at length from a variety of conditions, including leprosy. Finally the cure of this patient is described, beginning with the non-naturals, during the description of which Torrella assured him that "with the help of God he would be completely well within a few days." After an extended description of the details of this patient's therapy, Torrella exclaims,

And thus with the help of omnipotent God and the most glorious Virgin Mary, not only did he continue freed from the disease but also, I hope, will be preserved. And afterwards, I determined to turn to other matters and to bring these *consilia* to a conclusion. There remains a prayer that Saint Damian was wont to say on bended knees for all draughts administered by him. Let him, whose words are as follows, conclude this treatise: "Omnipotent, eternal God, who have given medicine for curing the infirmities of men's bodies, give your sacred blessing from heaven upon this medicine, so that in whatever body it enters it may be efficacious in effecting health of mind and of body. Through Christ our Lord, who lives and reigns for ever and ever. Amen." Indeed, if anyone says this prayer in the presence of the patient, after any devout priest has said mass for him, the virtues of the medicine will increase and the patient will be cured more quickly.[79]

Bruce Thomas Boehrer, who apparently was unaware that Torrella was not only a physician but also a priest and bishop, remarks,

This early treatise on syphilis is distinguished both by its close, useful observation of the disease and by the patron to whom it is dedicated: Cesare Borgia, cardinal and archbishop of Valencia. Indeed, subject and patron are inextricably connected, for Torrella's medical clarity derives in part from Borgia's own excesses; by 1497, Torrella had treated the young cardinal (then twenty-one) for syphilis, together with at least seventeen other patients drawn from the Borgia family and the papal court *within a single two-month period* [Boehrer's emphasis]. In at least this early and important instance, thus, the physician's duties can only be served by a potentially self-destructive double discourse. The authority of the cardinalate forces one to view disease as the just, ineluctable *flagellum dei;* and yet the body of the stricken cardinal himself demands that one somehow find a way to avoid the whip—preferably without registering any nervousness or ambivalence in the process.[80]

Boehrer would have us believe that Torrella found himself in a most uncomfortable situation. Hence, treating a cardinal of the church who was suffering from the "just, ineluctable *flagellum dei*" was, as it were, supposedly to be party to a significant contradiction, which, according to Boehrer, placed poor Torrella in a very compromised position and forced him to walk precariously on a tightrope "without registering any nervousness or ambivalence in the process." But, quite to the contrary, insofar as morbus Gallicus was seen as the *flagellum Dei*, which did not mark its objects as greater sinners than others, succoring them involved no contradiction, not even a paradox. Even after he had designated the disease as pudendagra, Torrella did not regard those suffering from it as having been rewarded with due recompense for their profligacy. Its venereal nature, as explicated by humoral pathology, had not yet rendered it a venereal disease. Soon that would change, and the distinctly venereal nature of the disease would become patently manifest. And Torrella would write on the disease with greater clarity three years later. We shall return to him shortly to see whether in the interim this physician, priest, and bishop changed his attitude toward those suffering from this disease in light of his increased knowledge of its typical mode of transmission.

An Ongoing Italian Academic Debate: Natale Montesauro and Antonio Scanaroli (1498)

In 1498 two more syphilographic treatises were published in response to the disputations at Ferrara. The first of these, directed against Leoniceno, was *De dispositionibus quas vulgares mal Franzoso appellant*, by Natale Montesauro of Verona.[81] His argument with Leoniceno centers on the latter's attacks against the reliability of the Arabic physician Avicenna. There is little in Montesauro's treatise that is worthy of comment. He insists that the *mal Franzoso* is not a new disease—in this he agrees with Leoniceno—and that it was known to the ancients as *bothor, asaphatus,* and *tusius.*

The causes of the disease are both extrinsic and intrinsic. "Certain of the extrinsic causes are due the physician's consideration; certain ones are not." Those that are appropriate for the physician to consider are such matters as humoral imbalances, the non-naturals, and so forth. Perhaps the stars exercise an influence, but that is not of concern to the physician.[82]

He insists that he has observed cases in which the genitals are not affected, for they are affected only if the disease is contracted through sexual intercourse. But even then, humoral theory explains why the bad humors are concentrated there.[83] His only other reference to sexual intercourse is in his discussion of evacuations, which, he insists, should be maintained, either by nature or by art, in accordance with the patient's custom. "Therefore, if one is accustomed to sexual intercourse, although nothing is more harmful than a mistake occurring in sexual intercourse, nevertheless we hold that such a person may engage in it moderately and as he is accustomed. He should not abandon it entirely lest the semen that is accustomed to being emitted in sexual intercourse be converted into something noxious and corrupt the principal members. For those who are accustomed to sexual intercourse but do not wish to engage in it," the appropriate diet and medication will effect the evacuation of the semen.[84]

Montesauro's attack on Leoniceno via his defense of Avicenna aroused the indignation of one of Leoniceno's former students, Antonio Scanaroli of Modena, whose *Disputatio utilis de morbo Gallico, et opinionis Nicolai Leoniceni confirmatio contra Natalen Montesaurum Veronensem, eandem opinionem oppugnantem* was printed in March 1498.[85] He agrees with Leoniceno that it is appropriate to call this disease an epidemic because "the cause is universal and not remote, as perhaps the theologian or the astrologer maintain, but immediate such as is proper for the physician to advance as an explanation."[86] In reference to the involvement of the genitals, Scanaroli writes that Montesauro avoids the question of why the disease begins in the genitals and,

denying sense and reason, he maintains that unless the disease is contracted through contagion in sexual intercourse, [the genitals are not affected]. Nevertheless, we ourselves have seen, and all know this, that also very many boys and virginal girls, as well as the elderly, who never have engaged in sexual intercourse, when they are seized by this disease, first experience its inception in the genitals. On account of this most common occurrence, that most distinguished man, Gaspar Torrella, bishop of Saint Justa, in his book about this disease that he wrote not less learnedly than splendidly, called this very disease by the sensibly tasteful name *pudendagra*, because even if two or three out of a hundred were found in whom this disease began elsewhere, this says nothing against Leoniceno[,]

who maintained that this disease could not be *asaphatus* because the latter is typically first manifested on the head.[87] Scanaroli then presents the standard arguments for the collection of bad humors in the genitals of one suffering from morbus Gallicus even if the disease was not contracted by sexual intercourse.

If it was Scanaroli's intention to refute Montesauro point by point, in the most erudite fashion, regarding the latter's understanding of the nature of the morbus Gallicus, without contributing anything new to the understanding of this disease in the process, he succeeded admirably.

Francisco Lopez de Villalobos' Treatise (1498)

The next treatise on morbus Gallicus, and the first by a Spaniard, is a poem of seventy-four stanzas, *Sumario de la medicina en romance trovado con un tratado sobre las pestiferas bubas*, also published in 1498, from the pen of a twenty-four-year-old licentiate in medicine at the University of Salamanca, Francisco Lopez de Villalobos.[88] In stanza 3, convinced that this disease, which was exceedingly horrible, was entirely new, he exclaims,

> It was a pestilence ne'er to be found at all
> In verse or in prose, in science or in story,
> So evil and perverse and cruel past control,
> Exceedingly contagious, and in filth so prodigal,
> So strong to hold its own, there is little got of glory;
> And it makes one dark in feature and obscure in countenance,
> Hunchback'd and indisposed, and seldom much at ease,
> And it makes one pained and crippled in such sort as never was,
> A scoundrel sort of thing, which also doth commence
> In the rascalliest place that a man has.

He then describes two theological explanations of the disease. The first is in stanza 4:

> Theologians will say[89] the cause of it doth lie
> In certain new-found sins that are rife in Christendom.
> Oh! Providence divine, oh! judgment from on high!
> Which ever hast in store a perfect penalty.

Howe'er we go astray, our folly is brought home.
Out of heaven Thou has seen all this schism and dissension,
In thy sons and thy servants, both churchmen and lay,
How for mere opinion's sake and the lust of contention,
With shrewd swelling taunts and vehement intention,
They make appeal to arms in disorderly array.

God has sent this new disease as punishment for new sins. Gaskoin, in his note on this stanza, writes, "At this time schism was raising its head in Christian Europe. Savonarola was laying the foundation of a new sect at Florence, the *Piagnoni*. Scepticism was rampant in Italy; the world was stirred to new modes of thought, the gradual swelling of the storm before the Reformation. The writings of Erasmus at a period a little subsequent are full of lamentations over this wretched state of affairs."[90]

Villalobos, in the next one and one-half stanzas (5 and 6), speaks in the divine first person, switching back to normal first person usage halfway through the sixth stanza.

Since now ye turn aside from fighting the good fight
Of faith against the infidel at my behest,
And those brave faculties which I thought right
To furnish you withal are used to my despite,
With much of scandal to the church and joy to the unblest,
An Angel I will send, with skill to strike and lame
Each faculty, your waywardness I shall chastise.
Nor part that stirs, nor arm nor limb can 'scape the touch of
    shame
For all aggression impotent, disfurnished, dull, and tame,
And rack'd with cruel throes anon in very fearful wise.

And in seeing those go free that have headed the rout,
Don't go to believe that my messenger shall spare,
That he neither sees nor cares what each is about,
For he strikes as a' finds, both within and without,
And full well he knows who the ill intentioned are.
When in Egypt God sent such a one to destroy
His enemies' first-born, with terrible amends
For cruelty to Israel, He saved from annoy
The houses of the Jewish folk, by causing his envoy
To know by a clear sign the doorposts of his friends.[91]

An additional new sin has now been specified: they have turned from war against the infidel. Hence, for this new sin and the ones enunciated in the preceding stanza, God has sent this new disease. But an objection can be raised: many suffer from this new plague who are not responsible for, or participants in, these new sins. He has answered this concern in part in stanza 6, above. He now introduces a new dimension in stanza 7:

> And although as for me I read not the mystery
> Why sheep are made to pay for the shepherd's naughtiness,
> As seen in that great prophet who wrote the psaltery,
> Half the nation has to die for his shocking adultery,
> And my lord all the while goes free from sickness;[92]
> But seeing this complaint 'mong Christian folk prevail,
> And how that Church troubles have got the dominion,
> And the Schism to be new no less than what they ail,
> We must know the two alike to judge the matter well,
> I confirm as being good the aforesaid opinion.

Having endorsed this first theological explanation of the final cause of *las bubas*, he gives a second (stanza 8):

> But some to *lujuría*,[93] and all of wanton sense,
> To which the world is giv'n do refer the same.
> The ailment, say they, is a just and proper sentence;
> According to the sin so is the repentance,
> And the part that suffers most is the part most to blame.
> And this seems borne out by a passage in Scripture,
> Chapter XII, Genesis, where we read of Egypt's king,
> Pharaoh, engrossed by excellence of feature
> In Sarah. God struck him in his nature
> With this same disease, or some such other thing.

He had previously maintained unequivocally that las bubas was a new disease, after he had given the first theological explanation of this disease—a new disease for new sins—a position of which he expressed unhesitating approval. Now, having introduced a second theological explanation, he hedges on the question of whether las bubas is indeed a totally new disease, as we see in the last two lines above. He then proceeds to endorse this second theological explanation as well (stanza 9):

> And thus you'll surely see that those who do them keep
> From sharing in this sin do not become its drudge;
> But those who press the cup of pleasure to the lip,
> Do barely as by power of some miracle escape,
> Through righteous judgment of an all-righteous Judge.
> And so it is indeed the men have turned so chaste,
> They dare not now draw near to any woman, as we see.
> O mystery of God! that all are so straight-laced
> And humbly penitent wherein they have transgress'd,
> Because we could not do it in a moderate degree.

The sarcasm of the last three lines seems to be directed not against this second theological explanation but rather against the hypocrisy and inconsistencies of his fellow men in the sphere of *lujuría*.

In crediting both theological explanations, Villalobos is not particularly inconsistent. He appears to have regarded them as not mutually exclusive, but possibly as complementary. Of course it was not necessary for him to juxtapose the two and choose one over the other. He, after all, was not a theologian. So he turns from the final cause to the intermediate and immediate causes. Astrologers attribute the disease to the conjunction of Saturn and Mars, and physicians attribute it to celestially generated miasma affecting the humors. Hence the physicians, according to Villalobos, agree with the astrologers but are, as physicians, directly concerned with proximate causes, whereas the astrologers deal with intermediate causality. Ellis Hudson remarks that, although Villalobos accepted an astrological miasmatic intermediate origin, he specifies proximate causes such as "bad air, bad food and bad health habits, such as melancholic foods, excess in sex, gluttonous eating, inebriation, cold, draught, and lack of exercise. All of these, he said, produced 'adustion of the humors.' He listed sexual excess coordinately with other excesses, and did not attribute *las buvas* to venery *per se*."[94] The sexual organs are typically beset first, of course, because of the weakness of the genitals relative to the other organs, not because of sexual transmission. Hudson explains, "Although he recognized that the eruption appeared first on the genitals, he did not ascribe this to sexual contact, but to 'weakness' of the genitals relative to the other organs. He seems to have missed the point that the genital sore was the place where the infection entered the body."[95] Villalobos' only mention of sexual intercourse in his discussion of therapy is in the context of regimen of the non-naturals (in stanza 69):

> From all trashy food he should utterly abstain,
> And keep from loose thoughts and especially from women,
> From passion and rage, vexation and moan.

In *A History of Syphilis*, Charles Clayton Dennie, discussing Villalobos, writes, "The idea of ascribing the cause of this pestilence to a divine source was the accepted one and, due to the ignorance of the physicians, this was accepted for many years."[96] Dennie's misunderstanding of Villalobos springs from a twofold ignorance. First is a seriously distorted, but common, view of the perceived role of God in natural disasters and sickness in historical Judeo-Christian monotheism. Second is a failure to read carefully the very sources that he was analyzing, namely, the early syphilographic literature, in which, as we have seen and will continue to see, divine causality, regardless of the extent to which speculation about it might fascinate individual physicians, was compartmentalized and regarded as irrelevant to the concern of the physician *qua* physician, that is, immediate causes.

Petrus Pinctor's Treatise (1499)

Meanwhile, back in Italy, another of Pope Alexander VI's physicians was addressing the same disease. In 1499 Petrus Pinctor dedicated to Alexander VI a lengthy treatise entitled *Tractatus de morbo foedo et occulto, his temporibus afflingente*.[97] This, the most tendentious and verbose of the treatises thus far addressed, is also the most astrological in its orientation. Its preface begins with a discussion of the innate desire of all creatures to avoid death and the pernicious effects of disease. Pinctor then asserts that the further each thing is from its *principium*, the more vulnerable it is. Hence, the human race, now far removed temporally from Adam or from God, has been significantly weakened since the time of the antediluvians, whose individual life spans were extremely long. This brings Pinctor to the subject of medicine.

I am certain, most clement Pope Alexander VI, that you are not unaware how essential for humanity is the knowledge of medicine, which the ancients not unreasonably thought the immortal gods had invented. For it seems to be something divine rather than human to understand the varied *dispositiones* of the human body. In short the physician's work is divine or at least very close to a divine work. So, of course, the greatest diligence must be devoted to this field because our life as human beings is continually troubled (owing to the imperfection of *complexio, compositio,* and *unitas*) by diverse and almost innumerable species of diseases, just as at the present time the human body is being attacked by unknown sicknesses.[98]

One of these "unknown" diseases "evidently from the year 1494 even to the present year 1499" had been torturing a multitude of nations with a variety of symptoms. The name popularly given to it by the Romans was morbus Gallicus, but it was called by a wide variety of names by diverse peoples. "Nevertheless, the most learned doctors of medicine," Pinctor laments, "have said nothing about this disease, neither have they written about its cause, nor have they put in writing its cure."[99] There are at least three possible explanations for this remarkable statement: (1) Pinctor is yet unaware that any other physician has written on morbus Gallicus. (2) He knows that many, or at least several, have done so, but he does not regard them as being among "the most learned doctors of medicine." (3) No one yet had actually written on the correct disease because all thus far had misidentified it. Both the first and the second seem to be quite unlikely. The last will prove to be the most likely explanation.

Still in the preface, Pinctor briefly describes the astrological origins of the disease in question, and then remarks on the seriousness of the challenge facing the best and the brightest of the medical community and prays that "God, the regulator of nature, the only healer of diseases, may, by the unction of his Spirit, make complete my explanation of the cause of this unknown disease and of its cure, make famous the intellect of my old age, and illuminate my genius."[100] Then, after a discussion of the philosophical foundations of scientific inquiry into disease quiddity and causality, he returns to the subject at hand, reiterates much that he had already said about the spread of morbus Gallicus, refers to it as a contagious disease, argues that it does not spread only through contagion but is caused primarily by the "influence of erratic stars," laments once more that no one has ever said anything accurate about the appropriate name and quiddity of the disease, discusses its supposed identification with a wide variety of diseases, and ends his preface with an outline of the contents of the treatise to follow. Finally, in chapter 1 of the treatise, after detailing why it cannot be any of the various diseases with which others have identified it, he reveals its true identity: the third species of variolae, that is, *aluhumata*.[101]

In chapter 2 he notes that aluhumata is sometimes found in fetuses, never in young children, and only rarely in the senectuous.[102] Nowhere yet has he even alluded to sexual intercourse or any involvement of the genitals. His understanding of aluhumata is thoroughly formulated by an astrologically oriented humoral pathology. He argues on astrological grounds in chapter 4 that this disease actually had begun in 1483. Fortunately it will end in 1500. In the meantime, because of the conjunction of various planets, "this disease itself begins on peoples' genitals, typically on the glans penis of males and in the vulva of females, because Scorpio has his dominion in those realms."[103]

Pinctor has much to say about preservation from the disease. "First is to return blessing and glory to God and to the Virgin Mary, and so forth."[104] In the course of a sustained discussion of the six non-naturals, he mentions sexual intercourse under the rubric of exercise. Stressing the prophylactic importance of moderate exercise, he quotes Galen, that "those who are unable to exercise, ought to have mild massages and just slightly warm baths and engage moderately in natural acts of sexual intercourse." Pinctor then asserts that "bathing and sexual intercourse are indeed kinds of exercise" and cites Avicenna as additional authority for such a suggestion.[105]

After exhausting the prophylactic utility of a rational regulation of the non-naturals, Pinctor emphasizes, "This *morbus aluhumata* is contagious." Hence, "when being in a place infected by this disease, you should immediately flee. However, if you linger there very long, flight will provide little security." Very importantly, three things must be observed in flight. "The first of these is that whenever in any place or villa or city you see men who are infected with this disease, you should flee immediately. The second is that you should flee to places far away, safe places where men are not infected by such a disease as this. The third is that you should come back cautiously lest you go where *aluhumata* is attacking a multitude of men."[106]

Pinctor next describes some astral effects that produce environmental factors conducive to aluhumata. The safest places are those in which the air is *grossus*. "For the incarcerated, men who are confined, religious women who are confined, and those living . . . in marshy places that have air that is *aptus* or *grossus*, are safe from this *morbus aluhumata*." But once the disease has been brought into an otherwise safe environment, that area must be avoided. "For one man who has been infected with this disease can infect men even conversing with him or being in his presence. He can even infect the air of the room and the home and thus the disease passes from one man to another and from one house to another and that evil air is carried throughout the entire city and thereby the men of that city are infected by this contagion." Then, after discussing the type of contagion that is not conveyed by direct, physical contact with the infected, he writes,

Nevertheless, we assert that this sickness is quite contagious by means of sexual intercourse with a woman who has this *morbus aluhumata* and especially one with whom a man who has this disease has had sexual intercourse. For on account of a man's warmth and the openness of the pores of the *membrum virile* the vapors, when corrupted by matter and having increased, corrupt him quite quickly. For this cause and reason, intercourse must be avoided with a woman who is suffering from *morbus aluhumata*. A woman, however, is not thus infected, unless perhaps from frequent intercourse with an infected man, since her matrix is cold and dry, dense and very little receptive to damage. Indeed the semen of one suffering from *aluhumata,* once it has been received by her, is quite quickly ejected or, if retained, is quietly destroyed.

It is as though Pinctor has intentionally combined observations or ideas of Widmann, Gilinus, and Torrella. More likely he is quite independent of them, since humoral pathology easily conduced to such explanations. Pinctor next comments that although the authorities "say that this happens in lepers, we, however, also assert that it occurs in those who are suffering from this disease. For through experience we have seen it happen in such a time as the present, that this disease tortures men through contagion, especially from sexual intercourse with a woman infected by this disease."[107]

A More Experienced Torrella (1500)

In 1500, three years after writing his *Tractatus cum consiliis contra pudendagrum seu morbum Gallicum,* Torrella published a second treatise on pudendagra, *Dialogus de dolore tractatu de ulceribus in pudendagra evenire solitis,*[108] the first half of which is a fictitious discussion between a physician and a layman on the nature of pudendagra, with the major emphasis on the internal pains that typically are manifest in those suffering from the disease, and the second half being an analysis of the nature and treatment of the external sores that pudendagra causes.

The *Dialogus* opens with a description of the scope of Torrella's earlier *Tractatus.* Now he is directing his attention to the cause and the means of alleviating the excruciating internal pains of the disease. He stresses here, as he had in his earlier treatise, that it is essential that one know the nature of a disease to be able to treat it. He laments that the unskilled, stubborn, illiterate rabble had been publicly proclaiming that the science of medicine was vain and imperfect, because no physician was able to help those suffering from this disease. Indeed the learned were causing this criticism by fleeing from the task at hand and admitting that they themselves knew nothing about the nature of this sickness. Torrella writes:

And therefore dealers in spices, herb-gathers, certain mechanics, and vagabonds and imposters in these times declared themselves to be the true and perfect healers of this disease, and because they know nothing, they are in doubt about nothing, and promise marvels. If you heard them you would believe that they raise the dead but in a little while hope proves worthless. For a sudden and unexpected death cuts their patients off. Indeed bandits or murderers or poisoners kill men inhumanly. Such men, however, most humanely, courteously, and solemnly terminate them. And if anyone, nature helping or God permitting, gets better, they claim that they were cured by the benefit of their ointments, and they wish to be endowed not only with praises but also with rewards. Such men, being ignorant of medicine, misuse medicine, and they make a show of a distinguished and nearly divine art which they have never learned.

He goes on to assert that the physician can eradicate and thoroughly destroy the false reasoning of the rabble and urges his audience to listen.

It is at this point that the actual "dialogue" begins. The layman says, "Most learned doctor of medicine, tell me why it is that the common people in different regions call this disease by different names."[109] The physician's extensive response includes the well-known reasons why it is called *morbus Gallicus* in Italy but *morbus Neapolitanus* in France. The Valencians, Catalans, and Aragonese, however, named it *morbus Sementi* after much research had convinced them that an old disease bearing that name was the same as the present affliction. So also in some of the French realm. "For just as the common people call leprosy *morbus Sancti Lazari* after Saint Lazarus, likewise the French call the *malum mortuum* the *morbus Sancti Sementi,* because very many are cured by imploring his help, and especially if they go by foot to his body as beggars. The body of this saint is in Britain, held in the greatest veneration." Torrella then describes the traditional manner in which pilgrims approach this saint's shrine for the healing that is typically bestowed. Torrella, as a priest, bishop, and physician, appears to have approved this practice. Torrella then says that in Further Spain, where the disease is called *morbus Curialis* because it attacks the *Curia* (that is, the court, whether ecclesiastical or royal), physicians, unable to understand the disease, relinquished it to empirics. In Paris and in other great cities of France, it is identified with *grossa variola,* which Torrella insists he has already proved to be a false identification.

The layman now asks about the contagious nature of the disease and comments that he has no faith in the opinions of astrologers since "they seem in the present situation to proceed from the effect to the cause, although they ought to have prognosticated before the arrival of this disease by proceeding from the cause to the effect."[110] Torrella feels compelled to come to the defense of astrology as a science approved by reason, utility, and experience. "If anyone wishes to understand natural effects, he must give attention to the motions of the stars" since they "depend upon the divine will." Astrology's only defects are in its modern practitioners who deceive thousands by their prognostications, "for very often the blessed God tests us to see whether we love him."[111] Torrella's argument is with predictive and determinative astrology, the failures of which he seeks to illustrate by historical examples.

Turning now to the contagiousness of the disease under consideration, he writes,

In my previous tractate I had said that it came through contagion, just as scabies, which infects through contact. In fact, most often the genitals are first infected, then the other members. For whatever is touched directly by the infection is infected. Hence if another member were to touch a sordid or virulent pustule, that very member is infected first. This is evident in nursing babies. In these the infection first appears on the mouth or on the face. This happens either from the infected breasts of the wet nurse or, since wet nurses very often are wont to kiss the infants, it comes from their infected faces or mouths. And very often I have seen an infant who is infected with this disease infect many wet nurses.[112]

Torrella then makes it abundantly clear that he has rejected the typical explanation of the genitals' usually being the first members that become pustulous. He urges that one not believe that the genitals attract the sordid or virulent matter from other parts of the body. He does not break with humoral pathology, however, but uses its principles to argue against the feasibility of the standard explanation of genital infection that he and other earlier authors had given. "Therefore it remains," Torrella insists, "that the contagion is multiplied by itself and finally infects these members, for the malignant matter itself, by its own malignity and corrupt property, corrupts and converts into its own nature anything that it touches."

The layman now asks whether any means of preservation could be found. Torrella replies, "I have said in my tractate on *pudendagra* that the best remedy is to beware of the infected as one avoids lepers. Nor is flight alone sufficient, for the disease is found everywhere." After remarking that "the infection does not begin immediately, but the principal members, as I have said, are infected over time, and finally the whole body," he suggests that the reader turn to the end of his *Tractatus de ulceribus*, where the subject of preservation is treated at some length. There we find,

I have decided to place at the end of this work the chapter on the manner of preservation from so foul and contagious and so destructive a sickness as *pudendagra* is, although the true preservation is to beware of those who are infected (for this sickness is contagious, just as scabies that infect through contact) and especially to beware of prostitutes and so forth. As I have said in the first tractate, usually the genitals are first infected, then the other members, for whatever is immediately touched by that which is infected is itself infected.

This passage continues as a nearly verbatim repetition of his earlier statements on infants and wet nurses and his insistence that one must not give credence to the theory that the genitals attract the fetid matter from elsewhere in the body. For anyone who is infected in the genitals and "wishes to be preserved from falling into a worse condition" Torrella then prescribes a variety of procedures, including various medications to be applied to the pustules on the male genitals.[113]

We see that a change has occurred in Torrella's understanding of the nature of the disease and its transmission—a refinement, as well as a narrowing of focus. This is well illustrated by the following exchange in the *Dialogus*. The layman asks, "Is it possible for this disease to be eradicated from our midst?" The physician responds, "It is, indeed, possible with the help of almighty God and of his mother, the most glorious Virgin Mary." Then, in answer to the layman's question regarding how this could be accomplished, the physician says, "The rulers, such as the pope, the emperor, kings, and other magistrates, should appoint *matronae* who would carefully examine prostitutes especially, and those whom they find to be infected they would confine in a place appointed by either the community or the magistrate, and there they would be cured[114] *a medico seu chirurgico deputato,* and in this manner will this disease be eradicated without fail [*infallibiliter*]."[115]

Another change that Torrella had undergone warrants reference. In the *Tractatus* he had recommended the external application of mercury in the treatment of pudendagra, although he had not even mentioned it, much less prescribed it, in any of his five consilia. In the dedicatory epistle to a second edition of the *Tractatus* he had warned against and condemned the use of mercury on those suffering from pudendagra.[116] In his *Dialogus* he is even more outspoken against the use of this drug. He inveighs against charlatans and quacks who were thus seriously harming, even killing, some of their patients, and he urges physicians to intervene in order to compel such irresponsible practitioners to desist.[117] At the end of the *Dialogus* he credited the deaths of two members of the Borgia family and a Spanish cardinal to mercury therapy.[118]

The failure of Bishop Torrella, physician to the pope and the Borgia family, in his *Tractatus* of 1497, to make a moral judgment on the contracting of the disease was not simply diplomatic. It was entirely consistent with the view that those affected during epidemics were no greater sinners than those left unscathed. And even after the predominantly venereal nature of the transmission of pudendagra had become clear to him, which it surely had by 1500, he did not see the venereal character of the disease as evidence that it was punishment for sexual sin.

Antonio Benivieni's Treatise (before 1502)

Antonio Benivieni, a Florentine physician who died in 1502, had left the manuscript of a work that was published posthumously under the title *De abditis nonnullis ac mirandis morborum et sanationum causis* (On some hidden and remarkable causes of disease and recovery).[119] The first chapter, entitled "De morbo quem vulgo Gallicum vocant," begins with the statement that in the year 1496 "a new kind of disease crept over Italy and nearly all Europe. It began in Spain, and spreading thence far and wide, first over Italy and then through France and the other countries of Europe, attacked most [*plurimi*] of the inhabitants."[120] His description of the symptoms begins with the observation that "pustules of various kinds broke out first on the genitals (sometimes it might be on the head, but this rarely)." Throughout this chapter he warns against "*imperiti medici* who, in complete ignorance of the causes of this disorder, hasten with their mixtures of ointments to cure it in its first stages. Thus they often bring their patients to their death or to a worse or even completely incurable state."[121] But "*peritissimi medici* claim to undertake a cure with these very drugs (which also cure *lepra*) if a disease of this type has spread over the whole body."[122] He then describes his own method of treatment of the disease at its various stages.

This short syphilographic piece is more interesting for what it fails to address than for what it does address. Although he recognized that the first evidence of morbus Gallicus appeared on the genitals, Benivieni says nothing about the transmission of the disease. Nor does he give any advice on how to avoid it. He makes no judgmental assessment of those who suffered from this affliction. He avoids speculation about intermediate and final causes. In making no comment about final cause, he sidesteps theological considerations entirely. Does this tell us anything directly about his theological, as distinct from his professional, views? When Leoniceno *appeared* to have dismissed the possibility of divine agency in the advent of morbus Gallicus, it elicited from Anna Foa her hearty approval, as we have seen above. However, even Leoniceno did not deny the possibility of a divine final cause. Rather, as a physician, he concentrated on proximate causes. But whereas Leoniceno seems generally to have been quite humanistic, Benivieni was a deeply spiritual man,[123] as is unequivocally demonstrated by the accounts of miraculous cures that he includes in his posthumously published manuscript.[124]

Even a cursory reading of these accounts should impress one that Benivieni's religious devotion was obviously personal and deeply cherished. Nevertheless, he apparently felt no inclination *as a physician* to link sin and sickness or to speculate concerning divine purposes regarding the epidemic of morbus Gallicus. Villalobos, the tone of whose work evinces much less personal piety, did not hesitate to devote considerable space to theological speculation, yet without making any moral judgments against individuals who suffered from the disease. So also with the next author to be considered.

Juan Almenar's Treatise (1502)

Juan Almenar of Spain, *artium et medicinae doctor,* in 1502 published his *De morbo Gallico libellus.*[125] Almenar appears to have been a man of personal piety. In the preface to his treatise, he writes that, compelled by piety, in the face of the suffering of those afflicted by this disease, grieving over the extent of physicians' ignorance of how to treat the ill,

I implored the assistance of the highest Craftsman. Insofar as he will illuminate my mind for writing, to that degree will the remedies that I shall give in the following pages prove able to cure, and he will lavishly bestow favor on the ill by restoring them to health. Therefore, I shall endeavor to deliver to you a treatise by which you may teach the healthy how to guard against *morbus Gallicus,* and thus you may free the ill so that the disease will never return. . . . May praise and glory be given to God! And as the wages of my labor, may it be pleasing to you and to those, who will benefit from my labor, to pray to him. In supplication we entreat you, God, that whoever does this favor for us would himself be strengthened by your favor, so that he and we also would be free from misery, both of soul and of body. Amen.[126]

Almenar was convinced that the origins of morbus Gallicus were astral, but that since its inception the disease had been transmitted by contact with infected people. Miasmic infection, however, must still linger on. How else, he asks, can we account for cases of the disease among the religious (i.e., among those who lived in religious houses, such as monks and nuns)? But acquiring the disease in this manner was, by then, he asserts, extremely rare.[127] He felt that the most common form of transmission was through sexual intercourse, although he believed that the disease might also be contracted through kissing and breast-feeding of infants.[128] Although Almenar was well aware that the disease was contagious and was contracted primarily though sexual intercourse, nevertheless he, like so many other contemporary syphilographers, never argued that infected patients should abstain from sexual intercourse because of the risk of infecting their sexual partners. Hence in his discussion of the cure of the disease, when considering the non-naturals, he writes, with reference to emotions, "Sexual intercourse, however, should be moderate" and should take place only after digestion is complete.[129]

Morbus Gallicus, Almenar remarks early in chapter 1, according to certain wise men "ought now to be called *patursa,* which is interpreted *passio turpis saturnina, turpis* [which means disgraceful or filthy as well as ugly or unsightly] because it causes women to be regarded as unchaste and irreligious, and generally it disfigures all. It is saturnine because it had its origin from Saturn on account of its entrance into Aries."[130] Later in chapter 1, after identifying the efficient cause as celestial, the formal cause as a bad physical constitution *(mala dispositio),* and the material cause as "when it is said to be in one's members," he writes, "But the *medicus corporalis* does not involve himself [*non se intromittit*] with the final cause. The *spirituales medici,* however, assert that it has arisen as punishment of sins [*peccata*]. And therefore, whoever would be freed from this or would avoid it, let him guard against transgressions [*delicta*] so that he may devote his mind to God. For God alone heals sicknesses."[131]

Almenar returns to this subject in chapter 5, "Concerning Precautions for Avoiding Morbus Gallicus," where he writes,

Let those who would avoid *morbus Gallicus* especially be on guard against transgressions [*delicta*]. Wherefore it is typically said that misfortunes [*adversa*] occur on account of sins [*peccata*], and especially they ought to be on guard against the sin of *luxuria,* for it is said in Job that *luxuria* is a fire that continuously devours to the point of destruction,[132] and *spirituales medici* say that different sicknesses occur on account of different sins, such as quotidian fever on account of the sin of pride, gout on account of sloth, leprosy on account of *luxuria,* and so on concerning others. Therefore, since this disease resembles leprosy, it must be attributed to *luxuria.* But because these things pertain *ad alium medicum* [i.e., to the *spiritualis medicus*], what has been said must be sufficient. Therefore let us say what is important for us, that a man, of course, should guard against associating very much with the infected, and chiefly against sexual intercourse with an infected woman, for this disease is contagious.[133]

A little later in the same chapter he says that "there is a certain category [of sickness] that passes from one thing to another, such as leprosy, scabies, variolae, and pestilential fevers, also *apostemata putrida*. Since this sickness [sc. *morbus Gallicus*] is fashioned similarly [*conformatur*] to leprosy or scabies, it is proper to call it contagious." At this point he gives some specific advice about how to protect oneself against contagion. For example: "If it happens that a blemish occurs on the penis on account of sexual intercourse, immediately it must be met with the following lotion." After giving the recipe for this lotion, he recommends that "for greater safety, when a man and a woman have completed the act of sexual intercourse, let them wipe very thoroughly around their genitals" with particular types of cloths. The man is then advised to beware of contact with the cloths that such women [*ipsae mulieres*, probably prostitutes] have used for this purpose "since they [sc. the cloths] have been contaminated." Then "for greater safety still, let him wash the area" in the prescribed manner.[134]

Almenar's treatise is especially fascinating. He appears to have been a man of deep personal piety. He certainly seems to have been sincere in his conviction that miasmic infection must account for the fact that cloistered religious sometimes contracted the disease. He also suggests a theologically based linking of individual sicknesses with the "seven deadly sins," a late medieval aberration that represented a minority position among theologians, not to speak of physicians. Nevertheless, he not only recommends moderate engagement in sexual intercourse rather than abstinence for his infected patients, but also gives advice to the healthy about how to engage in "safe sex." Almenar is an outstanding, albeit somewhat extreme, example of the harmonious congruence of what may strike the modern reader as discordancies and incongruities.

A Very Changed Joseph Grünpeck (1503)

In 1503 we hear again from Joseph Grünpeck, who, after he had himself contracted syphilis, wrote a subsequent work on the disease, *Libellus de mentulagra alias morbo Gallico*.[135] In 1498 he had traveled to Italy and viewed firsthand soldiers who were suffering from the disease laid out in a field; according to his misiatric biases, they were shunned by physicians owing to their putridly disgusting sores and left untreated except by some well-intending and compassionate rustics. His account of their suffering and specific symptoms is unmatched except by his terrifying description of his own physical and mental anguish when he was similarly afflicted.

How Grünpeck perceived that he had contracted the disease himself is unclear. In the preface to the *Libellus* he writes that "on the occasion of a banquet I had arranged at Augsburg . . . at which not only Bacchus and Ceres, but also Venus, were present, there intruded into the midst of the revelry, that nurse of human pestilences, Contagion, bearing countless darts of infection. Terrified, we all abandoned our feast and took to our heels. But scarcely had I set foot on the countryside beyond the gate of Augsburg . . . when a cruel deity [*infelix numen*], assaulting me unawares from behind, wounded me most grievously."[136] The preface continues with a confession that nothing recommended in his earlier treatise proved helpful now; as well as with accusations of incompetence and greed against the physicians and surgeons at whose hands he had suffered, a short description of the techniques that he devised whereby he had cured himself, and finally the suggestion of a name for the disease—*mentulagra*, because it afflicts the *mentula* (Latin for penis).

The *Libellus* proper is a fascinating mixture of descriptions of the disease and denunciations of the motives and competence of nearly everyone who attempted to treat it. Grünpeck maintains that his penis was so swollen that only with difficulty could he encircle it with both hands. He movingly describes how shame *(verecundia)* had caused him to remain hidden and not disclose the nature of his affliction even to his closest friends. "Finally, prevailed upon by their entreaties, I made known, with certain reservations, the troubles that were besetting me, namely, that I had been attacked by a certain disease that people call *morbus Gallicus* or *Francicus*. No sooner had I uttered this word than my dearest friends took to their heels as if an enemy with naked weapons were at their backs. From thereon, they did not observe the obligations of hospitality or friendship."[137] Although he excoriates the friends who had fled from him in fear, there is, in all his extensive, vitriolic vituperations against physicians, surgeons, pharmacists, empirics, quacks, and rustics, no suggestion that any of them ever refused to treat him.

A question that Grünpeck raises, while contemplating his wretched state, is why this disease, more cruel and horrible than all others, had beset humanity at this time. His answer is that even in the best of times God sends numerous afflictions, including pestilence, to expiate people's sins, which he regards as an act of mercy on God's part. But the present age is one in which honesty has given way to vice, crime is being praised, religion is held up to mockery, justice is replaced by vengeance, good faith by violence, solemn oaths by fraud, innocence by guilt, courage, temperance, and all other virtues are held in contempt. Indeed, that alone is considered good, upright, and honest among men which is the perpetual enemy of goodness and honesty. Nor does the stupidity of mankind fear the whirlwind of punishment which the Heavenly Father, up to now so merciful, has inflicted because of the sins committed against Him. Therefore He hurls down new destruction, the cruelty of which is such that, should mankind not repent and should a worse plague follow, it is reasonable to believe that the whole world is doomed. Should anyone wish to deny this, he will at once be confronted by the following argument. There has never been a century so pure and guiltless that it has remained free from the hardships of adversity and affliction. In past times, the common excesses of human frailty, insolence, greed for money, lust and malice were expiated by special punishments such as floods, conflagrations, plagues of locusts and rats, famine, slaughter and pestilence. At present our sins are being expiated not only by these punishments, all of which are at present prevalent amongst us, but also by far crueler miseries and sufferings. Whence it necessarily follows that our life is being sullied and depraved by sins more wicked than those of our forefathers. Because of this depravity, this cruel disease, most horrible of all, is being visited upon us.[138]

After Grünpeck had described the regimen and medications by which he had ostensibly cured himself, he thus concludes his treatise:

But lest I pass by in silence divine medicine, than which there is nothing more useful, health giving and efficacious to human frailty, I exhort all mortals, not only those already defiled by these foul calamities and afflicted with these unspeakable agonies, but also those who have not yet tasted of the bitterness of this vile filth, that they appease with devout prayer the stern avenger of crime, God Almighty, Who inflicts this destruction upon humanity because of those base crimes into which all men have submerged themselves. This He does that He may snatch them, ensnared in crime and the evils of this disease, from the storms of ill health and restore them to the peaceful and safe haven of good health and keep the innocent and those still free from the disease safely on the shores of security. Surely the Prince of Pity, Who does not measure out health according to the greatness and seriousness of one's deserts, but according to the magnitude of His divine grace and compassion, aware even of the slightest ray of devotion, penitence and contrition on the part of miserable sinners, shall immediately pour forth health, giving medicines which shall not only preserve human bodies from this poisonous pest, but shall immediately destroy it.[139]

It should be noted that Grünpeck apparently was aware that the disease was most typically contracted through sexual intercourse. His obscure and highly literary style precludes our knowing even whether he knew how he himself had been infected. His mention of the banquet at which not only Bacchus (wine) and Ceres (food) were present, but also Venus (sex), suggests that he viewed the latter as responsible, although his being "assaulted unawares from behind by a cruel Deity" hardly renders the situation more perspicuous. This is further obfuscated by this statement later in the treatise by which he describes his contracting the disease: "That foul disease . . . attacked me unexpectedly while strolling about the countryside of Augsburg and implanted its poisonous arrow in my glans penis."[140] Even if he knew that he had contracted the disease by venereal contact with an infected woman, it was not the manner in which he was afflicted with morbus Gallicus but its very extreme priapic manifestation that appears to have caused him such shame that he was loath to reveal the nature of his ailment. The flight of his friends when he finally did disclose his condition to them was obviously precipitated by fear, not of direct venereal infection but of being infected by merely being in his presence. Given a century and a half of intermittent plague and the fear of miasmic contagion in the face of any disease that had even an ostensible affinity with plague—that is, any disease that was popularly viewed as epidemic and highly communicable—their reaction is not surprising. It is clear that they were not shunning him as one contaminated by a disease that was specifically sexual in its nature and transmission. Nor did Grünpeck regard himself as being punished with this disease for sexual sin or, for that matter, for any specific sin. Rather, as is obvious from the extended quotations above, he believed that his sickness had resulted from God's just anger against Grünpeck's contemporaries in general and not against Grünpeck in particular.

Jacobus Cataneus's Treatise (ca. 1504)

Jacobus Cataneus de Lacumarino, *doctor artium et medicinae* of Geneva, published his *De morbo Gallico tractatus* circa 1504.[141] In various ways, it is the most theologically oriented of the treatises we have thus far encountered. Cataneus begins with a short account of the origin of morbus Gallicus, which he was convinced was a new disease brought into Italy in 1494 by the invading French army. He calls it a monstrous disease that "disfigures women and men" and is accompanied by excruciating pains and "so attacks the human race that any kind of death whatsoever is preferable. It is indeed contagious, sparing neither sex nor age nor region . . . seizing princes, nobles, and common folk equally. A certain man has called it *pudendagra* because it begins on the genitals through sexual intercourse with an infected girl. . . . We affirm that it is a new disease by which angered Jove himself deployed his just wrath against us."[142]

Cataneus is especially interested in the causes of morbus Gallicus, to which chapter 3 of his treatise is devoted. He writes: "Some causes of *morbus Gallicus* are superior and incorporeal. I call those incorporeal that through celestial influence and not through contact act against these inferior things. Other causes are inferior and corporeal. These act against human bodies through contact, by infecting them. . . . Its cause is universal, which it is not proper to say unless the cause is a celestial influence. It is, I say, universal" because it has afflicted people in all regions. Cataneus wishes, however, to disassociate himself from determinative astrology:

A wise man will rule over the stars. Although, of course, the stars resolutely incline us to good and evil, nevertheless they do not compel. For by free will we are able to direct ourselves, irrespective of the stars, in all things. And therefore we believe that this disease was sent down by the sovereign God against mortals because of their sins in order to punish those who continually and indiscriminately pursue adulteries and sexual unions forbidden by law, and live in the manner of brute beasts. As the prophet says, "They have been made like a horse or a mule, in whom there is no understanding."[143] This insight, since it is true and universal, is corroborated by the sayings of the pagans, as it is by the lyric poet in his songs: "Through our sin we let not Jove lay down his bolts of wrath."[144]

Cataneus then refers to Thucydides' remark (in the account of the plague in his *Peloponnesian War*), that while the pestilence was raging, some recalled that it had been presaged by the prophetic verse "A Dorian war shall come and pestilence with it."[145] This leads Cataneus to Pliny's description of *colum*, a disease that had occurred during the principate of Tiberius and had first attacked the emperor himself. He then quotes Pliny: "What are we to say that this means? Or what wrath of the gods? Were the recognized kinds of human disease, of which there are more than three hundred, too few, so that they must be increased by new ones to add to men's fears?"[146]

In spite of Cataneus' fascination with divine causality, he immediately asserts that these matters are not connected with the art of medicine. "For in the present situation, since we are acting as a physician, let it suffice for us to describe only proximate and inferior causes." He then describes six immediate causes of morbus Gallicus, introduced by the unequivocal insistence that "this disease is contagious." The first and usual cause is transmission "through sexual intercourse with an infected woman or with an infected man. The membrum virile or the vulva is first infected by contact with an ulcer on the same members." The second cause is sexual intercourse with a woman who has no ulcer in her vulva. In this case the infection is caused by "an evil ulcerative quality present in the vulva." The third cause is the "*sperma* of the girl, said to be *gutta,* because, coming down from the veins of the whole body, it can infect the membrum virile by contact. . . . We have seen very many men who were healthy in reference to their membrum virile . . . but sanguinously inclined to this disease. These, by sexual intercourse with a healthy woman, were infected and this does not happen except by contact with the woman's *semen* when it is infected by an evil ulcerative quality." The fourth cause is "sexual intercourse with a healthy woman, while the *semen* of an infected man who has recently had sexual intercourse with her is still present in her matrix."

Only the fifth and sixth causes do not involve sexual intercourse. The fifth cause is living for a sustained period in close proximity with an infected woman or with an infected man. "For we have seen very many mothers, who cared for and ministered to their sons who were infected with this disease, in due time incur this infection themselves. Also we have seen in this manner very many infants, who were infected with the disease, in turn infect very many wet nurses." The sixth cause is the milk of an infected woman on whose body there is no cutaneous eruption. "On this account I advise that infants not be given to wet nurses who are suffering from this disease, unless they have been very well cared for, and if possible they should be entirely avoided, for this disease is most easily contracted."[147]

Now Cataneus asserts that there is considerable variation from person to person, depending on each individual's *dispositio.*

For I have seen very many who do not decline sexual unions with unclean women and rush precipitously into filth and sexual licentiousness, and nevertheless do not become infected from this. But it happens in this disease, just as in epidemics, that probably those who keep their bodies healthy and clean do not suffer from these things, as Avicenna says. All the same, it is safer to abstain and to be cautious, "because it is written, 'You shall not tempt the Lord your God.'"[148] Even as the lyric poet says, "Rarely does Vengeance, although of halting gait, fail to overtake the sinner, though he have a head start."[149]

In chapter 5, "Concerning the Prognosis of *Morbus Gallicus,*" Cataneus distinguishes various categories of people with reference to the degree of difficulty involved in effecting a cure. The first category that he mentions consists of "adulterers and brothel-keepers and those who are given to sexual licentiousness." These are more liable to this disease than others. "Youths are more easily cured, for the most part, than the elderly."[150] In answer to the question Who is more susceptible to this disease, a man or a woman? Cataneus replies, "It must be said that a man is, because he is warmer and consequently the pores of the glans penis have more openings through which this poison can easily enter and run through the entire body and infect the sanguinous mass. A woman, however, since she is cooler than a man, is not as easily infected except by frequent sexual intercourse with an infected man, and that is because the matrix, being cold, dry, and dense, resists more effectively the exterior causes." This, as we have seen, is quite standard. Cataneus, however, goes on to say, "Nevertheless, I have seen very many women who have been infected from a single instance of sexual intercourse with an infected man, as they themselves affirm."[151]

In regard to prevention, Cataneus begins his advice at the most basic level: "If anyone wishes to be preserved from this disease, let him note the causes that produce this disease, and, as much as he is able, let him flee from them. . . . And since this disease usually is contracted by sleeping with an infected woman, therefore, above all else, sexual intercourse with infected women and with prostitutes must be avoided."[152] Then, after discussing various ways to strengthen one's constitution to render one less susceptible to contracting morbus Gallicus, he devotes considerable space to the treatment of those who are infected. He strongly advocates the use of mercury and criticizes Gaspar Torrella for his condemnation of the use of this therapeutic substance.[153]

Cataneus was a man of very strong opinions. He does not mince his words when describing the conduct that most conduces to contracting morbus Gallicus. His disapproval of sexual looseness is patently conjunctive with his religious convictions. Yet he never questions the appropriateness of treating those suffering from morbus Gallicus, irrespective of the manner in which they contracted it, and he clearly regarded sexual intercourse as the dominant means of infection. Not only did he unequivocally believe that divine purpose behind the disease is not within the purview of the physician, but also he was convinced that God was distinctly interested in successful treatment being effected through Cataneus' treatise. In fact, midway through the tractate he writes, "If those things that I have said and will say prove to be well said, let all praise be ascribed to almighty God to whom I give great praise, because he has taught me these things and he has chosen me to be the proclaimer of these discourses."[154] He concludes the treatise with the prayer, "Let these things that I have said be sufficient, to the praise of the sovereign and eternal God, who is blessed for ever and ever. Amen."[155] And throughout the treatise there are parenthetical asides such as *Deo dante, Deo duce, Deo concedente, nutu Dei,* and *auxiliatus Dei.*[156]

Cataneus was indeed a deeply religious physician and morally sensitive to the sexual licentiousness that he regarded as most responsible for the spread of the disease. Nevertheless he was thoroughly convinced that his divinely directed role as a physician was to care for the ill who suffered from this disease, irrespective of the exact circumstances surrounding their contracting it.

Conclusions

Although there are numerous minor differences among the authors of the treatises written before 1500, they are similar on the major areas of interpretation. Morbus Gallicus, whether a new disease or an old one that had reappeared, was contracted by contagion, as contagion was then defined, that is, it was contracted miasmically by the effects of one's immediate environment, or physically by contact with the infected. One means of contact was sexual intercourse. But sexual intercourse conduced to certain diseases even if the act itself was not the immediate means of contracting the disease, because sexual intercourse, by certain types of people or under a variety of circumstances, could affect the humors adversely, rendering one more susceptible to contracting disease either miasmically or by contact with the infected. Nevertheless, according to some authorities, those who were accustomed to sexual intercourse needed to continue that form of evacuation lest their health be jeopardized by retention of the semen. Some others held that sexual intercourse, if engaged in moderately, was a salutary form of exercise. And yet others endorsed it for some patients since it was pleasant and hence involved a salubrious emotion. Why did the pustular manifestation of the disease typically occur first on the genitals? Because the bad humors typically concentrated in the weaker members.

There is considerable disagreement among these authors regarding the relevance of intermediate astral causality for the physician's understanding of the disease. They disagree little if at all about the relevance of final, that is, divine, causality for the physician. It is extremely unlikely that any of them would have denied that God's sovereign will effected and affected temporal and material affairs. There would have been some dispute among them, as among other segments of their society, regarding the extent to which God's purposes were specifically identifiable. They vary among themselves in the degree of their interest in questions regarding divine causality. But one constant is this: in the final analysis, final causality was entirely irrelevant to the physician's understanding of immediate causality, prophylaxis, and cure.

They most certainly did not see the disease as punishment specifically for sexual sin. Intercourse with an infected woman was simply one way of contracting the disease. Nor did they imply that those afflicted, regardless of how they contracted it, were especially sinful. In short, by the end of 1499 the medical writers on morbus Gallicus, irrespective of the substantial interpretative differences that prevailed among them and in spite of the ostensible tidiness of Torrella's creation of the name *pudendagra,* had not yet come to see this disease as being in a category that conveys the nuances that are basic to such designations as venereal or sexually transmitted disease. Nor did any stigma yet attach to those who suffered from this variously named disease.

There was no spectacular change in the understanding of morbus Gallicus marked specifically by the year 1500. Nevertheless, the syphilographic treatises written during the next five years differ in some ultimately significant ways from those composed earlier. There is little reference in these later treatises to the humoral explanation of genital pustules, that is, that the genitals, being the weakest members, attract the putrid humors. This theory had thoroughly conditioned the earliest explanations of the disease. The modern reader who is unaware of the underlying humoral theory, however, can easily see in the treatises on morbus Gallicus that were composed prior to 1500 something that simply is not there: a recognition by the authors that the disease was primarily transmitted through sexual intercourse as a *direct result* of that act. Even those very earliest syphilographers, who emphasized both that the disease was highly contagious and that it was very frequently contracted through sexual intercourse with the infected, viewed both through a humoral pathoanatomical grid that did not readily conduce to explaining genital pustules as originating from direct genital contact with the genital pustules of the sexual partner. But in the treatises written from 1500 to 1505 we see a recognition of the primarily venereal nature of morbus Gallicus, in other words, a recognition that this was (to use a modern expression) primarily a sexually transmitted disease. Recourse to the earlier explanation of genital pustules was primarily taken in order to account for their presence on people who either could not have contracted the disease through sexual intercourse (e.g., infants) or, in the opinion of the syphilographer, would not have (i.e., the cloistered). It is in reference to the latter that Almenar piously resurrected miasmic contagion, a very important explanation of morbus Gallicus for the very earliest syphilographers, which had by Almenar's time fallen mostly into desuetude.

The treatises on syphilis that were composed from 1500 to 1505, however, have much in common with those written earlier: (1) In spite of the later authors' recognition that the disease was typically transmitted through sexual intercourse with an infected partner, the role of sexual intercourse in the regimen of the six non-naturals remains essentially the same as before. (2) The later syphilographers also disagreed among themselves about the reality of intermediate astral causality. Those who believed in its reality differed among themselves on its relevance for the physician. (3) In regard to the final cause, it is extremely unlikely that any of the syphilographers who wrote from 1500 to 1505 would have denied the sovereignty of God over the affairs of nature. But like the earlier syphilographers, they ranged from those who made no mention of divine involvement in morbus Gallicus to those who were eager to explicate it. Even the latter, however, explicitly state that such matters are not the business of the physician. (4) Even though the venereal nature of the disease had become conspicuously evident, and some theologically oriented syphilographers expressed strong moral disapproval of those who, because of their sexual conduct, were most liable to contract the disease, these factors appear not to have affected even slightly the syphilographer *qua* physician's attitude toward the patient who had contacted the disease by promiscuous behavior. None of the syphilographers' advice on sexual intercourse in their regulation of the regimen of the six non-naturals is affected in any way by religious or moral considerations. And interestingly, Almenar, one of the most manifestly religious authors, who linked the sickness quite specifically to sin, also prescribed methods for "safe sex."

Not once does any author advise the infected patient (assumed to be male) to refrain from sexual intercourse lest he infect his sexual partner (assumed to be female). Of course, owing to the supposed coldness, dryness, and denseness of the female reproductive organs, women were much less apt to contract the disease than men. Accordingly, women rarely were infected sexually except by frequent intercourse with infected men. A man, by contrast, could be infected by a single act of coitus with an infected woman. Hence, assuming that these authors did in fact believe that what they wrote was true, in their opinion the women who transmitted the disease to men were those who had been sexually active with a variety of partners. Of these, the preponderance would have been prostitutes.

Some scholars cannot resist the temptation to focus on, and view aspects of, late medieval and Renaissance society—such as discriminatory treatment of women, persecution of Jews as scapegoats for various ills, efforts at quarantine, attempted suppression or regulation of prostitution, the closing of public baths, and the sometimes blatant disregard of the sick poor—exclusively through the grid of syphilology or venereology. They argue that these social features were either the result of, or were significantly amplified by, prejudice against syphilitics in general or against particular categories of syphilitics because of the diseases's being primarily transmitted sexually. To make such an argument, and many modern historians do so, is to distort all aspects of the questions addressed, at least for the first decade of the syphilis "epidemic."

Quétel, when discussing Torrella's earliest treatise, asseverates, "It is always the male sex for which the doctor feels pity, the woman being strictly confined to the role of contaminator."[157] This, as we have seen, is only partially true. But there is enough truth in Quétel's assessment to elicit the following observations. If the understanding of syphilis was then significantly affected by misogyny, then the syphilis "epidemic" provides merely another illustration of a mind-set already strongly present before the outbreak of that "epidemic." Granted, late-fifteenth- and early-sixteenth-century European society was, in many ways, blatantly misogynistic and male dominated. But the medical understanding of the role of women in the transmission of morbus Gallicus was not the *direct result* of that misogyny. It was, at the very most, the *indirect consequence* of a very old misogyny. And the latter is true only if humoral pathology itself had, nearly two millennia earlier, been formulated by principles that were conditioned by misogyny. Why were women regarded as the contaminators? Because men were thought to contract the disease much more easily than women. The woman's matrix, being cold, dry, and dense, was regarded as significantly less susceptible to contracting the disease. The membrum virile, being warm and moist, and having open pores, was viewed as being exceedingly vulnerable to infection. So, whereas a man could easily contract the disease by having sexual intercourse with an infected woman, or even with a healthy woman with whom an infected man had recently engaged in coitus, a woman, by contrast, could generally contract the disease sexually only by frequent intercourse with the infected. It follows that women who were infected sexually were promiscuous and that the majority were prostitutes. No wonder Almenar called this disease disgraceful "because it causes women to be regarded as unchaste and irreligious."[158] Sad indeed was the plight of the woman who contracted the disease extragenitally or through a single act of sexual intercourse with an infected man. At least one of our syphilographers, Cataneus, asserts that he had "seen very many women who have been infected from a single instance of sexual intercourse with an infected man, as they themselves affirm."[159] In conceding this, he is, in a significant sense, questioning a fundamental aspect of the contemporary understanding of sexual transmission of morbus Gallicus. And in taking these women seriously, Cataneus displays a sensitivity to the untenable situation in which many women undoubtedly found themselves. Nevertheless, it is in the very nature of humoral pathology that women were the contaminators. Not women generally, however, but typically only those women who were sexually loose, and most specifically prostitutes. Hence the obvious concern of syphilographers with the role of prostitutes in the spread of syphilis has undergirding nuances that are not so obvious at first sight.

If it can be demonstrated that the syphilis "epidemic" significantly exacerbated misogyny, especially medical misogyny, the very act of documenting and explicating this exacerbation will identify a time frame during which this venereally stimulated misogyny increased. There is, however, no evidence in the syphilographic treatises that any indigenous medical misogyny was exacerbated by syphilis in the period that extends from 1495 to 1505.

But was there a perceived duty to treat those whose actions had brought disease upon themselves, especially if their actions were popularly or religiously perceived as immoral? What was the moral response of the authors of medical treatises to syphilis and to those suffering from this disease, especially as its primarily venereal nature became patent? How early in the history of syphilis could an attitude like Dr. Solly's be found in the medical community? It is reported in *Lancet* in 1860 that Samuel Solly, author of *The Human Brain* (1836), council member of the Royal College of Surgeons, Fellow of the Royal Society, and later to be elected president of the Royal Medical and Chirurgical Society (for 1867–68), "far from considering syphilis an evil regarded it, on the contrary, as a blessing, and believed that it was inflicted by the Almighty to act as a restraint upon the indulgence of evil passions. Could the disease be exterminated, which he hoped it could not, fornication would ride rampant through the land."[160]

Although the undergirding theology of the ethos that included the syphilographers who wrote before 1505 typically viewed natural disasters, epidemic disease, and personal sickness as blessings in the sense that such occurrences both expiated sin and turned communities and individuals from sin, nevertheless these authors fervently desired to disseminate their understanding of morbus Gallicus and their therapeutic methods so that more and more patients could be cured, until the disease would be extirpated. Indeed, Cataneus, arguably the most theologically oriented and the most vocally moralizing of these syphilographers, devoutly expressed his conviction that God had anointed him for this purpose.[161] Were Solly's attitudes shared by any physicians or laymen during the first decade of the "epidemic" of morbus Gallicus? If any physicians then had that perspective, they must not have been vocal in expressing it. Otherwise the syphilographers, especially those who expressed both moral and theological views of the disease, would surely have made some response, some defense, in justification of their seeking to cure it and to instruct others in how to treat those suffering from it.

Such an apologia, however, was eloquently and forcefully written in 1673 by that giant of British medicine, Thomas Sydenham:

As a preliminary, however, I must remark that I have met with many persons who, either from the praiseworthy desire of terrifying the unchaste by the fear of future trouble, or for the sake of claiming credit for continence on their own part, have not hesitated to argue that the cure of the venereal disease should not be taught. With such I disagree. If we reject all cases of affliction which the improvidence of human beings has brought upon themselves, there will be but little room left for the exercise of mutual love and charity. God alone punishes. We, as we best can, must relieve. Neither must we be too curious in respect to causes and motives, nor too vexatious in our censorship. Hence I will state what I have observed and tried in the disease in question; and that not with the view of making men's minds more immoral, but for the sake of making their bodies sounder. This is the business of the physician.[162]

Let us note that Sydenham expressed a personal, moral view by referring to the "desire of terrifying the unchaste" as "praiseworthy." In asserting that "God alone punishes" he expressed a theological position. With both of these Solly would undoubtedly have been in agreement. Likely all, or at least the vast majority, of the syphilographers whom we have considered also would have been. Nevertheless the same fundamental line that divides Sydenham from Solly also separates the early syphilographers from Solly.

Were any of those against whom Sydenham felt compelled to argue in defense of writing about the cure of venereal disease physicians? And if so, did they represent a small or a significant minority, or even a majority, of the medical community? How early in the history of syphilis can one find physicians who shared Solly's views? Perhaps as early as the British surgeon William Clowes, who in 1579 also felt compelled to justify treating syphilitics and writing about syphilis.[163]

Owsei Temkin, in his profoundly insightful essay "Medicine and the Problem of Moral Responsibility,"[164] gave Sydenham as an example of a negative answer to the question "Should the physician reckon with the moral responsibility of his patient?" Temkin had just cited the French physician Jacque de Béthencourt as an example of one who gave an affirmative response to that question. In 1527 Béthencourt had published his *Nova penitentialis quadragesima, necnon purgatorium in morbum Gallicum sive venereum.* The title strongly suggests that Béthencourt had a rigorous and judgmentally moralizing attitude toward his syphilitic patients. Is that, however, a correct appraisal? I do not think that in the final analysis it will prove to be.

But Béthencourt is beyond the temporal parameters of the present study. He wrote just over a decade after 1516, the year in which the first verifiable reference was made to a new cure for morbus Gallicus: guaiacum, holy wood, imported from America. During the next year, Luther posted his ninety-five theses, which retrospectively marks the beginning of the Reformation. And Luther was by no means silent about syphilis. Nine years later, in 1526, the first documentable suggestion was made that the disease itself had also been first imported from America by Columbus' crew. But such developments occurred well after the end of the period under consideration in the present study.

By 1505 there was as yet no suggestion in the medical literature that any voices had been raised within the medical community against seeking to cure those who suffered from what, by the turn of the century, had become generally recognized as a disease that was primarily transmitted sexually. At no time during the period under consideration did any physician or surgeon, to the best of my knowledge, refuse to treat a patient for syphilis *because of its venereal nature.* Granted, some physicians were accused of not treating syphilitics owing to ignorance of how to treat the condition. Furthermore, in some regions, physicians, because of their aversion to any manual procedures, relegated syphilis, along with many other conditions, to surgeons or barbers. But such disdain had nothing to do with the venereal nature of the disease. The only ethical debate in the syphilis literature of this period was not whether to treat but how to treat. This debate sometimes became very heated because it typically involved as one option, and often the dominant approach, a dangerous therapy—the use of mercury. But was there any prejudice expressed against syphilitics by medical authors specifically owing to the venereal nature of their disease during the period under consideration? Yes, but only in the sense that those syphilographers, who evince a theological and moral judgment, regarded the disease as being spread primarily by sexual promiscuity. Yet even those physicians appear to have been convinced that such considerations were irrelevant to their role as physicians.

NOTES

Abbreviations

Gruner.   Christian Gottfried Gruner, *Aphrodisiacus, sive de lue venerea* (Jena: Chr. Henr. Cunonis Hereder, 1789).

Luisinus.   Aloysius Luisinus, *De morbo Gallico omnia quae extant apud omnes medicos cuiuscunque nationis* (Venice: Jordanus Zilettus, 1566).

Sudhoff.   Karl Sudhoff, *The Earliest Printed Literature on Syphilis, Being Ten Tractates from the Years 1495–1498,* adapted by Charles Singer (Florence: R. Lier, 1925).

All translations in this chapter are my own unless otherwise indicated.

1. To say that there is a vast literature devoted to the history of syphilis is an understatement. Nearly from the beginning, the majority of treatises or books written about syphilis addressed various questions about the origin and history of the disease. Few readers of the present paper will be unaware of at least some significant fruits of modern scholarship on the history of syphilis. For some recent discussions in English, see Allan M. Brandt, "Sexually Transmitted Diseases," in *Companion Encyclopedia of the History of Medicine,* ed. W. F. Bynum and Roy Porter (London: Routledge, 1993), 562–84; Jon Arrizabalaga, "Syphilis," in

The Cambridge World History of Human Disease, ed. Kenneth F. Kiple (Cambridge: Cambridge University Press, 1993), 1025–33; Ann G. Carmichael, "Syphilis and the Columbian Exchange: Was the New Disease Really New?" in *The Great Maritime Discoveries and World Health,* ed. Mário Gomes Marques and John Cule (Lisbon: Escola Nacional de Saúde Pública, Ordem Dos Médicos, Instituto de Sintra, 1991), 187–200; Claude Quétel, *The History of Syphilis,* trans. J. Braddock and B. Pike (Baltimore: Johns Hopkins University Press, 1990); Yehudi M. Felman, "Syphilis: From 1495 Naples to 1989 AIDS," *Arch. Dermatol.* 125 (1989): 1698–1700; Francisco Guerra, "The Dispute over Syphilis: Europe versus America," *Clio Medica* 13 (1978): 39–61; Kenneth M. Flegel, "Changing Concepts of the Nosology of Gonorrhea and Syphilis," *Bull. Hist. Med.* 48 (1974): 571–88; Alfred W. Crosby, "The Early History of Syphilis: A Reappraisal," *Am. Anthropol.* 71 (1969): 218–27; Derek J. Cripps and Arthur C. Curtis, "Syphilis Maligna Praecox: Syphilis of the Great Epidemic? An Historical Review," *Arch. Intern. Med.* 119 (1967): 411–18; and C. J. Hackett, "On the Origin of Human Treponematoses," *Bull. World Health Org.* 29 (1963): 7–41. There are also many studies of the historiography of syphilis.

2. It is important to be aware how easily we can read back into premodern discussions of disease, presuppositions conceptually formulated by current nosologies and interpretations of contagion and infection. There is a rapidly expanding literature on the history of theories of disease transmission. A foundational starting point is Vivian Nutton, "The Seeds of Disease: An Explanation of Contagion and Infection from the Greeks to the Renaissance," *Med. Hist.* 27 (1983): 1–34. For a fascinating case study of the application of contemporary theories of contagion in an institutional setting, see Ann G. Carmichael, "Contagion Theory and Contagion Practice in Fifteenth-Century Milan," *Renaiss. Quart.* 44 (1991): 213–56.

3. I could easily have said, "who range from the very religious to the thoroughly humanistic." One must beware of assuming that classical humanism and Christianity were opposites in the late Italian and early northern Renaissance. The ethos of the Renaissance was in its very marrow Christian. A resurrected Greek or Roman would have felt only slightly more alien in a medieval environment than in the atmosphere of Renaissance Italy. And the predominantly Christian presuppositions that undergirded nearly all artistic and intellectual endeavors would have been the cause of his sense of alienation. The Christocentrism of the Renaissance was considerably stronger than the enthusiastically celebrated anthropocentrism that much later generations read back into that milieu. Human dignity—the worth of the human being, which was such a hallmark of the Renaissance—was inextricably bound up with the concept of the imago Dei, a concept entirely alien to classical philosophies and pagan religions.

4. Chap. 1 of this volume includes a discussion of the two major themes that recur with regularity in these essays, as well as some musings about the refinements and modifications of my position on at least some of the nuances of these themes.

5. This date is supported by Karl Sudhoff, *Aus der Frühgeschichte der Syphilis* (Leipzig: Johann Ambrosius Barth, 1912), 8–9, and by various of his subsequent

publications. Because the blasphemy edict is important for scholars who argue either for or against its actually dealing with syphilis, its date as well as its integrity have been much disputed. See Alfred Martin, "Are There Any Proofs That Syphilis Existed in Italy and North of the Alps before the Invasion of Italy by Charles VIII of France?" *Urol. Cutaneous Rev.* 27 (1923): 497–98, who argues for a date of August 1496. See also Han Haustein, who, in *Archiv für Dermatologie und Syphilis* 161 (1930): 255, maintains that the original document, in the words of David Riesman (to whom I owe this citation) "referred to blasphemy and to the coining of gold coins and the making of wine and not to syphilis. The passage applying to syphilis was added . . . probably not before January 1497." David Riesman, *The Story of Medicine in the Middle Ages* (New York: P. B. Hoeber, 1935), 291.

6. The German text reads *die pösen Plattern* (sc. *bösen Blattern*), that is, "the evil pox."

7. The relevant portions of both the Latin and German texts are printed in Sudhoff, xix.

8. Theodor Rosebury, *Microbes and Morals: The Strange Story of Venereal Disease* (New York: Viking, 1971), 168.

9. Richard Palmer, "The Church, Leprosy, and Plague in Medieval and Early Modern Europe," in *The Church and Healing*, ed. W. J. Sheils (Oxford: Blackwell, 1982), 83.

10. Bruce Thomas Boehrer, "Early Modern Syphilis," *J. Hist. Sexuality* 1 (1990): 203.

11. Ibid., 205.

12. Anna Foa, "The New and the Old: The Spread of Syphilis (1494–1530)," in *Sex and Gender in Historical Perspective*, ed. Edward Muir and Guido Ruggiero, trans. Margaret A. Gallucci, with Mary M. Gallucci and Carole C. Gallucci (Baltimore: Johns Hopkins University Press, 1990), 27.

13. The Latin text is in Gruner, 55–57, and a facsimile is in Sudhoff, 29–33. For a discussion and translation see William Renwick Riddell, "Sebastian Brant: *De pestilentiali scorra sive impetigine anni XCVI*," *Arch. Dermatol. Syphilol.* 20 (1929): 63–74.

14. Quétel, *History* (n. 1), 13.

15. A facsimile of the 1495/96 printing of the Latin is in Sudhoff, 3–22. The text also appears in Gruner, 40–47.

16. On Wimpheling see Lewis W. Spitz, *The Religious Renaissance of the German Humanists* (Cambridge: Harvard University Press, 1963), 41–60.

17. In antiquity, Insubria was the designation of the territory around Milan.

18. The Latin here is *abstrusae vires*. I assume that Wimpheling is referring generally to the occult potencies of substances used for medicinal purposes.

19. I take *res a se conditae* as including, but not necessarily limited to, the art of medicine.

20. Boehrer gives Schellig as an example of "the byzantine processes of literary patronage" that, he claims, also "inform every other work published on syphilis for the first century of its recognized existence," and of the "indisputable (and highly conventional) connection between the apparatus of government and the earliest publications on syphilis." Boehrer, "Early Modern Syphilis"

(n. 10), 205. Literary patronage, to include scientific patronage, need not be twisted into an ugly and insidious conspiracy between "the power elite" and "the Renaissance medical profession radicalized in service of the ruling classes" (202) to deepen class distinctions and oppress the masses. Boehrer and ideologues of his ilk are, of course, themselves typically the objects of literary patronage, usually by the state, an irony to which they appear not to be sensitive.

21. Roger French, "The Arrival of the French Disease in Leipzig," in *Maladie et société, XIIe-XVIIIe siècles: Actes du Colloque de Bielefeld* (Paris: Editions du CNRS, 1989), 134.

22. For discussions of the non-naturals in ancient and medieval medicine see, in order of ascending complexity, Nancy G. Siraisi, *Medieval and Early Renaissance Medicine: An Introduction to Knowledge and Practice* (Chicago: University of Chicago Press, 1990), 101; Per-Gunnar Ottosson, *Scholastic Medicine and Philosophy: A Study of Commentaries on Galen's Tegni (ca. 1300–1450)* (Naples: Bibliopolis, 1984), 253–70; Peter H. Niebyl, "The Non-Naturals," *Bull. Hist. Med.* 45 (1971): 486–92; and L. J. Rather, "The 'Six Things Non-Natural': A Note on the Origins and Fate of a Doctrine and a Phase," *Clio Medica* 3 (1968): 337–47.

23. Sudhoff, 6; Gruner, 41.

24. Sudhoff, 15–16; Gruner, 44.

25. Sudhoff, 17; Gruner, 45.

26. A facsimile of a 1498 printing of the Latin text is in Sudhoff, 23–68. The text also appears in Gruner, 54–63. I have followed the translation by William Renwick Riddell, "Joseph Grünpeck of Burckhausen and his *Tractatus de pestilentiali scorra sive mala de Franzos,*" *Arch. Dermatol. Syphilol.* 22 (1930): 430–61.

27. Quétel, *History* (n. 1), 16.

28. For the motif of plague as a "stepmother," see chap. 10, above.

29. Boehrer, "Early Modern Syphilis" (n. 10), 205.

30. Ibid., 201–2.

31. A facsimile of the Latin text is in Sudhoff, 261–78. The Latin text also appears in Gruner, 72–75.

32. Sudhoff, xlii.

33. *Inauditum* also means "unheard of before."

34. Sudhoff, 265; Gruner, 72.

35. Sudhoff, 269; Gruner, 73.

36. Sudhoff, 272–73; Gruner, 74.

37. Facsimiles of the entirety of one early printing and the introductory paragraphs of another printing are in Sudhoff, 235–49, 350–52; the Latin text also is in Gruner, 47–52. As for the nomenclature of the disease, which Widmann prefers to call *mal de Franzos*, he remarks that it is popularly called *malum Franciae* or *morbum Sancti Meui* (Sudhoff, 235; Gruner, 48). On the identification of this saint, Sudhoff remarks that this is "probably only a printer's error for Sancti Meni a saint whose name was especially associated with syphilis" (xxxviii). Sudhoff gives as other spellings: Saint Meen, Saint Mein, Saint Main, Saint Maenus, Saint Menus, and Saint Minus (xxxviii, n. 1).

38. Pliny, *Historia naturalis* 7.168.

39. Sudhoff, 235; Gruner, 47.

40. Sudhoff, 235–36; Gruner, 48.

41. See, e.g., Pearl Kibre, "Giovanni Garzoni of Bologna (1419–1505), Professor of Medicine and Defender of Astrology," *Isis* 58 (1967): 504–14; Siraisi, *Medieval and Renaissance Medicine* (n. 22), 67–68, 134–36, 189; and French, "The Arrival" (n. 21), 136–38, and the secondary literature that French cites in n. 8.

42. This treatise appears not to be extant.

43. Sudhoff, 240–41; Gruner, 49.

44. Sudhoff, xxxv.

45. Ibid., xxxix.

46. On Leipzig, see French, "The Arrival" (n. 21), 138–41.

47. A facsimile of the 1497 printing of the Latin text is in Sudhoff, 117–78. The Latin text is in Luisinus, 1:14–35. On Leoniceno see Daniela Mugnai Carrara, "Fra causalità astrologica e causalità naturale: Gli interventi di Nicolò Leoniceno e della sua scuola sul morbo gallico," *Physis* 21 (1979): 37–54.

48. Sudhoff, 123; Luisinus, 1:15.

49. Sudhoff, 124; Luisinus, 1:15.

50. Foa, "The New and the Old" (n. 12), 29.

51. Sudhoff, 166; Luisinus, 32.

52. W.P.D. Wightman, *Science and the Renaissance: An Introduction to the Study of the Emergence of the Sciences in the Sixteenth Century* (Edinburgh: Oliver and Boyd, 1962), 1:273–74.

53. A facsimile of the 1497 printing of the Latin text is in Sudhoff, 251–60. The text is also in Luisinus, 1:296–99. I have followed the translation by Cyril C. Barnard, "The *De morbo quem Gallicum nuncupant* [1497] of Coradinus Gilinus," *Janus* 34 (1930): 97–116.

54. Sudhoff, 253; Luisinus, 1:296; Barnard, *"De morbo"* (n. 53), 102.

55. Sudhoff, 253; Luisinus, 1:296–297; Barnard, *"De morbo"* (n. 53), 103–4.

56. Sudhoff, 253; Luisinus, 1:297; Barnard, *"De morbo"* (n. 53), 104.

57. Sudhoff, 256; Luisinus, 1:298; Barnard, *"De morbo"* (n. 53), 107.

58. Sudhoff, 298; Luisinus, 1:259; Barnard, *"De morbo"* (n. 53), 110.

59. A facsimile of the 1497 printing of the Latin text is in Sudhoff, 182–232. A somewhat abridged version is printed in Luisinus, 1:421–76. It should be noted that Torrella's *Tractatus cum consiliis* underwent several printings and revisions, was soon retitled *De morbo Gallico cum aliis*, and was followed in 1500 by his *Dialogus de dolore tractatu de ulceribus in pudendagra evenire solitis*. Luisinus begins his edited version of Torrella's syphilographia with a somewhat altered version of the *Tractatus* without the *consilia* (421–29). He next reproduces the *Dialogus*, treating *De ulceribus in pudendagra* as if it were a separate work (429–69). He concludes with an abridgment of the consilia that originally formed the conclusion to the *Tractatus*. See Ernest L. Zimmermann, "An Early English Manuscript on Syphilis: A Fragmentary Translation from the Second Edition of Gaspar Torrella's *Tractatus cum consiliis contra pudendagram seu morbum gallicum*," *Bull. Hist. Med.* 5 (1937): 461–82. Cf. Jon Arrizabalaga, "*De morbo gallico cum aliis:* Another Incunabular Edition of Gaspar Torrella's *Tractatus cum consiliis contra pudendagram seu morbum Gallicum* (1497)," *La Bibliofilia* 89 (1987): 145–57.

60. Sudhoff, xxxiv.

61. Sudhoff, 187. In Luisinus, 1:421, the first question reads, "What is this pestiferous sickness, named by some *morbus Sancti Sementi,* by the French *morbus Neapolitanus* or *grossa variola,* and by the Italians *morbus Gallicus?*"

62. As a corrective to the commonly encountered misunderstanding that by the late Middle Ages members of the clergy per se were ipso facto forbidden to practice medicine, see chap. 8, above.

63. Sudhoff, 190; Luisinus, 1:423.

64. Luisinus here inserts an enlargement of the astrological explanation that is not in the first edition as reproduced by Sudhoff.

65. Luisinus has "Alvernia."

66. Sudhoff, 192; Luisinus, 1:423.

67. Sudhoff, 193; Luisinus, 1:424.

68. Sudhoff, 201–2; Luisinus, 1:427.

69. Sudhoff, 207; Luisinus, 1:429.

70. I.e., Nicolaus Florintinus, Avicenna, and Galen.

71. Torrella appears to be thinking of Seneca, *Phaedra* 249, which reads, *Pars sanitatis velle sanari fuit.* Torrella has added *Maxima* at the beginning and has substituted *credere* for *velle,* the second being a significant change to favor his argument here. There is no evidence that I can find in the manuscript history of Seneca's *Phaedra* for *maxima* and *credere.* Torrella probably was quoting from a poor memory rather than intentionally altering the line.

72. Sudhoff, 208–12; Luisinus, 1:469–70.

73. Sudhoff, 212–17; Luisinus, 1:471–72.

74. Sudhoff, 217–19; Luisinus, 1:472–73.

75. Sudhoff, 219–21; Luisinus, 1:473.

76. Sudhoff, 221–30; Luisinus, 1:474–76.

77. Zimmermann, "Early English Manuscript" (n. 59), 476.

78. The theme of tensions and compatibilities between Christianity and secular medicine appears in most of the essays in this volume. See the discussion in chap. 1, above.

79. Sudhoff, 230; Luisinus, 1:476.

80. Boehrer, "Early Modern Syphilis" (n. 10), 206.

81. A facsimile of the Latin text is in Sudhoff, 279–312. The Latin text, with some significant deviations, appears in Luisinus, 1:100–109.

82. Sudhoff, 288–91; Luisinus, 1:103–4.

83. Sudhoff, 286; Luisinus, 1:102.

84. Sudhoff, 293; Luisinus, 1:106.

85. Sudhoff, 313–46; Luisinus, 1:110–22.

86. Sudhoff, 318; Luisinus, 1:110.

87. Sudhoff, 322–23; Luisinus, 1:112.

88. The Spanish text is in Francisco Lopez de Villalobos, *El sumario de la medicina, con un tratado sobre las pestiferas buvas,* ed. Eduardo Garcia del Real (Madrid: J. Cosano, 1948). A translation that, in spite of being in rhymed English verse, is remarkably accurate has been made by George Gaskoin: *The Medical Works of Villalobos* (London: Churchill, 1870). I have followed Gaskoin's translation with minor variations. On p. 371 of the fifth edition of *Morton's Medical*

Bibliography: An Annotated Check-list of Texts Illustrating the History of Medicine (Aldershot, Hants, England: Scolar, 1991), we are told, "For English translation [of Villalobos' work] see *Bull. Inst. Hist. Med.*, 1939, 7, 1129–39." The article in question, however, proves to be only a short discussion of Villalobos in which several stanzas of Gaskoin's translation are quoted.

89. I have departed here from Gaskoin's translation. I am at a loss why he here renders *dirán* as "pretend." *Dirán* is the future tense of *decir*, "to say." My colleague Walter Suess, who was living in Spain when AIDS first appeared, relates to me that people commonly remarked about this new affliction, "Dirán que el SIDA es un castigo justo de Dios," that is, "They will say [i.e., it is expected from them, you would not expect anything else] that AIDS is a just punishment by God." Villalobos is not saying that the theologians give an explanation that they know is not correct, which "pretend" suggests. The force is probably more present general than future hypothetical.

90. Gaskoin, *Medical Works* (n. 88), 133.

91. The reference, of course, is to the first Passover as recorded in Exod. 12.

92. Villalobos is confusing two incidents. The plague came upon the Israelites not because of David's adultery but as punishment for his making a census of the people. See 2 Sam. 24 and 1 Chron. 21.

93. The Spanish *lujuría* is the equivalent of the Latin *luxuria*, that is, lust or concupiscence.

94. Ellis Herndon Hudson, "Villalobos and Columbus," *Am. J. Med.* 32 (1962): 582.

95. Ibid.

96. Charles Clayton Dennie, *A History of Syphilis* (Springfield: Charles C. Thomas, 1962), 31.

97. The Latin text is in Gruner, 85–115.

98. Ibid., 86.

99. Ibid.

100. Ibid.

101. Ibid., 88.

102. Ibid., 90.

103. Ibid., 91.

104. Ibid., 95.

105. Ibid., 97.

106. Ibid., 102.

107. Ibid.

108. On which see above, n. 59.

109. Luisinus, 1:430.

110. Ibid., 1:431.

111. Ibid., 1:431–32.

112. Ibid., 1:432.

113. Ibid., 1:467–69.

114. *Curentur*, of course, can also mean "be cared for" or "be treated." Since Torrella thought that, if properly treated, pudendagra could be cured, it seems preferable to render it "be cured."

115. Luisinus, 1:445. See Zimmermann, "Early English Manuscript" (n. 59), 477–78; and Quétel, *History* (n. 1), 66.

116. See Arrizabalaga, *"De morbo gallico"* (n. 59), 153.

117. See ibid., 152; Zimmermann, "Early English Manuscript" (n. 59), 476–80; and Quétel, *History* (n. 1), 31.

118. Luisinus, 1:453.

119. It was printed posthumously in 1507. The Latin text with an English translation on facing pages was published as Antonio Benivieni, *De abditis nonnullis ac mirandis morborum et sanationum causis,* trans. Charles Singer (Springfield: Charles C Thomas, 1954). I have followed Singer's translation with some minor modifications.

120. Ibid., 8–9.

121. Ibid., 12–15.

122. Ibid., 14–15.

123. See the qualifying statements in n. 3, above.

124. Benivieni, *De abditis* (n. 119), chaps. 9, 10, 45.

125. The Latin text is in Luisinus, 1:310–19.

126. Ibid., 1:310.

127. Ibid., 1:311. Some scholars have thought that Almenar was being sarcastic in suggesting that "the religious" who have contracted morbus Gallicus must have been infected miasmically. This, however, seems unlikely owing to the highly religious tone that permeates his treatise.

128. Ibid., 1:311–12.

129. Ibid., 1:314.

130. Ibid., 1:311.

131. Ibid.

132. Almenar is probably thinking of Job 31:12.

133. Ibid., 1:316.

134. Ibid.

135. The Latin text is in Gruner, 63–69. I have followed the translation by Ernest L. Zimmermann, "Joseph Grünpeck's *Libellus de mentulagra alias morbo Gallico* of 1503," *Am. J. Syphilis, Gonorrhea, Venereal Dis.* 24 (1940): 364–85.

136. Gruner, 63; Zimmerman, "Grünpeck's *Libellus*" (n. 135), 370–71.

137. Gruner, 65; Zimmerman, "Grünpeck's *Libellus*" (n. 135), 375–76.

138. Gruner, 66; Zimmerman, "Grünpeck's *Libellus*" (n. 135), 378.

139. Gruner, 68–69; Zimmerman, "Grünpeck's *Libellus*" (n. 135), 385.

140. Gruner 65; Zimmerman, "Grünpeck's *Libellus*" (n. 135), 375.

141. The Latin text is in Luisinus, 1:123–48. I accept Quétel's dating; Quétel, *History* (n. 1) 25, 26, 31.

142. Luisinus, 1:123.

143. Ps. 32:9.

144. Horace, *Odes* 1.3.39–40.

145. Thucydides, *Peloponnesian War* 2.54.2.

146. Pliny, *Historia naturalis* 26.6.

147. Luisinus, 1:123–24.

148. Matt. 4:7 and Luke 4:12, quoting Deut. 6:16.

149. Horace, *Odes* 3.2.31–32.

150. Luisinus, 1:132.

151. Ibid., 1:133.

152. Ibid.

153. Ibid., 1:144.

154. Ibid., 1:131.

155. Ibid., 1:148.

156. E.g., ibid, 1:133, 136, 137, 145.

157. Quétel, *History* (n. 1), 23.

158. See text to n. 130, above.

159. See text to n. 151, above.

160. *Lancet* (1), 1860:198, as quoted in Peter Fryer "Introduction," in *Prostitution*, by William Acton (1857; reprint, New York: Frederick A. Praeger, 1968), 7.

161. See text to n. 155, above.

162. *The Works of Thomas Sydenham,* trans. R. G. Latham (London: Sydenham Society, 1850), 2:32–33, as cited and quoted by Owsei Temkin, "Medicine and the Problem of Moral Responsibility," in *The Double Face of Janus* (Baltimore: Johns Hopkins University Press, 1977), 56–57.

163. William Clowes, *A Short and Profitable Treatise Touching the Cure of the Disease Called Lues Venera* (1579).

164. Temkin, "Medicine and Moral Responsibility" (n. 162).

Indexes

These indexes were compiled by Otto W. Mandahl, Jr.

Index of Subjects

Cross-references from this index to the Index of Names are indicated by "(n.)."

Health: and the Christian, 27, 77;
church fathers on, 76; defined by
World Health Organization, 4; in
fifth-century Athens, 33; and heaven,
139; Jerome on, 84; and prophylaxis,
2; sinful means to restore, 202–3,
205, 266–68; Ullmann on, 183; when
restored only delays death, 142–43
Hemlock Society: founded by Humphrey, 15–16; endorsement of *A Noble
Death* (Droge and Tabor), 15–16
Henotheism, 128
Heresies: Arian, 175; and Catholicism,
176; difficult to define, 5–6; Donatist,
109; Ebionite, 94–95; Elkesaite, 94–
95; Encratite, 147, 158; Gnostic, 78–
80; Manichean, 83–84, 131–33; Mar-
cionite, 83–84, 134, 146; Messalian,
85–86, 150; and Montanism, 78–80;
rejection of secular medicine by
some, 151; and Tatian, 158
Hermeneutics: and Alexandrian fathers,
130–31; and Antiochine theologians,
131–32; and Cappadocian fathers,
130–31
Hippocratic Corpus: and abortion, 38–
40; *Ancient Medicine*, 45–46; *Aphorisms*,
46; *The Art*, 33, 45, 308; and assisted
suicide, 38–39; *Decorum*, 46; *Diseases*,
45; *Epidemics*, 35; *Internal Affections*,
45; *Oath*, 16, 38–40; *On Fractures*,
35–36, 46, 308; *On Joints*, 35–36, 45,
46; *Precepts*, 44, 45; and preventing
advancement of disease, 35; *Prorrhetic*, 46; and refusal to treat, 33–34;
Regimen, 45; and religion, 36–37;
and treatment to advance the art,
36–37
Historians: as frustrated anthropologists,
sociologists, and psychologists, x; and
presentism, x
HIV and AIDS: and *Cardiovascular News*,
23; and communicable diseases, 22; as
divine retribution, 23, 370; and *pax
antibiotica*, 22; Suess on, 370; and
syphilis, 24, 311, 370
Homicide: abortion as, 199, 200; contraception as, 199, 200
Homosexuality: Catholic condemnation
of, 185; condemned by Christian apologists, 100, 101
Hospitals: called xenodochia, hospitia,
hospitalia, 195; as houses of charity,
199; and Knights Hospitallers, 198;
and laicization, 199
Humanity: concepts of worth and rights

of, in pagan antiquity, 50–53; —, in
Christianity, 62–65; in a fallen state,
6; and humanitarianism, 53; Rist on,
50, 53–54; Tatian's view of, 164–65

Imago Dei: and Augustine, 64–65; basis
of sanctity of human life, 63; and
Clement of Alexandria, 78; and Tatian, 164–65
Infanticide: church fathers on, 63; condemned, 56; and exposure, 56; and
Greek customs, 57–58, 60; opposed
by Christian apologists, 63, 70, 71,
100, 101; and Roman law, 58; and sacrifice of children, 63; Valentinian's
statute on, 50
Insanity, 186
In vitro fertilization, 5
Irish Canons, 215

Jews and Judaism: and Catholicism, 176;
as cause of plague, 313; and Christian
perception of medicine, 151; and Ecclesiasticus, 144; and Greek philosophy, 90, 128, 144; Jewish medical
practitioners, 144; persecution of,
360; as praeparatio evangelica, 128;
raised all their children, 56; on role
of physicians and medicine, 144–45
Judgment of Clement, 215

Kenoma, 147
Knights Hospitallers of St. John of Jerusalem, 198

Laicization: of Europe, 178–79; and
hospitals, 198
Lemans, Council of, 223–24
Leprosy and lepers, 210, 321, 324, 327,
331, 343, 344, 345, 347, 349, 350
Licensure: and guilds, 17–20, 30, 43,
247–49, 291–94; marks change in
practice of medicine and surgery
from right to privilege, 17–20, 247–
48, 291–94, 306; none in classical antiquity and early Middle Ages, 31,
290–91; and unlicensed practitioners,
206, 289–302; and witchcraft, 205–6;
and women, 206
Life: Christian view of inherent value of,
75; pagans' lack of belief in inherent
value of, 54; physician's obligation to
prolong, 12–13, 16–21, chap. 2 passim,
263–65; respect for, 18, 41–42; right
to live, viii; spiritual greater than
physical, 74; and state, 50

Library of Congress Cataloging-in-Publication Data

Amundsen, Darrel W.
    Medicine, society, and faith in the ancient and medieval worlds / Darrel W.
Amundsen.
        p. cm.
Collection of previously published essays.
Includes bibliographical references and index.
ISBN 0-8018-5109-2 (hc : alk. paper)
    1. Medical ethics—History.   2. Medicine—Religious aspects—Christianity.   3. Medi-
cine, Medieval.   4. Medicine, Ancient.   I. Title.
    [DNLM: 1. Religion and Medicine—collected works.   2. Ethics, Medical—
history—collected works.   3. Christianity—history—collected works.   4. History of
Medicine, Ancient—collected works.   5. History of Medicine, Medieval—collected
works.   W 50 A5315m 1996]
R725.56.A48   1996   610'.9—dc20   DNLM/DLC
for Library of Congress   95-11759